Triumph and Tragedy 1991 - 2016

The Wokingham Mental Health Crisis House Twenty-Five Year History

by

Pam Jenkinson

Illustrations by Anna Felice Cook

The Jun

First published in 2016

by The June Press Ltd

UK distributor
The June Press Ltd
PO Box 119, Totnes
Devon TQ9 7WA
Tel: 44(0)8456 120 175
Email: info@junepress.com
Web: www.junepress.com

ISBN 978-0-9927501-3-8

Contents

Our Befriending Service

Part Four

'Blew Him Up With Dynamite, But Him They Could Not Kill'

The Battle For The Crisis House

Awards 1996 - 2016

Part Five

'Felix Keeps On Walking, Keeps On Walking Still. Miles up in The Air He Flew. He Just Murmured 'Toodle-oo'. He Landed Down In Timbuctoo. And He Kept On Walking Still.'

Introduction

By Pam Jenkinson

I am, essentially, an educationist. I have a degree in education from London University, and, for many years, I ran mental health education programmes for the National Schizophrenia Fellowship. These ranged from grass-roots work on welfare benefits, to international research conferences at Imperial College, and at the Royal Society of Medicine.

Then twenty-five years ago, I set up the Wokingham Mental Health Crisis House, as a model of excellence, in response to the urgent need for local, voluntary, mental health services – to be established - in the wake of the wholesale closure of the old, Victorian, mental asylums. Running the crisis house absorbed most of my time and energy, thereafter, though I did continue to contribute articles to journals, and chapters in mental health publications, throughout the rest of the nineteen-nineties.

Twenty-five years on, I have, with this book, returned to my first love. I hope that it will be a valuable contribution to mental health education, and so to the reduction of stigma.

Stigma, however, does persist, so all names of service-users – throughout the book – have been changed completely – in order to ensure their anonymity, and thus, their protection.

Volunteers, many of whom are former service-users, are mentioned by first names, only. Dignitaries, patrons, and benefactors, are the only ones referred to by their full names, and titles.

I hope very much that my readers will enjoy the book, and that it will inspire others to set up small, local, volunteer-run, crisis houses – and thus offer the chance of a return to normality – through self-help – to a greater number of people throughout the UK, and not just in Wokingham.

Acknowledgements

This book is dedicated to all those people, who, through self-help, and the support of the Wokingham Crisis House, have turned their lives around, for the better.

Foreword

By Christopher Hoskin

I became interested in the whole field of mental health because I had a low period in my life in my twenties. I went to a psychoanalyst who helped me enormously and set me right. As the years went by, I realised that my good fortune was far from being the lot of all those with mental health problems who were dependent on the state mental health services. I researched the subject of the latter, and wrote a book about it. In the course of my researches, I came across an article by Pam Jenkinson entitled, 'The Duty of Community Care: The Wokingham Mind Crisis House'. This impressed me greatly, and I got in touch with Pam. I started coming to the Wokingham Crisis House, and have been coming once a fortnight ever since.

The Crisis House is furnished like a private house. It is decorated with lots of china ornaments and pictures, and has two cats, a fishtank, and a budgerigar. The whole atmosphere is totally non-threatening and designed to make people feel at home. The people with problems who drop in, come into a relaxed place, where they are accepted for who they are, and there is no pressure on them of any kind. They can be sociable, or not, as they please. In all the time I have been coming to the Crisis House, there has never been any hint of violence or unpleasantness from anybody. There is a bar open at lunchtime where everybody who has paid their subscription is allowed one alcoholic drink. Upstairs there is a room where people can play snooker, a library, and another room where they can just go to be quiet.

Over the years, I have developed a tremendous admiration for Pam. She is a true respecter of human beings, and possessed of unequalled common sense. She is also a jolly person with a great sense of humour – as well as having great intelligence. She has fought like a tiger for the Crisis House, and has been constantly willing to do the work required to keep the place as it is. She has also been ever ready to help those who come to the Crisis House in practical ways. Unlike most people, she is unfazed by the pretentions of the authorities, and is ever willing to think outside the box. Her achievement in creating and running the Crisis House is all the greater in that over the whole country it is probably unique. I am sure that you will very much enjoy her book, and come to feel the same admiration for her and the Crisis House – as do I and many others.

Christopher Hoskin has a degree in philosophy from Cambridge University, and is a published author on a number of subjects of social importance.

PART ONE

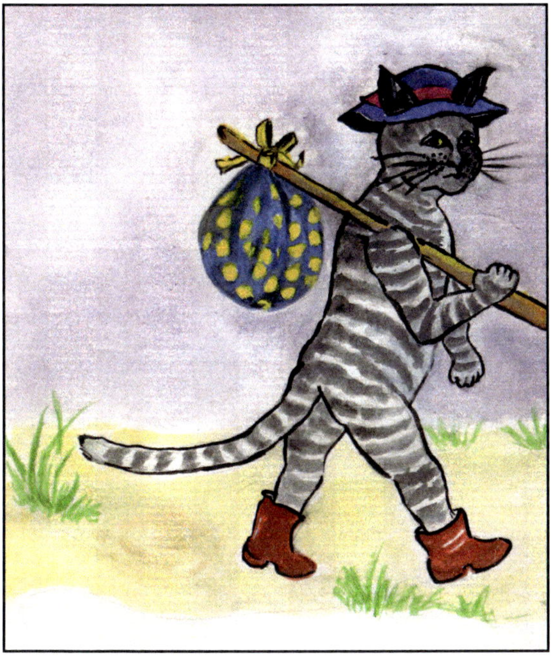

'Felix keeps on walking, keeps on walking still.
With his hands behind him, you will always find him.
Blew him up with dynamite, but him they couldn't kill.
Miles up in the air he flew,
He just murmured "Toodle-oo!"
Landed down in Timbuctoo, and kept on walking still.

Felix kept on walking, kept on walking still.
By a train at Dover, had his tail run over,
On the rail he left his tail, it gave the folks a thrill,
Still for that, he didn't care.
Though he had no rudder there,
Wagged his "nothing" in the air, and kept on walking still.'

'Felix Keeps On Walking, Keeps On Walking Still'

*'There's No Strings Upon This Love Of Mine,
It Was Always You From The Start'*

Chapter 1

It Was Always You From The Start

Why would anyone want to get involved in mental health? The answer is that – in the majority of cases – one does not choose. One's involvement is personal – either as a mental health sufferer, or as the relative, or friend, of one. It is the last thing on earth that anyone would choose to be!

The public, commonly say, laughingly, about psychiatrists – that they become psychiatrists, because they are, themselves, a bit mad! Funnily enough, in my opinion, the group of mental health professionals LEAST likely to get involved for personal reasons – are psychiatrists. The public perception of a psychiatrist is, in any case, generally, erroneous.

What they are visualizing is, in fact, the psychoanalyst – with the mental patient lying on his couch! This image may have some accuracy in America, but in England, psychiatry is simply a branch of medicine – its treatment the control of symptoms with medication. The doctors who practise it are, therefore, just like any other doctors. To them, treating schizophrenia with quetiapine, for instance, is not substantially different, from treating diabetes with insulin!

Psychiatry is of low status, in the hierarchy of medical disciplines – so choosing it in order to obtain quicker promotion - may well be one of the motivating factors, for doctors pursuing their careers. So I don't think that it is, generally, the case with psychiatrists, as it is with some other mental health professionals, that they go into mental health, in order to solve their own problems.

Most people, who, like me, were ricocheted into mental health on a personal basis, decide, if they then wish to work in mental health, to seek a professional position within it – usually training either, for psychiatric nursing, for social work, or for psychotherapy, or counselling. I have yet to encounter a psychiatrist who did so.

But we have had 'graduates' of the crisis house, who have done, precisely, that. We have also had befrienders who were pursuing this route.

I chose not to. I started in mental health at the tender age of seventeen, on a personal basis, and I am still involved, on a personal basis, at the age of seventy!

Traditional psychoanalysts advise, 'Make the disadvantage, an advantage. Turn the crisis into a triumph.' That is what I determined to do – firstly, with my educational, and support, work for the National Schizophrenia Fellowship, and, for the past twenty-five years, with the Wokingham Crisis House.

When one finds oneself in the situation – as a relative of someone with a very severe mental, or physical illness - one feels alone, and unique.

In fact, one's situation is the common lot of humanity! From the highest in the land – Camilla Parker-Bowles, Duchess of Cornwall, for example, who chose to become Patron of the Osteoporosis Society, because her mother suffered from this disease, or Brian Rix – who became a Patron of MENCAP – because his daughter was mentally handicapped – down to humble you and me. We get involved in, and dedicated to, a particular cause – because it has touched us personally.

When I was seventeen, I was very unhappy. I considered that seventeen-year-olds should have stars in their eyes, but I did not. My father was, then, terminally ill, and my brother and sister were, already, ill, with schizophrenia. Nobody that I knew, seemed to have a happy life.

When one has no effective parental guidance, one becomes like a cork, bobbing about on life's bewildering sea.

The teachers, at school, were not happy. They were frustrated spinsters. But the families that I knew, including my own, were not happy either.

I turned to a Christian Church for guidance. 'What do you do?' I asked them. 'You win renown, and gain a victor's crown. Then at His feet, you cast it down,' was their reply. Such is the symbolism of Evangelical Christianity, that I didn't really understand what they meant. Nevertheless, I did what they said. 'You win renown?' I did that all right!

I considered everybody that I knew. I could identify only one person – a lady in that church – who seemed to be happy with her lot in life.

She was happily married to a scientist, did not need to go out to work, had no children, and spent her life, doing voluntary work.

They lived in a big, four bedroom, house. They had linen, antimacassars on the backs of their chairs. The house had an old fashioned, white bath, not built in, but standing on little feet. There was always a tablet of Wright's coal tar soap, in a dish, on the wash basin.

As I sit here, writing this. I am happily married to a scientist. Having had no children, I haven't needed to go out to work for many years now. I spend my life doing voluntary work.

We live in a big, four bedroom house. We have linen antimacassars on the backs of our chairs. Our house has an old-fashioned, white bath, not built in, but standing on little feet. The tablet of Wright's coal tar soap is, duly, in its dish on the wash basin.

You would not think that anyone would take it as far as the soap, but, as far as the soap, I have taken it.

At seventeen, I concluded, that, if this lady could be happy with such a life, then so could I be, and I am. This lady was what she, as a practising Christian, would have called a 'witness'. Psychologists call her a 'role model'. To me, she was simply, an 'example'.

Love Changes Everything

'Love changes everything, hands and faces, earth and sky.
Love changes everything, how you live, and how you die.
Love makes fools of everyone – for the rules we make are broken.
Love changes everyone – live or perish in its flame.
Nothing in the world will ever be the same.'

If you asked me, 'What are the strongest human emotions?' High up there on the list - with sexual passion, and jealousy, I would include, gratitude.

Close to forty years after my decision, at the age of seventeen, to follow in her footsteps, I attended this lady's funeral – even though it was held, miles away, in another county.

She had continued with her voluntary work, until she died, at the age of eighty-six. The song that she chose for her funeral service, was 'Love Changes Everything', and no-one joined in singing it more heartily, than me!

Chapter 2

What's It All About?

For people who have no knowledge or experience of mental health at all, a good premise on which to start their education, is that mentally ill people want the same things, in life, that everybody else wants. Frequently, due to illness, they have been robbed of ordinary things, but the aspirations remain the same.

That is why I have created the Wokingham Crisis House, as an ordinary environment. Mental illness is not infectious, so there is no need whatsoever, to create for people, an environment that resembles an operating theatre. On the other hand, if, due to illness, their personal environments are chaotic, squalid, and deprived, that is all the more reason to enable them to experience well-organised and comfortable normality in their crisis house.

Then the aim – through support and self-help – is to enable people to attain, or, in some cases, to regain, a normal, worth-while life. Such a life includes work, a decent place to live, relationships, friendships, and a social life, and full participation in the local community - through taking up hobbies and interests. Skills – such as cooking, shopping, laundry, and household maintenance, may, in some instances, also need to be acquired.

In the summer of 1990, a few months before I set up the Wokingham Crisis House, I revisited a National Schizophrenia Fellowship Support Group in North London. I had previously visited this group in the summer of 1985.

To describe the second visit as, '*déjà vu*', would underestimate the experience. They were exactly the same people – complaining about exactly the same problems – as those whom I had visited, five years previously. What was particularly sad, as well, was that I knew that this group had worked hard to raise a lot of money for the national organization.

In five years, there had been no progress, nor any improvement in their situation, whatsoever. What do these national charities do with the money raised, and donated? I have answered this question elsewhere in this narrative. The answer, all too frequently, is - spend it on fat salaries, cars, and pensions, for the failed social workers, whom they employ in soft-option jobs!

I determined that this would not happen with the crisis house, and it never has. By contrast, after five years, one observes the most remarkable progress in individuals.

What it is about, is striving – with the person – and taking into consideration their limitations – to get back, as far as is possible, to normality. A good example of a mentally ill person doing just this, can be found in Chapter 45: 'Lucy's Story'. Another excellent example – albeit with the limitations imposed by a chronic schizophrenic illness, can be found in Chapter 8: 'She Ticks all the Boxes.'

Chapter 3

What Is Needed For Mental Health

When we opened the crisis house, twenty-five years ago, the old mental asylums were in the process of closing. All are now closed. During the decade of the 1990's, there was, therefore, tremendous interest in community alternatives – crisis houses being one – hence our chapters on 'Spreading the Word'. The Wokingham crisis house is a hugely successful project, but it is, most emphatically, NOT an alternative to a mental hospital.

By contrast, it fits in, as it should, with a wide range of community facilities, which are needed for mental health. A hospital, as a clinical centre, is still needed. Structured community centres are needed. Supported housing is needed, and, now that care is in the community, it is even more important for general practitioners, to receive better training in mental health.

One thing that is now woefully deficient, is sheltered employment. Some individuals who have suffered a breakdown, eventually move back into full-time employment, in the open market, but most do not. There is, therefore, a great need for the provision of part-time and sheltered employment.

There is, currently, a lot of criticism of Iain Duncan-Smith's reform of the benefits system. Claims are being made, that people who cannot work, are being forced back into work. I do not agree. With the old system of mental health care, in mental asylums, the patients certainly did work – in workshops, market gardens, and farms – on the hospital site.

This is what needs to be duplicated in the community – sheltered work for the mentally and physically disabled. There is practically nobody, who is incapable of any work at all, but it must be tailored to the needs of disabled people, and take note of their limitations.

The great benefit of work is that one's colleagues give one a realistic view of one's capabilities, and thus keep one grounded in reality. If totally unemployed, one sits about fantasising the most grandiose future jobs for oneself. Such is not good for mental health!

On 10th October 2015, World Mental Health Day, I took part in a Berkshire Radio broadcast in which employment and mental health was discussed. The view expressed was that employers need to do more to support employees with mental health problems.

I agree for those temporarily, or less severely, affected. For those with long-term, and severe, disorders, open market employment is not a realistic option. Some degree of shelter is necessary.

Since I started working in Wokingham, nearly thirty years ago, mental health services, have, unfortunately, deteriorated. Is it that the local authority thinks that, as with homelessness, there can be no such problem in Wokingham? Facts refute this. Statistics reveal that one in four people in Wokingham, will suffer from mental illness!

Furthermore, mental illness is no respecter of persons. Its sufferers range from Royalty to the destitute! When mental illness first strikes an individual, and thus, vicariously, his/her family, they think that they are alone in this experience. Eventually, as Bob Dylan has it, 'She finally sees that she's like all the rest!'

Until recently, there was, for decades, a mental health day centre on the Reading Road – now demolished, to make way for the new Station Link Road. For twenty years, there were two mental health hostels, on the London Road – now closed!

People still speak, with nostalgia, of the days when Jim ran these hostels. Jim was a trained mental health nurse, of the old school.

One hostel was high support, and one was low support. Patients, on discharge from hospital, who still had considerable rehabilitation needs, would be admitted to the high support hostel. Jim then, had a programme, where all would participate, in planning and budgeting for meals, shopping, cooking and serving. Essential daily tasks – such as laundry and cleaning – would also be taught.

If residents did well in this system, they could then progress into the low-support hostel – which was self-catering, but residents still had access to the staff next door, if they felt the need. In due course, if they made sufficient progress in the low-support hostel, residents would be considered for independent flats, in the ordinary community. What you might call a traditional, and effective, rehabilitation scheme!

The first service to be removed from the high support hostel, was the night cover, and then the service diminished, and diminished, until it was closed completely. All residents were moved into ordinary flats in the community. As a result of the consequent lack of support, they have relapsed into acute illness, and, in some instances, have been re-admitted to hospital under Sections of the Mental Health Act.

Wokingham mental health services have never been good. As I told one of their former social services officers, in a conversation in which she was trying to defend them, 'You come bottom every year in the league tables!'

However, in those days, poor though they were, they did, at least, exist. Now, they are virtually non-existent! At least the authorities failed to close our crisis house. With it having received the nation's top awards, that would, indeed, have been vandalism!

But there is still the sad tale of the demise of our crisis beds – a most useful service, these. A mentally ill person could have immediate access to a bed, and stay, until more permanent arrangements were made. Through using the beds, we got mentally ill patients, stable enough to move into flats, drug addicts, off heroin, and back to useful lives, and battered women, away from abuse, and back to safety.

Despite this, in 2007, we were told that our two thousand pounds, per year, funding for the beds, would cease, and that there would be no further referrals from the community mental health team. No further referrals, that was, until Friday afternoon - when the community mental health team, were eager to get off early, for a nice, relaxing, weekend!

The homeless mentally ill man, turns up at the team's office. The community psychiatric nurse, telephones me, on her boss's advice. 'Could this homeless man come and stay at the crisis house?'

'Alas, no, the beds – like their funding – have vanished!' It is peanuts that charities run on, and not fresh air! And I would swear that they are miffed. All that effort – either to take over, or to destroy. Then the failure to destroy. We are still here, but self-funding, and we will not use our funding, to get them off the hook!

In July 2015, a local Police Officer, had occasion to visit the crisis house. He nearly wept. It is so obviously what is needed everywhere – and the former beds, even more so. The Police have the duty of imposing 136 Sections, the 'Place of Safety' Section, of the Mental Health Act.

As he explained, the mentally ill people, obviously disturbed in public places, whom the Police are obliged to arrest, do not like going to the cold, clinical, setting of the mental hospital, and, in any case, hospital beds are at a premium, so patients are only accepted in the most extreme circumstances. They would greatly prefer staying at the crisis house.

Well, they could have, couldn't they? The service was highly successful. In twenty years, we never had a suicide on the premises. We thought that Nigel Hills had committed suicide: [Chapter 23: A waste of a young life'.] But the coroner disagreed. His verdict was 'Open' – with a drug-related accident being the most likely scenario. Such could happen anywhere, and HAS happened in the private homes of local heroin addicts.

We never had significant self-harm. We never had a homicide, nor violence. Furthermore, the model could have been replicated. In Berkshire, you could do with a four bedroom crisis house in Hungerford, another in Newbury, two in Reading, one in Maidenhead, one in Windsor, two in Bracknell, and two in Slough – all catering for the individual needs of those, very diverse, communities.

As I pointed out to our political leaders, when the crisis house was under threat of closure, to give people choice, by having entirely voluntary services – completely separate from statutory ones – is within the political philosophy of conservatism – which Wokingham constituents vote for consistently! By contrast, to have only one service – controlled by the State – is a product of the, failed, political philosophy, of socialism!

This brings me to relate, an incident, and you will find many of them in this book, where the poignant, and the funny, were intertwined. When fighting for the crisis house, I took the matter up with our MP, as well as with Wokingham Borough Council.

There are some things, in life, which one does not expect to have to do. I never thought, that I, would ever have to sit in the former Cabinet Minister, and Wokingham MP's, surgery, at the Conservative Association's office, in Rose Street, and instruct him, and the Chairman of the Conservative Council – in the fundamentals of the political philosophy of conservatism!

I started running voluntary mental health services in Wokingham – nearly thirty years ago – because a colleague, who knew of my work for the National Schizophrenia Fellowship, asked for my involvement. She was employed on a three-year fixed contract, with Wokingham Borough Council, to get volunteers in the community setting up voluntary sector mental health services.

I agreed to do so – provided that they actually were voluntary services. No way, would I, ever consider having a paid post, or working in an organization where people were paid. I also insisted that any services in which I became involved, banned mental health professionals in their constitution.

The Council would be well-advised to thus encourage voluntary work, once again. If they provided minimal funding, and encouraged volunteers to run things, there would be a chance of sustainability, and the stability, and security, in services, which the mentally ill so desperately need.

Chapter 4

Know Your Enemy

'No coward soul is mine, no trembler in the world's storm-troubled sphere'
Emily Bronte

When embarking upon an exciting and valuable new project, it is somewhat daunting, to know, before one starts, that people will be out to destroy it, but this is, nevertheless, essential knowledge to have.

Forewarned is forearmed! If you know, in advance, that you will be faced with ruthless, and persistent attempts at destruction, you do then, stand at least a chance, of surviving them. I knew, when I opened the Wokingham Crisis House, in March 1991, that they, the mental health establishment, would try, persistently over years, to destroy us, and I was right!

One of our service users, years ago – a lady with a somewhat jaundiced view of life, said to me, that I always got Trustees for the Charity, who would agree with what I do! I cannot deny it. Fighting the enemy is exhausting enough, without having to fight the allies as well!

I come now to my favourite author, Agatha Christie. I have read all her books – some of them – hundreds of times. A recent survey of her fans revealed that their all-time favourite, is the book, now known, as 'And Then There Were None'. Agatha Christie: [Published: Collins: 1939.]

I concurred with this universal choice. The quotation from 'And Then There Were None', which has been most useful to me in my twenty-five years in the crisis house is this: 'His quick brain was working. Which way – which method? All his life Lombard had taken the risky way. He took it now.'

Agatha Christie's lesson is that you will never change people. In twenty-five years, I have observed, that of the people who have come through the crisis house, those who have made the most successful recoveries, have been those who were successful in life before they suffered mental breakdown!

Such psychology explains so much in mental health. People never change. They mature, but they do not change. In crisis, they become, even more, themselves. Thus, a person in crisis, will, for instance, revert to his mother tongue – even if he is fluent in other languages, and has been speaking them for years.

People in distress talk of 'working on autopilot'. This phenomenon also explains the common situation where people, previously academically successful, can pass examinations whilst in a state of mental breakdown, but then are unable to cope in the jobs for which the examination passes qualify them, because this would require the mastering of new skills, which they are incapable of doing!

Throughout this book, I have selected passages from twenty-five of Agatha Christie's works, to mark the twenty-five years, that I have been using her psychology, for my work in the crisis house.

I recognise in myself, for instance, some of the characteristics of Miss Bulstrode, Headmistress of Meadow Bank School: [Please see: 'Cat Among the Pigeons': Agatha Christie; Published: Collins: 1959.]

Remonstrating with a parent, who wanted to take her child out of school, during term time, Miss Bulstrode said, in reply to the mother's plea, 'She's my child!' 'Exactly, but it's my school.' Miss Bulstrode went on to explain, that if this parent took the child out in term time, then she would not be allowed back. 'You wanted my school for your daughter, didn't you? But it's take it as it is, or leave it. Like that very charming Balenciaga model you are wearing. It is Balenciaga, isn't it?'

Mind you, Miss Bulstrode was confident in her knowledge that Meadow Bank enjoyed having the reputation of being the best girls' school in the United Kingdom – patronised by Royalty, and, as Agatha Christie explained 'You paid through the nose, but you got what you paid for!'

Equally confident, that - as Chris Hoskin says in his 'Foreword' to this book, our service is probably unique in the United Kingdom, 'Take it, or leave it', has always been the stance, upon which the Wokingham Crisis House has been offered!

It is not on Social Services' terms, or, indeed, on anyone else's terms. It is on MY terms, but that is not to say that other people ideas, and suggestions, are not taken on board . They are.

One example is the Games Room. I had always rejected the idea of having a Games Room at the Crisis House, because I thought that the rooms were too small, and that it would be too institutionalising. Service users should be encouraged to participate in the normal community, and would be better off, playing pool and darts, in the pub, next door, or joining the St Crispin's Sports Centre, which is well equipped, for a wide range of sports.

However, once we discontinued the beds, rooms became available, and members argued that there was a case, for service users who had lost all confidence, to build up some skills, gradually, using a room at the crisis house, and then graduating into community facilities, once their confidence was restored.

Thus overruled, I established a Games Room, and very well-used, and popular, it has proved to be – achieving precisely what our members envisaged – the acquisition of some basic skills, and confidence, and then moving on to better facilities in the ordinary community in due course!

I hardly came green to the crisis house project. I was then forty-five years of age; now I am seventy.

I had then been involved in mental health for thirty years, and had spent the previous twelve, as a local voluntary co-ordinator, for the National Schizophrenia Fellowship. In addition to running their education programmes, I had served, for some ten years, on their national Council of Management, and was well-versed in political manoeuvres!

Most separatist, user-run, crisis houses, fail to get off the ground; of the few that do, most are, inevitably, destroyed by the mental health establishment. We have survived. Something that lasts for twenty-five years has survived. It has passed the test of time. It may not, of course, last for ever – very few things do. But in terms of survival, as a radical, separatist, crisis house, it has made it!

By contrast, things that do not fulfil their *raison d'être*, do not last. I have seen it happen. When I was tied in London, looking after my mother, and my brother and sister, I was unable to take a full-time teaching post, because I had so many hospital appointments to keep, and so much to do, on their behalf. So I did some temporary teaching, not by choice, but due to geographical convenience, in Inner London Education Authority schools.

Among its many, awful, schools, one, particularly, stands out in my memory. The Head Teacher, besides arriving at school, obviously unwashed, and in dirty clothes, was unable to read and write, and was also, a pathological liar! 'Impossible!' You will say. No, they are always, there, crawling about in the woodwork, and nothing is impossible – once standards are allowed to slip.

I have always let this experience, be a lesson to me! As someone commented, at the time, 'If you let in the wind, you will reap the whirlwind!' What intrigued me, about some of my colleagues at the time, is that they failed to see that the writing was on the wall! They would talk of the positions that they would be holding, with the Authority, in ten years time. 'This won't be here, in ten years' time!' I remonstrated. It wasn't!

The Inner London Education Authority, was established, in order to provide education. It failed to do so, and it was abolished! I shall hail the day - when statutory Social Services go the same way! In fact, I detect signs, the early warning signs, that this is already happening.

Certainly, in Wokingham, local welfare is already being delivered by charities, such as the Salvation Army, while the statutory services get worse, and worse, and more and more negligent. Our, tiny little, Association is currently dealing with two, major negligence cases. Is the answer to improve statutory Social Services? No, the answer is to abolish them!

In contrast to the failure of the Inner London Education Authority, I also recall, forty-five years ago, undertaking, Post Graduate, a Montessori Teaching Course.

At one lecture, the tutor was demonstrating the teaching of language skills, to infants, using flash cards. She said, 'Of course, there will be afternoons, when you put it all away.' In other words, when everyone is too tired. 'But you mustn't do that too often', she added.

How right she was! To run anything – whether it be a mental health crisis house, or an education authority, or a welfare service, one has to be completely conscientious – if not one hundred per cent of the time, then, at least, ninety-nine, point nine, per cent of the time! Otherwise, all quickly goes to pot.

When I left the service of the Inner London Education Authority, thirty years ago, it had gone, yours truly, to pot! The, right, [no pun intended], decision to close it down, was taken by Margaret Thatcher's returning government, one year later.

I.L.E.A.'s problems stemmed from a combination of factors. First, the high price of property in London, drove experienced teachers out into suburbia. So, I.L.E.A., was reliant on many of its staff coming straight from college – the blind leading the blind!

Add to that, a misguided and idealistic political philosophy, at its heart – which took no account of the realities of human nature. Thus, the authority acquired the unfortunate reputation, that they would take anybody, as staff!

At yet another of their schools, one teacher actually said to me, 'I know that I am useless, and people told me that I.L.E.A. would take anybody, so that is how I got the job.' What a reputation to have! Where is the Inner London Education Authority, now? Relegated to the dustbin of history – at one with Nineveh and Tyre!

By contrast, Montessori Schools flourish, internationally, to this day. We had an excellent Montessori Mother and Toddler Play Group, run by Bonnie Perry, at the crisis house.

The comment in our Visitors' Book, made by Teresa Winship, when she visited this play group, from the Royal Berkshire Hospital, was, 'Absolutely fantastic!' Note: it was Bonnie Perry who ran it, not me!

Dal, our recent crisis house psychotherapy student, has a niece in a Montessori School. Another such school, flourishes, on the Wokingham Road, not a stone's throw from where I live, and there is yet another, highly successful, Montessori School, out in Hurst, in West Wokingham. Most recently, in January 2016, a new one has opened in Windsor.

The reason for Montessori's success, and for I.L.E.A.'s failure, is that Montessori is not about politics. It is about teaching; it is about education! So, it has passed the acid test; it has lasted!

An anecdote about Montessori teaching, illustrates an important, philosophical, point about services. A colleague had an eleven- year-old in his class who was completely unable to read and write. He asked to borrow some of my Montessori apparatus, to help him, because he feared, that if this child entered a large secondary school, unable to read and write, he would never catch up, and would become an adult illiterate.

I offered to teach this child during my lunch-times, and had him reading, and writing, fluently, within six weeks!

Now the important point! On 'Parents' Evening', my colleague brought this child's mother in, to thank me, which she did, with tears of relief running down her cheeks. What I said was this: 'You should not have to come and thank me. If a primary school fails to turn its pupils out – literate, and numerate – it has failed to do what society set it up for. We would not even be earning our money!' This philosophical point applies to all services which society sets up to meet all social needs – including mental health!

The lesson, for mental health services, is that Social Services came from an erroneous political stance. Welfare should be about care, and not about politics. It is about practical help and facilities, and not about psycho/social babble! So it needs to be restored to the voluntary sector.

You have waited for the joke, readers, and I shall not deprive you of it. Montessori, was, by far, the best teacher training course, that I ever undertook. Yes, you have guessed it. That is the one that the statutory authorities don't recognise – so all Montessori schools, are private schools!

Chapter 5

Background To The Crisis House

'I'm just an old-fashioned girl – with an old fashioned mind – not sophisticated – I'm the plain and simple kind'

One of my problems – when envisaging setting up the crisis house – is that I'm the plain and simple kind. If an organization states publicly that it wants something, being plain and simple, I assume that they want it – otherwise, why say so?

A quarter of a century ago, MIND, the National Association for Mental Health, had a Manifesto. Statement number one on the Manifesto was this:

'By the year two thousand, MIND wants to see all Victorian Mental Asylums closed, and replaced by services which users value – such as crisis houses in the community.'

Considering such a Manifesto, and its declared first priority, you would think, and we certainly thought, that for a MIND affiliated local association, to set up one such, pioneering, crisis house, would be hailed with delight, and warmly embraced by the national organization.

We also assumed, that, if we proved ourselves to be successful, over – say, a five year period – then, we would be used as the model for the development of such crisis houses, throughout the UK.

Not so! From the outset, they expressed fears, about the risks involved in such a project. We did receive some support from them, in terms of Awards, but this was largely, because the service users who were on the Awards Committee, insisted. They insisted because crisis houses in the community were what they, themselves, wanted as a mental health service. From the national organization, we never detected total support, for our user-run crisis house.

At one juncture, when we were undergoing our regular 'review' with one of their officers, I pointed out to her, 'The Wokingham Crisis House is the sort of place that is, all jokey on the surface, and all very carefully run, underneath – hence our immaculate record!' I think that she took my point.

We decided, however, to sever the connection with MIND, in 2004 – having reached the conclusion that we simply did not share their values – their true values, that is, not what they said on the tin!

I recall a radio interview, in which the presenter asked me – in response to my views on this subject – 'If national charities have no relevance to local mental health, why are they there?' 'To provide soft option employment, for failed social workers', I replied. 'Harsh words!' he said. I don't think so.

One such MIND employee, on yet another review, visited us. I asked the reasonable question, 'What is your background in mental health?' Her reply was, 'I worked in a hospital as a social worker – clearing beds for Consultants, and having to get people into the community, but....' now my words .... 'It was too much like work, so I thought that I would get a cushy little job with a charity. People think that charity workers are volunteers - but I am paid handsomely. I knew that I would not have to meet any targets, nor have any real responsibilities, but I could just go around telling voluntary groups like yours what to do, so here I am!'

Harsh thoughts of mine? I don't think so!

An important point to note, is that these 'professionals' who escape into employment with voluntary organizations, in order to shirk responsibility, inevitably bring some of their rubbish with them. Thus they will impose upon you 'Complaints Procedures' and 'Confidentiality Documents'. Why complain about something that is an alternative choice? If you don't like it, don't use it, or, as Agatha Christie would have it, leave the Balenciaga model hanging in the boutique!

As for confidentiality, whenever was a community confidential? The best communities have a healthy grapevine, and thus ensure that everyone within them, is looked after!

So incensed have I become, over the years, by the failure of national MIND, to implement any of its policies, or, indeed, to provide anything for mental health, that I was actually stimulated to write the following letter to the Press, and this was published in the *Wokingham Times* in February 2013.

Newspaper article: - 'Why are there not better services?'

"I refer to the letter that local mental health crisis care is in crisis, and that MIND [The National Association for Mental Health] is campaigning for better services [The Wokingham Times, *Wednesday, February 6th, 2013.]*

Why are they not providing them? MIND has existed for 67 years [NOW 70], and has an annual income of more than one hundred million pounds, yet, certainly in Berkshire, they provide no mental health services whatsoever, nothing.

There is a MIND charity shop on the Oxford Road in Reading. Where does the money raised there go? It certainly does not go to a

Reading MIND mental health service. There isn't one.

Until recently, sat comfortably in front of their computers, in their plush London Headquarters, paid MIND staff were passing the Berkshire buck to me. So I pointed out to their handsomely remunerated chiefs, that local people with mental health problems can easily access our service details, for free, in Wokingham library. They don't need to contact a redundant, but costly, MIND information line – only to be boomeranged back to us.

Furthermore, we cannot realistically provide a crisis service for places as far away as Newbury and Hungerford. Since we include 'West Berkshire' in our title, we have no objection to people from these towns using our services, but it is unacceptable that mentally ill people should have to travel so far to get a service.

One of our own service users, a Wokingham resident, recently rang the MIND information line - just to see what they could offer her of their own services. They referred her to Guildford!

Seven decades, and millions of pounds on, a national association for mental health, should either be providing a fully comprehensive network of services, including crisis care, in every locality throughout England and Wales, or cease to receive 'charitable status' and funding."

This was written in the context that MIND, by then, had no services left in Berkshire at all, and, in addition to passing the buck to me, were referring Berkshire people, to associations as far afield, as High Wycombe, in Buckinghamshire, and to Andover, in Hampshire.

More recently, in December 2014, Wycombe Mind became so incensed at, thus, being imposed upon, being expected to accept referrals from the Berkshire towns of Reading and Slough, that they contacted me – to see whether I would help support a re-launch of MIND in Berkshire.

I would not. Once bitten is twice shy. In my view, the way forward, for voluntary mental health services in Berkshire, is for each town to have its own, small, independent, mental health association – just as we have in Wokingham. A centralised, county-based, organization would not meet the need.

Hungerford – at the extreme west of the county – probably has, for instance, somewhat different needs, from those of Bracknell – which – again – has different needs from Slough – the latter having an enormous, ethnic minority, population.

But that is not to say, that a place like Hungerford, can't have severe mental health problems! Michael Ryan, being severely mentally ill, went berserk on the streets, and he went berserk on the streets of the nice little Berkshire town of Hungerford!

On the very day that I am writing this narrative, in September 2015, I have received an e-mail from a lady referred to me by MIND. This lady wanted me to provide an advocate, to attend a PIP [Personal Independence Payment] Assessment with her. Why cannot MIND, with its multi-million pounds income, provide such an advocacy service, the length and breadth of the UK? Why do they have to refer to me – unpaid, and unfunded?

Why A Separatist Crisis House?

Why, twenty-five years ago, did I want to set up a separatist, user-run, mental health crisis house? I had no personal experience of treatment within the main-stream mental health services. My experience of them was very limited, and second-hand, through members of my family. My own experience of mental health, was all through self-help and empowerment – so successful in my case – that I had a strong commitment to it being offered - at least as a choice - to other people.

Furthermore, my years of experience, in running support groups, for the National Schizophrenia Fellowship, led me to the conclusion, that it would be nice to have something more substantial to offer people, than tea and sympathy! A crisis house – with beds and a day-time drop-in centre would achieve this.

Luck has come into my experience. What was, then, the Wokingham MIND Local Association, was given the opportunity to take a lease on a house. Prior to 1991, we had only, for two years, a hired hall, as a drop-in centre. I have no doubt whatsoever, that the plan of the local statutory mental health service, was that they would get us taking the lease on the house - which was owned and funded by Wokingham District Council, and would then move in, and take over our Association.

This is precisely what happened with another local MIND Association with which I had been involved. [Now, of course, defunct!] In the initial stages, community volunteers are used to get something going, and, once they have, the idea is that local mental health professionals, will take over the committee – having all the decision-making power – and the community volunteers are then simply relegated for use as free labour!

Depending on what level they are at, the attitude of mental health 'professionals', towards volunteers, varies. High level professionals, such as Dr Anna Higget, [Chapter 12: 'Embroidered on silk!'.], are admiring, and appreciative. There is also the point that people like Dr Anna Higget, are highly intelligent. They see, immediately, what a service is about. In fact, I have always found doctors, in general, to be OK.

I worked with two very distinguished psychiatrists, when I chaired a National Schizophrenia Fellowship Working Party, on the Closure of Mental Hospitals – way back in the early 1980's.

I mentioned to one that I was 'Top of the Class', in a course that I was undertaking. 'I have no doubt, he replied, that that has always been the case, with you, wherever you have been.' Thus, observing that an individual is gifted, they will know that that individual has creative ideas for a separatist, and excellent, mental health service, and will not get involved with, low-grade, people in the main stream.

Both these psychiatrists shared my views about Social Services. I lamented that they were bringing in more training for social workers, 'So, it will be even more . . . .Yes, even more theoretical!' one finished, for me. The second, like me, lamented the demise of hospital almoners. These high level doctors prescribe excellent medical treatment for the mentally ill, but are so frustrated, that they can't get basic welfare services, to complement this.

By contrast, low grade 'professionals', are, frequently, outright rude and offensive.

My first real experience of this, occurred thirty-five years ago, when I was Local Voluntary Co-ordinator, for the National Schizophrenia Fellowship, in Ilford, Essex. The National Schizophrenia Fellowship, in those days, was a totally separatist, self-help, organization, so I rarely encountered any mental health 'professionals'.

I encountered this one, at a meeting about community care. He laughed in my face, and then declared, that I had no power. 'Social workers, he asserted, have definite powers, within the Mental Health Act. With you, the mentally ill can be as disturbed, and as violent, as they like. There is nothing you can do about it!'

It transpired, that he was a nurse at a local day centre, with an attitude typically to be found among the low grade! He spoke of his patients with utter contempt. Thus, it is so important to provide alternative, separatist, services. How awful, if a demeaning, and demoralising day centre, run by the likes of him, is the only service available to people!

That was my first bite of the cherry, but I have come across similar attitudes, perhaps not quite so pugnacious, quite frequently, ever since. In fact, he was talking nonsense. Social workers have no power. All that they can do, is to apply for a patient to be Sectioned – as, indeed, can the patient's nearest relative. Beyond the emergency Sections, then, two doctors, must agree that the patient should be detained, and there is, always, recourse to a Mental Health Review Tribunal.

Throughout my, successful, separatist stance, I have been told that I must co-operate with the Social Services, because they have the power and the money.

I always respond with my analogy to the Roman Catholic Church, not that I have anything against this institution. I even applaud some of its practices - such as celibacy for the priesthood. But, my analogy is a good one.

No one can deny, that the Roman Catholic Church, has enormous power, and vast riches. It owns the art treasures of the world! It has enormous influence over its millions of adherents. But, for the other millions, who don't believe in the Roman Catholic creed, it is all as nothing! I am the same with Social Services!

Voluntary organizations, in fact, have a lot of power, but it is power of a different kind – the power to do good! We are free to go to Parliament, and campaign for improvements, in the way that statutory organizations, are not. For instance, I recall seeing the Health Minister, when Severe Disablement Allowance, was to be introduced.

I emphasised to him, that it should be clearly established, that this benefit was to be available to the mentally, as well as to the, physically, disabled, and I was so pleased to see, that when the leaflet explaining this benefit, was published, it stated 'For the mentally, or physically, disabled' – giving mental disability the priority.

The Health Minister, furthermore, had his finger on the pulse. 'A medical examination will be required, he said, to establish a person's qualification for this benefit. Doctors are used to making objective judgements. But social workers . . . . .' and he shook his head!

Before setting up the Wokingham Crisis House, I was involved, briefly, with another local Mind Association. Local, low level, mental health professionals, were involved. They actually thought that they were going to tell the volunteers what to do, and to control them. This amused me. I thought, 'if they get control of Pam Jenkinson, they will be the first ever to do so!'

I have some memories of their awfulness. One social worker, when we were setting up the mental health centre, laughed, and said, 'Of course, after we have messed people up in the 'care' system, [Children's Social Services], then they often turn up in the adult mental health services!' I did not reply. I could hardly reveal my private thoughts, which were, that it would serve him right, if one of those whom he had 'messed up' in the care system, returned to the adult mental health services, and murdered him.

One of the Social Services' employees, in this MIND organization, was, almost unbelievably, incompetent. She used to flap around, losing things, and a regular activity for the service users, was 'hunt the handbag'. She had lost her handbag, again!

In the early days, she was supposed to be driving a group of us, over to Surrey – to see some, established, drop-in centres, there – with a view to getting some ideas for the drop-in centre that we were just setting up.

She overslept – leaving the group stranded. Finally, having intended to follow a full day's programme, carefully prepared by the Surrey people, we arrived after lunch. She had wrecked the whole day's schedule.

This woman had a colleague, an occupational therapist, who appeared to us to be just about as intelligent as one of her baskets! The service users had nick-names for this pair – Fanny Flapdoodle, and Dopey Dora!

Their colleague in this organization, the social worker who was expecting to encounter the people whom he had 'messed up' in 'care', turning up in the adult mental health services, said, of these two's deficiencies, 'It's difficult to get people.' The implication was, that any old rubbish, would do for the mental health voluntary sector!

If you watch the DVD that accompanies this book, you will observe that I regard COMPETENCE as the overall essential feature in a crisis house. One must be punctual, reliable, clean, tidy, and predictable. The house must be clean, tidy, neat, well organized. We are dealing with the chaos and confusion that go, inevitably, with mental illness. We do not wish to compound it!

I have never found it difficult to get good people. Over the twenty-five years, in the crisis house, we have recruited some excellent befrienders.

Some time after I had left that association, and had set up the crisis house in Wokingham, [ensuring legal protection from Social Services' infiltration, by banning them in the charity's Constitution], the incompetent social worker, telephoned me.

'Social Services, she explained, were running a 'Carers' Day'. Had I any carers in my Schizophrenia Fellowship Group, who might attend?'

I reflected, that any carer who got her, as a social worker, would end up, looking after their sick relative, and looking after her, as well! By contrast, none of the people whom we have befriended, over the twenty-five years, have had to look after their befriender!

By the time that the social worker was boasting, that he 'messed up' children, sufficiently, to drive them into adult mental health, I had already decided to leave this association, to go over to my colleague in Wokingham, and to set up a separatist service there. A fellow volunteer decided to stay.

After I had left, she laughed, on the telephone. 'You would have been furious, she said. We, [the remaining volunteers], voted to allow the Social Services to take over the Association – because that is the only way that we will get any funding. So I voted for this, because I wanted the mentally ill people to have a centre to go to.'

It is important to note, here, that the motivation, was excellent, the intentions, misguided, but good! This conversation took place in August.

Early in September, I received a second, hysterical, telephone call from this lady. She said that the Social Services had noticed that her daughter, who suffered from schizophrenia, was friendly with a man in the day centre, so they had placed them in a house, together. How stupid can you get?

On the Saturday, prior to Bank Holiday Monday, this man had committed suicide, and her daughter was left there – with the corpse. Because it was a holiday weekend, she could not get the services out. This horrific event had triggered another breakdown, and her daughter was, now, Sectioned, back into the mental hospital.

When Gavin Morton made his most recent visit to the crisis house, [Chapter 10: 'Step by step to success'] he questioned the wisdom of placing a number of severely mentally ill people in a block of flats together. That is where he, when seriously mentally ill, had been placed, and it ended in disaster.

I had a friend, some years ago, who came up with a better solution. His Housing Association had a number of individual flats – within a housing estate, but distributed throughout it, so no 'mental health' ghetto was created.

To return to my story, the following week, the local Press had telephoned the MIND Association, to see whether they had any comments, to make, about this tragedy. MIND, stated on its tin, that it stood up for the rights of the mentally ill, so the Press expected some adverse comments about the way that these patients had been treated!

This mother had plenty to say, and of a very critical nature, but the Social Services' employee, who was now established in the office, said that they had no comment to make!

The lady complained to me that the Social Services' employees were saying, 'Let's get these volunteers under control'. They can't control you if, like us, you won't let them through the door!

This lady was wailing, and weeping on my shoulder, but she failed to see that it was too late. Once they are in, you have lost your independence, and you will never get rid of them. If readers detect a certain lack of sympathy on my part, that is only because we must take the consequences of our actions! It would be nice if someone could wave a magic wand, and reverse everything stupid that we do, but they can't!

Since those days, I have suffered rudeness from a nurse at the [now defunct] mental hospital, and a nurse at the [now defunct] day hospital, but I have so little to do with them, and this is even more the case, now that we have closed the beds, that I have virtually eliminated their presence from my life!

In 2015, there was an attempt to re-involve me with local mental health 'professionals' – through the Wokingham Homelessness Forum, but, as Lewis Carrol would have it:

'The eldest oyster winked his eye, and shook his heavy head – meaning to say he did not choose to leave the oyster bed!'

As I tell crisis house service users regularly – 'They can only do to you what you let them'. They could not move in, and take over in Wokingham, because we, by unanimous vote, banned mental health professionals in the Association's Constitution, before we ever set up any services at all! I told the group of mental health users and carers on day one – 'You either vote to ban them tonight, or cry for the rest of your lives! Once they are in, you will never get rid of them.'

Of course, one can see the quandary for the uninitiated. To people with no previous experience of running mental health services, it seems so sensible, to have the local Consultant Psychiatrist, and Head of the local Mental Health Team, on your committee – to give their professional support. I told my fellow volunteers, that I would resign if the psychiatrist came on our committee, and I told the Head of the Mental Health Team, that we did not want his 'professional' support.

One of my points did go home, and probably persuaded people to the unanimous vote that was achieved. 'Can't you see, I said to them, that, having used statutory services, yourselves, if Social Services had any intention of providing anything worthwhile, they would already have done so? Why would they wait for us to come along? All that they want us for, is free labour, and a convenient dumping ground for people whom they are too lazy to deal with!'

I recall a local, grass roots, psychiatrist, visiting the crisis house, in our early days, with a desire to join our committee. She was grass roots – not like my distinguished friends, of my Schizophrenia Fellowship days.

When I explained that we were user run, and would not allow professional intervention, she maintained that she was only looking for a suitable place for her post natally depressed patients to come to, and did not wish to interfere in our running. In that case, why not simply refer her patients to us, and leave our committee alone? They say that they don't want to interfere, but they do!

I told her, bluntly, that the only relevance that mental health professionals could have to voluntary organizations, was when those at a very high level could provide us with specialist knowledge. 'How high do you have to be?' she asked. 'Higher than her', was the answer!

They went away, very angry, and no doubt thinking that, within a few weeks, we would have fallen apart, or experienced some dreadful incident, in our amateur-run crisis house. Twenty-five years on, we have done neither!

We had a very funny incident, at the crisis house, in these early days. Agatha Christie, never fails to come up with a parallel in her books – demonstrating her wonderful grasp of human nature

Twenty-five years ago, an official from the [defunct] Shire Hall was coming to see the crisis house. One of our number was so terrified that this official would see, and condemn, our use of the house for mentally ill residents, that she, bodily, lifted a wardrobe from a bedroom, and heaved it into the library, next door!

This has always reminded me of the scene in 'Hickory Dickory Dock': [Agatha Christie: Published: Collins: 1955.] Patricia and Nigel are arguing over a missing bottle of morphia. Patricia had removed it from Nigel's sock drawer, and hidden it in her own underwear drawer.

'Really Pat, said Nigel, your logical thought processes beggar description! What was the point?' 'I felt it was safer there.' 'My dear girl, either the morphia should have been under lock and key, or, if it wasn't, it couldn't really matter whether it was among my socks, or your handkerchiefs.'

My sentiments, at the time, coincided exactly with those of Nigel Chapman, in 'Hickory Dickory Dock'. The Crisis House either, was, or was not, being used as a residential crisis house, and if it was, whether you placed the wardrobe in the bedroom, or in the library next door to it, made no difference!

If the battle were over then, when we first told them that they were banned, life would be relatively trouble-free, but, alas, it is not. The undermining, and intent upon destruction, goes on and on. Fortunately, so does time. It dawned on them, one day, that five years had actually passed, since we set up the crisis house, and no disaster had happened. They were then, intent upon destruction, before it was too late.

My experience of main-stream mental health services is very limited, because I am a separatist. On the rare occasions that I have visited any of them, they invariably remind me of 'One Flew Over the Cuckoo's Nest'!

My efforts to make the Wokingham Crisis House a physically beautiful, as well as a user-friendly, place, are described in detail in other publications [Please see: 'This is Madness': PCCS Publications: Herefordshire: 1999.]. Suffice to say here, that we offer it as a CHOICE.

I obtained my ideas for my mental health service, from Agatha Christie's books, and the following two passages describe, exactly, what I have tried to create, in the Wokingham Crisis House.

Firstly, from 'The Pale Horse': [Published: Collins: 1961.]:

'The vicarage sitting-room was big and shabby. It was much shaded by a gargantuan Victorian shrubbery that no one seemed to have had the energy to curb. But the dimness was not gloomy for some peculiar reason. It was, on the contrary, restful. All the large shabby chairs bore the impress of resting bodies in them over the years.

A fat clock on the chimney piece ticked with heavy comfortable regularity. Here, there would always be time to talk, to say what you wanted to say, to relax from the cares brought about by the bright day outside.'

Then, from 'Dumb Witness': [Published: Collins: 1937.].

'The drawing room conjured up memories of the past. A faint fragrance of potpourri hung about it. The chintzes were worn, their pattern faded garlands of roses. On the walls were prints and water colour drawings. There was a good deal of china – fragile shepherds and shepherdesses. There were cushions worked in crewel stitch. There were faded photographs in handsome silver frames. There were many inlaid work-boxes and tea caddies. Most fascinating of all to me were two exquisitely cut tissue-paper ladies under glass stands. One, with a spinning wheel, one with a cat on her knee.'

These two passages reflect exactly the atmosphere and environment of the crisis house. It is good to see mentally distressed people do exactly that. They come in from the stressful world outside, relax, have a real cat climb onto their lap, and experience asylum!

If you actually prefer to sit on a broken plastic chair – with cigarette burns in it, [one of our members insisted that I include the cigarette burns]: if you want to gaze at a bare, dirty, wall, at a five years out-of-date calendar, and at a plant dying in its pot, because no-one has been funded to water it, by all means go to your local Social Services day centre. We're not stopping you!

The things I can guarantee you in statutory services, are plastic chairs and bare walls! Our crisis house has a thousand pictures. By contrast, I remember, over twenty years' ago, visiting a mental health day hospital [fortunately, now closed], which had only one picture on its grimy walls – 'The Scream' – by Edvard Munch!

Now, like me, you may legitimately prefer Constable to Turner, but both are, at least, suitable! Amongst our thousand pictures, we do have one Gauguin. I can't say that I go much for Gauguin, but his stuff is, at least, within the bounds of the acceptable.

Very important for mental health, we have Vermeer. I always held that this artist's work is therapeutic. My view was confirmed at the time that ethnic Moslems were being persecuted by Serbs in Bosnia. One of the officials charged with dealing with the atrocities, made a point, in the evenings, of visiting a Vermeer exhibition that happened to be showing at that time. He found that it relieved his mental distress.

'The Scream' – no! If you were not disturbed when you arrived at that awful place, I can guarantee that you would be, once you had walked through the door!

One of our service users, Peter Black, had received treatment for anxiety, at this awful day hospital. He tells the amusing story of how they attempted to make their service look scientific, and professional.

On admission, his anxiety levels were measured on a scale. On discharge, they were measured again. His levels were higher on discharge, than they were on admission. Hardly surprising if you have to sit looking at 'The Scream'! It is, in any case, all nonsense. Human emotions, like anxiety, are immeasurable!

Chapter 6

A Therapeutic Environment

'Home, home, sweet, sweet, home.
Be it ever so humble, there's no place like home!'
John Howard Payne

Once you have banned the professionals – with their environments that resemble either rubbish dumps, or operating theatres, it is advisable to think about mental illness, and what are the features in an environment, that mental health service-users actually need.

They are depressed and disturbed. They need things that are bright, cheerful, cosy, comfortable, interesting, stimulating, and, above all, safe. One of my current service users, laments the fact that we don't have open coal fires. The Crisis House is a Victorian building, with chimneys, but, like most people in the twenty-first century, we have gone in for electric fires, that only look as though they have glowing coals.

This service-user appreciates greatly all our efforts, and would like them to be even more authentic. My problem is that I have such a lot of work to do anyway, that I don't feel able to take on scuttles of coal, and clearing up ash!

People with severe mental health problems, don't always find it easy, to initiate conversation. Beautiful objects stimulate this. On the very day before I was writing this narrative, a service-user, a sufferer from chronic schizophrenia, came into our drop-in lounge, and commented that some figurines displayed on the centre table, were the work of Jack Vetriano.

I had not realised this when I bought them, but liked them, because they were full of life and movement. As well as mental health books, we have, in our library, art books – including one on Jack Vetriano. We looked at this, and found that our service user was right, and this stimulated further discussion about Vetriano's work. By contrast, sitting in a Social Services day centre, one can't discuss a bare wall!

If you want some of the features of civilization – animals, fresh flowers, hand-embroidered table-cloths, comfortable chairs and cushions, original paintings, and a well-stocked bar, come to us!

Wokingham, largely because of the high property prices, and the fact that the Thames Valley is the epicentre of the high technology industry, is the kind of place that is full of successful professional, and business people.

It must be so demeaning for them if, unfortunate enough to have suffered mental health problems, they have to attend dreary and infantilizing services. The kind of person who, without us, would have fallen foul of such services, was Malcolm Chase. [Chapter 9: 'Manners makyth man'.]

Malcolm Chase was a Cambridge science graduate, had been a successful businessman, a multi-millionaire. How awful, if, now poverty stricken due to mental illness, nothing was available to him – other than the standard mental health service.

If you go into statutory services, a dozen identical chairs, ordered, without thought, from a catalogue, confront you. Frequently, they are all low, and without arms. So, on occasions, if you sit down, you struggle to get up! A drop-in centre needs chairs for fat people, and chairs for thin people, high chairs and low chairs, chairs to snuggle into, hard chairs, and soft chairs!

We have one, elderly service user, who has recently undergone a, not altogether successful knee replacement. He is most appreciative of a chair recently donated, especially for him, by one of my brothers. This brother, now retired, was highly successful in professional life, as an accountant. He has always been very supportive of the crisis house, has visited on numerous occasions, and has donated many useful, and beautiful, items to us.

Indeed, all of my siblings who do not suffer from mental illness, have done very well in life. Coming again to Agatha Christie, Hercule Poirot explains, that, when young, he was poor, there were many brothers and sisters, and so he had to get on in life. If no one else is there to give one advantages in life, then one has to make it by oneself!

The chair donated by my brother is a comfortable armchair, but it is high, so our service user, who cannot bend his knee, does not experience agony when getting out of it. Such may seem very simple things, but they make all the difference!

Of all the features in our crisis house, our wonderful bar is probably the one that has raised most questions. I explain, patiently. In a place like Wokingham, you get a lot of people, who have been, overall, successful in life, but, due to work or personal problems, have suffered a mental breakdown. They are used to the adult freedoms, the adult choices, and our bar gives them that reassurance that all is not lost. Mental health problems, or not, you can still have a whisky and soda!

As I have already described earlier in this book, relentless efforts have been made over the years, to destroy the Wokingham Crisis House. On occasions, mental health service users have, themselves, been used, as a front, to assist in this destruction.

My only reprisal is to ban them from our premises – suggesting that main-stream services may be more suitable for them, since that is what they say they want. The main-stream services can hardly regard this openly as a reprisal, but, in my view, it is by far the worst punishment that anyone can possibly inflict.

Nothing can be more valuable, nor more telling, than the views of the service users, themselves. This article appeared in the *Wokingham Times* – on the occasion of Dr Anna Higget's visit in November 1999.

Article in local newspaper - 'It's The Homely Approach That Does So Much To Aid Recovery'

"Wokingham and District MIND [as we were then] offers a very different approach to helping those with mental health problems, compared to professional organizations like the NHS. Harriet Jones found this plays a key role in getting its users well again.

'One of the things I love about this place is there's no file on me, no labels are attached to me, I am just me.' Denise Grimsdell is a 44 year old service user of Wokingham and District MIND Crisis House. Mrs Grimsdell, who works as a care visitor to sufferers of Alzheimers disease, became a regular at Wokingham and District MIND, Station Approach, in April of this year.

She said, 'I'd been diagnosed as having post traumatic stress disorder. I was depressed. I needed someone who could understand the problems I was having. I found the atmosphere here was family-like – I was able to talk about the problems I'd had because it's relaxing and non-judgmental.'

Wokingham MIND offers something of a departure from the norm in terms of offering care to people with diagnosed mental health problems. Pam Jenkinson, who has worked tirelessly as a volunteer for the charity since Wokingham's branch of MIND was born ten years ago, explained its philosophy. She said 'We are a radical, separatist, mental health service. We don't work in partnership with the National Health Service or social services. It is written in our constitution that professionals are banned from any involvement – the only thing they can do is visit.' She added 'We're never going to change that stance.'

Mrs Jenkinson tours the UK speaking about the unusual stance Wokingham's branch of MIND takes. It was a recent lecture she gave which prompted the unusual visit of Government Policy Adviser, Dr

Anna Higgett. The senior adviser, on secondment from her routine work as a psychiatrist – was so impressed by what she heard of the crisis centre, she decided to see it for herself.

Dr Higgett agreed that the atmosphere in the cosy house was so relaxed it made it difficult to identify who exactly were the service users and who were the volunteers. She said: 'My visit has backed up my initial impressions – it works. But only with an awful lot of effort, good will and energy.'

The aim of the centre – which offers crisis beds to those in times of trouble – is to give people back their self-esteem. Mrs Jenkinson said: 'We want people to access their own strengths, and, with the support of others, get back to a normal life. It is not that we are against the services offered by professionals – we just don't share their philosophy.'

Philip Green, who is unable to work due to anxiety and depression, has been involved with Wokingham's branch of MIND since its advent. Over the last decade his involvement has changed, so much so, he is no longer simply a service user, but a carer as well. He said 'I still have treatment for my illness. With this type of illness, you have to learn to deal with it on your own – it's about tailoring your life to what you can manage, and learning to live within your limitations. But that does not mean that you can't have a fulfilling life, because I do.'

Philip attributes much of his happiness and ability to cope with living with mental health problems to the time he has spent with people at the crisis centre. He explained :'I've got my independence. I lived with my parents until I was thirty-seven, but MIND helped me to get my own place nearly two years ago. I've got a partner who I met here [one of the rare occasions when meeting at the crisis house proved a long-term success]. Being involved in this place is like being part of an extended family. To say this place has made my life a lot better is an understate - ment.'

Everyone involved in the crisis house stands firm in their belief that the care offered by Wokingham and District MIND is the way forward for mental health treatment.

Denise Grimsdell explained that she has a fierce loyalty to the centre after receiving what she terms 'rough treatment' at the hands of the NHS. She said: 'I support this place 100 per cent – I feel protective of this place.I feel this has got to be the way forward for mental health when everything else is failing."

NOTE: Dr Anna Higgett's comment is that the crisis house works because of the hard work, good will, and energy that goes into it. Is not that the reason, distinguished psychiatrist, that anything that works, works?

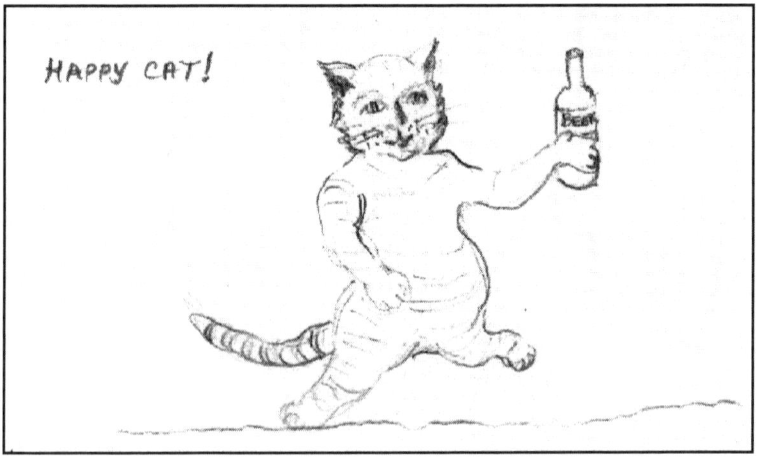

PART TWO

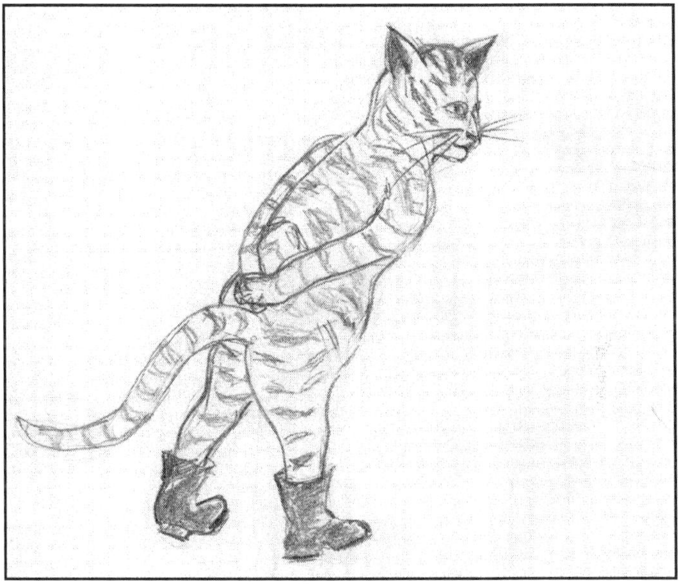

'With His Hands Behind Him, You Will Always Find Him'

Twenty-Five Crisis House Success Stories

In twenty-five years, any project will look back upon a mixture of results. We have had a number of spectacular successes, a handful of abject failures, and most results, falling somewhere between those two poles. I have selected, from the many available, one success story for each of the twenty-five years in which the crisis house has been operating.

It is a fact, that the crisis house has about it, that, '*je ne sais quoi*', that goes with success. One cannot define, exactly, what this is, but people coming to visit us, recognise it immediately, and I am so glad that this is the case, because mental health is, so frequently, associated with failure!

This is why I am such a fan of Susan Boyle – success, despite the mental health, success – even with the mental health. I play her wonderful rendering of 'I Dreamed a Dream' regularly, and it never fails to inspire me!

'I dreamed a dream in times gone by,
when hopes were high, and life worth living.
I dreamed that love would never die,
I dreamed that God would be forgiving.
For I was young, and unafraid, when dreams are made, and
used, and wasted. There was no ransom to be paid,
no song unsung, no wine untasted.

But the tigers come at night, with their voice as soft as thunder, and
they tear your hopes apart, and they turn your dream to shame.

I had a dream that life would be so different from this
hell I'm living, so different now, from what it seemed.
Now life has killed the dream, I dreamed.'

We have had people in the crisis house, who could sing this song from 'Les Misérables' – with Susan Boyle. Both Malcolm Chase, and Toby Warfield [Chapter 9: 'Manners makyth man' and Chapter 11: Why not enjoy life?'], described their childhood as idyllic, but, adult life, as full of problems.

Mind you, there are, also, people, like Maurice Santereau, and myself, [Chapter 10: 'What Starts as Disaster, can end as Triumph', and my Introduction: Chapter 1: 'It was Always You From The Start'], who find adult life, compared with early life, wonderful, beyond our wildest dreams! Agatha Christie always has her finger on the pulse of human experience. In 'Five Little Pigs', she recognised this truth:

'It occurred to him [Hercule Poirot], that of the five people in whom he had become interested as a result of his investigations, those who might have been said to start with the fullest advantages, were not those who had actually wrested the most success and happiness from life. Elsa, [the little pig who had roast beef], who might have been said to start with all advantages – youth, beauty, riches – had done worst. Cecilia Williams [the little pig who had none], to outward appearances , had no assets of which to boast. Nevertheless, to Poirot's eye, there was no despondency there, and no sense of failure. In Angela Warren [the little pig that cried 'wee, wee, wee, wee' all the way home], – that young creature – handicapped by disfigurement and its consequent humiliations, Poirot believed he saw a spirit strengthened by its necessary fight for confidence and assurance.'

Overcoming disadvantage, and disability, and fighting for confidence and assurance, is what the Wokingham Crisis House is, and has always been, about.

Chapter 7

Early Success: 1991 - 1996

When we took over the Crisis House, twenty-five years ago, the lease was awarded on condition that we would continue to welcome into the drop-in centre, a small group of chronically mentally ill people, who had been used to attending the Crisis House when it was the former statutory mental health facility. We agreed, gladly, to this.

1991 - 1992: Eileen Morrison: 'I wanted to be a nurse'

One of the group was Eileen Morrison. Eileen was a small, attractive forty-year-old - very neatly dressed, and with pretty blonde curly hair. She was diagnosed with depression, and had been trapped in the mental health system for several years.

Eileen illustrated perfectly the point that I am always making, and that Judi Chamberlin made before me. [Please see: 'On Our Own'. Publisher: MIND: London: 1988.] The mental health system will NOT sort your life out. Outsiders can see this so clearly – while patients and their families, trapped within the system, go on hoping in vain – just as Judi Chamberlin and her mother did for years.

Our Sadie Minton's mother, as an outsider, saw the truth immediately. [Chapter 8: 'She ticks all the boxes'.] Nearly thirty years ago, Sadie's mother came to see me at the system-run mental health day centre, which I was shortly to desert - in order to come over to Wokingham, and set up a separatist centre there. Of the system-run centre, she said: 'You start going to a place like that, and you could still be going at fifty!' How right she was!

Eileen Morrison told me that she had always wanted to be a nurse. She had done very well in grammar school – with excellent 'A' Level results – so her parents, dissatisfied with nursing as a career for her – insisted that she attend Law School. They also disapproved of her boyfriend of the time – whom she went on to marry, without their blessing. Eileen had a breakdown, and dropped out of Law School, after one year. Her marriage ended in divorce, but she had two daughters – suffering post-natal depression after each of the births. When I first met Eileen, the daughters were aged eighteen, and sixteen, respectively.

'Eileen, I said. You don't need to remain a chronic mental patient for the rest of your life. Now that your daughters are about to launch into their careers, why not launch into yours? Apply to work as a nursing auxiliary at a local nursing home. Prove yourself, by getting six months' experience, and a good reference under your belt. Then we can apply to colleges for nursing training.'

Eileen was turned down by all the colleges that we applied to – despite her experience and references – because of her mental health history. I suggested then, that she try to get in, through Clearing, and this she achieved.

She was top of her year in her final exams, went on to qualify as a community psychiatric nurse, and met her second husband while working in community nursing - taking his high-class, double-barrelled, name - as the icing on the cake! Eileen returned to celebrate with us on the tenth anniversary of the crisis house. Success story!

1992 - 1993: Peggy Taylor: 'Paddle your own canoe'

Peggy came to the drop-in centre – having suffered a breakdown. We gave her a lot of support and she made a full recovery – going on to train to be a counsellor – a success story.

Peggy's husband was so pleased that we had restored her to full health, that he wanted to show his gratitude. He ran a driving school for a living, and so offered, as a reward, to give me thirty, free, driving lessons.

I had never driven a car in my life, and never had any desire to do so. I thanked him for his kindness, but pointed out that I was technically and technologically challenged, completely uncoordinated, and not even able to operate a treadle sewing machine! I have my talents. I can write for England, and I also deserve a Nobel Prize for my ability to dispense with bureaucratic nonsense, and red tape! I can stand up and chair a conference of a thousand people – without turning a hair! But mechanics and machinery, no! He persisted, so, in the end, I gave in.

I took all thirty lessons. We started on a little blind road on the Bean Oak Estate – leading to a field. There was no other traffic on the road. What did I achieve in the thirty lessons? I was able to open the car door and get in. When I remembered, I was able to turn the ignition key. I never touched the pedals, but I did, in abject terror, learn to turn the steering wheel to the left, but never to the right.I refused to move the car at a speed of more than three miles an hour, so – not only was the engine likely to fail, but we agreed that one could walk faster. We never got off that little blind road!

In one of my lives, I recall, in my reading, coming across a cognitive psychologist – one Jean Piaget. He maintained that people absorb only the knowledge that is relevant, and needed by them. I agree with him. Furthermore, it is not a bad thing for people to know, that however brimming over with confidence one may be, everyone has their vulnerabilities!

After thirty lessons, I thanked William and said, 'Look, William. I am terrified of the roads. You are not. You run a Driving School. But you are terrified of the mentally ill! I am not. I run a mental health centre. Let us each paddle our own canoe. You stick to yours, and I'll stick to mine!'

Agatha Christie, among the many pearls of wisdom found in her works, gives the advice not to waste any time on something that one is never going to be any good at. I, at least since foolish youth, have always embraced this advice wholeheartedly!

1993 – 1994: Rosie Kalley: 'I don't ever want to go home anymore'

Rosie Kalley was one of the group of chronically mentally ill patients who had attended the Crisis House when it was a statutory mental health facility – prior to being taken over by us.

Rosie was the full-time carer of her husband of thirty-five years – whom she had married at the tender age of eighteen. For the past twenty-five years, he had suffered from multiple sclerosis. She was alone and isolated with his care – at times having to struggle up and down the stairs - with her husband balanced on a tray!

Rosie's life followed a predictable pattern. She would take regular overdoses of pills and alcohol, be admitted to the hospital, where they would de-toxify her, and then return her to her unbearable living situation. We decided to intervene. 'Can't you see, I asked her social worker, that one of these overdoses is going to be THE overdose – the one that kills her?'

In my experience, the tragic and the funny, so often go together. I recall the funny occasion when some of our befrienders had gone to see Rosie, and discovered that she was collapsed on the floor – having taken an overdose of pills and alcohol. They rang me for advice. 'She is still conscious, they said, shall we try talking to her?' 'No, I replied, you don't TALK to an overdose. Get an ambulance immediately, and, when she is discharged from hospital, recovered, THEN we can talk to her!'

In those glad old days of twenty and more years ago, the Disabled Living Foundation had available a Fund to pay for professional nurses to give round-the-clock care to patients such as Rosie's husband – thus relieving the informal carer. We arranged this, and admitted Rosie as a guest in the crisis house.

When the local Social Services questioned this, we made our position clear. 'How would you like to be nursed by somebody who is out cold, half the time, on pills and alcohol?' we demanded!! What we are doing is better for both the patient, and for the carer!' We resisted all attempts at emotional blackmail, and saw to it that Rosie was protected from them.

Rosie was an exhausted, spent, woman. When we admitted her, her knuckles were severely swollen with rheumatoid arthritis. This disappeared, as her stress levels abated. Rosie never went home. Her initial protests of 'I have to go home! I have to go home!', soon became 'I don't ever want to go home anymore!'

Rosie's actual marriage had broken down decades before, and all that she was, when she first came to us, was an exhausted and exploited care-giver – expressing her rage, and feelings of entrapment, in repeated overdoses.

When she was ready to move out of the crisis house, we found Rosie a lovely, rented flat in Rose Street – the most desirable part of Wokingham. She found a job, and a boyfriend, and, at the age of fifty-three, Rosie started to live again. Her former husband continued to receive proper, professional, nursing care, until his death some considerable time later. Had we not intervened, both would have died! Success story!

1994 – 1995: Edwina Schaley: 'Gentlemen prefer blondes'

When I met Edwina Schaley, she was a Sectioned patient in the mental hospital. She explained that she had a diagnosis of bi-polar affective disorder – an illness from which she had suffered since the birth of her two infant sons – now aged one and two.

Her Consultant Psychiatrist had said that he would have been prepared to lift the Section, and to discharge her home, but that her husband didn't want her back. He was having an affair with the resident nanny, who was looking after the two small boys in Edwina's absence.

I regarded Edwina as being extremely beautiful. She was tall and slim – with shining jet-black hair. Prior to marriage and motherhood, she had been a nursing sister.

I suggested that she come and stay in the crisis house, until her situation was resolved, so, with her Clinical Team's approval, she was admitted. Edwina worked hard on her problems from day one. Her husband was very critical of her, and, in particular, of her alleged neglect of the children. He brought the divorce papers, for Edwina, to sign whilst she was staying with us.

The nanny, a little blonde thing, who, in my opinion, was not a patch on Edwina, also visited with the children. How he could have preferred her, bemused me, but, as they say, 'Gentlemen prefer blondes!'

Edwina stayed for just over two months. In that time, she found a new boyfriend, found a private-sector rented flat, and found part-time work in Debenhams – from which, in due course, she graduated to Bank Nursing – with a view to getting back into full-time nursing, eventually. She also, through her solicitor, made arrangements for access, and, hopefully, for eventual custody, of the children. Step by step, up the ladder, as it always is, Edwina was a success story.

1995 - 1996: Rob Jenkins: 'Driving the bus'

When Rob came to us, he was severely underweight and depressed. His wife had divorced him, and he was homeless. He had been made redundant from his job as a refrigeration engineer, and was virtually destitute. Having always worked, he was largely unaware of the existence of welfare benefits.

Once Rob had settled into the crisis house, we sorted out his benefit claims, to ensure that he got an income. Our previous minibus driver had died, so we suggested that Rob drove the minibus - bringing people to the drop-in centre from all around Wokingham District.

Rob stayed for five months in the crisis house – recovering all the time. During this time, he saved five hundred pounds from his benefit money – a remarkable achievement. This enabled him to pay the deposit on a rented flat in the private sector. This flat was close to the crisis house, and, after leaving, he continued to drive the minibus for five years. A success story.

Sadly, Rob died, of motor neurone disease, at the age of sixty-eight, in October 2001. Why then, have I included him in 'Success Stories', rather than in 'Tragic Stories'?

This question brings me to a television programme, in which a neurosurgeon, from Oxford's John Radcliffe Hospital, explained that he measured his success, in getting the patient off the operating table, in good health, today, and not in terms of how that patient would be, in thirty years' time!

In the crisis house, we are endeavouring to get long-term, and sustainable, success, but, in some instances, even a further five, or ten, years of quality life, can be accounted a success – where previous circumstances were dire! A similar argument could be applied to Malcolm Chase. He died, from a stroke, in the summer of 2011, but he had achieved a better quality of life, for over nine years, after leaving the crisis house, in March 2002.

Chapter 8

Ongoing Success

1996 – 1997: Jack Hayward: 'All right in the sanctuary'

Jack Hayward's mother came to see me in tears. She explained that her son was severely mentally disturbed, and violent – having suffered a mental breakdown whilst at university. He had broken up the kitchen at their family home, so he had been staying temporarily with his grandmother, but he was now returning to the family, and his mother didn't know what to do.

I advised, first, that she consult a doctor, and get a proper diagnosis. The likelihood would be that he would then be admitted to hospital, and prescribed medication. This was done.

Once due for discharge from hospital, having received a diagnosis of schizophrenia, I suggested that Jack should come and stay in the crisis house until supported accommodation was arranged for him. 'But he will break up your kitchen', his mother remonstrated. 'He will not', I replied. 'The crisis house has an emotionally neutral ambience - whilst families have a high expressed emotion ambience - which people with schizophrenia cannot tolerate.'

He came to us – staying for six months, improving all the time, and presenting no problems. He then moved into a local supported flat - the family helping with carpets and furniture – to make an attractive home. Jack continued to improve – doing voluntary work – volunteer driving, and work with a local learning disabilities charity. His mother attended our Association's twenty-five year anniversary celebration – still grateful for our enabling of Jack to achieve success and a good quality of life.

One thing intrigued me about Jack. He explained that he had such lovely parents, and such a nice home, that he could not cope with aggression and hostility when he encountered it. He maintained that his illness, schizophrenia, had been triggered - because he was bullied at school - where he had been captain of the rugby team. The captain of the rugby team – bullied. Not in my young day, he wouldn't have been!

1997 – 1998: Adela Walsh: 'Use your talents'

Adela came to us in 1997 – having made a suicide attempt. She had lost the tenancy on her rented flat when admitted to hospital, and so, on discharge, was homeless. Adela was a talented music graduate. She had attempted to train for school-teaching – but without success.

Adela came from a very unstable background – her mother being diagnosed with bi-polar affective disorder – as was Adela herself. An example of the kind of things that her mother did, was forcing Adela to watch the film, 'Psycho' at the age of five! Adela stayed for some months in the crisis house – gradually getting herself back together. Eventually, it seemed appropriate for her to move out, so I told Adela's social worker that she was as ready as she was ever going to be.

The social worker found Adela a scruffy bed-sitter at the top of a house in the Red Light area of Reading. They visited the place, which was at the top of a narrow staircase. It was scruffy and depressing – with a defective electric heater. 'Ha, ha, ha, chortled the social worker. You have your own, personal, electro-convulsive therapy machine!' And you ask me why I want them abolished! The thought of moving into this awful place, daunted Adela, but she put on a brave face, and said nothing to me. It was Adela's boyfriend who put me wise.

Adela had a boyfriend, who would come and stay with her at the crisis house at weekends. He was fifty-two years old - to her twenty-seven years, and he had a very good job as a film director. He was divorced from his wife, but they had two teenage boys at public school. The boyfriend expressed concern to me about the awful place that the social worker had found for Adela. 'Could I do anything?'

'Well, I replied, the crisis room that she occupied is still vacant. Let her move back in, and we will then help her to find a better place.'

Adela sometimes lamented to me that, at times, she believed this boyfriend only wanted her, in order to get her knickers off on a Friday night. I was now able to be reassuring. 'Partly true, Clifford has been married, and has his boys, so he is not looking for marriage and a family, but he cared enough to come to me, when you were faced with the awful prospect of that bedsitter. So it is not the case that all men are bastards.'

Adela stayed awhile, and, eventually, moved into a very nice flat near to Reading University. She was able to get the high rent reduced, by giving the landlord's children free music lessons – a good use of her talents. In due course, Adela met a younger man, married him, and they had a little girl, Angela. Success story.

On the occasion that she visited the crisis house to find out what we were about, I explained to Adela's social worker that we were all unpaid – totally voluntary. 'Why then do you do it?' she said. I felt tempted to give the true answer, 'In order to protect them from people like you!'

There is a funny addendum to Adela's story. As I explain in 'Our

Befriending Service', I advise against befrienders inviting, those befriended; to their own homes. Adela and Clifford were the only ones, ever, that I invited to dinner at my house. Other service users were, naturally, curious. 'What was it like?' they asked.

'Very peculiar, Adela replied. The food was lovely, but you all sat around a polished oak, dining room table – with a lace table cloth, and you had linen table napkins, in silver rings, and wine, in crystal glasses. For a radical separatist, she sure does have conservative tastes!' *Chacun à son gout. Chacun à son gout.* I would not like to sit on a bean bag on the floor – eating dinner with my fingers, but if that is what you like to do, then, *chacun à son gout*!

I want to see social work abolished

The first 'professional' social work training course in the world, was instituted at the London School of Economics in the 1930's. Shame on you, Alma Mater! It was a product of the, flawed, political philosophy of socialism – then, very much, in the ascendant, and embraced by idealists. That is just the problem!

The ideal, was that society's welfare would no longer be delivered, haphazard, by Lady Bountiful. Instead, we would have trained, paid, agents of the State – employed to sort out your life! Thus were invented social workers, or, should I say, social shirkers?

The original criticism, was that Lady Bountiful was patronising to her beneficiaries. Did they think that paid, social workers would not be patronising? The difference is that Lady Bountiful was, at least, patronising with her own money. Social services are patronising with ours!

Since then, we have seen the scandals, of Maria Colwell, in the 1970's, of Jasmine Beckford, in the 1980's, and of Tyra Henry, in the 1990's. Continuing into the twenty-first century, we have seen the scandal of Victoria Climbie, of Peter Connolly, [Baby P.], and, more recently, of the little Polish boy – who literally starved to death. Now, in January 2016, the facts regarding the abuse and death of Poppi Worthington have finally been published. Police were criticised as well, but social workers claim child care as a 'Profession'.

In the 1980's, I actually attended the House of Lords debate - on Jasmine Beckford – led by the late Baroness Faithfull – former Head of Oxfordshire's Children's Services. She acknowledged the deficiencies, but, she thought that the answer was in better training. It isn't. It is in abolition, and give society's welfare back to volunteers, in charities.

Child protection should be restored to the National Society for the Prevention of Cruelty to Children, to Barnardo's, and to other children's charities, which, traditionally, assumed responsibility for child welfare. Age UK should have responsibility for the elderly, MENCAP, for the learning disabled, and so on. Most important, all this charitable work should be undertaken by volunteers. The role of social worker, a paid official, should be abolished.

The Post Mortem examination of Tyra Henry, revealed that the child had ninety human bite marks on her corpse! Do you need training to observe these?

Add to these high profile cases, all the other instances of neglect and incompetence, and the fact that the [now, abolished,] National Institute of Social Work, had, at one time, a notorious paedophile, as its Director, and how long will it take for society to grasp the nettle?

It is the fundamental concept that is faulty. A paid agent of the State is not going to sort out your life. Generally speaking, you are.

Of course, I accept that there are people who, either don't know how to cope with daily life, or who are too ill to do so. The former need teachers, the latter need nurses, and doctors. These are genuine professions – which have stood the test of time.

The ancient Greeks, for instance, had teachers and doctors! Evil people need to be sorted out by the Police, and the Criminal Justice System. Society does not need social workers, at all!

In the case of Baby P., it was quite obvious that the child's mother pretended to be co-operating with the social worker – while the social worker was looking, and went back to countenancing abuse, and torture, once the front door was closed. We are dealing, here, with evil, and not with ignorance. This brings me to the subject of Parenting Classes.

Whenever I hear about Parenting Classes, a naughty, little imp, pops up in my brain. What the naughty, little imp, tells me, is this:

'The kind of person, who will attend a Parenting Class regularly, who will listen to the child-care experts, who will read the books, who will try out the skills taught, and who will persevere patiently, if things don't improve immediately – is, wait for it, readers - the kind of person who would be a good parent anyway!!!!'

It would be all right if they had people, who, like me, are still listening to the Montessori tutor – forty-five years later, but they haven't!

The awful, and poignant, other side to this coin, is that Social Services take children away, when they shouldn't, just as frequently as they fail to take them away, when they should. For an instance of this malpractice, please see my chapter on 'Advocacy'.

One of our service-users, Edwin Huggin, was particularly bitter about Social Services' failure to do anything, when the removal of himself and his brothers, from his abusive family, was what was needed.

His parents were very well educated – a scientist, and a teacher. They systematically abused their children – both physically, and emotionally, but, because the children were not obviously, dirty, scruffy, and starving, and because the parents were well-dressed, well-spoken, and articulate, Edwin and his brothers were left to suffer the abuse.

Edwin asserted, that Social Services would only intervene, when the neglect was obvious. Maurice Santereau said the same thing. [Chapter 10: 'What starts as disaster, can end as triumph'.]

I tend to be even more critical. At times, they don't even intervene in cases of the most appalling, and obvious abuse. What is the answer? Get rid of them! As with the latest case of Poppi Worthington.

One of my favourite stories in Agatha Christie's Collection, 'The Hound of Death', [Published: Collins: 1933.] is called, 'The Fourth Man'.

In it, Dr Campbell Clark states. 'Felicie Bault was a Brittany peasant girl. She was the third of a family of five, the daughter of a drunken father and a mentally defective mother. In one of his drinking bouts the father strangled the mother and was, if I remember rightly, transported for life. Some charitable people interested themselves in the children and Felicie was brought up and educated by an English maiden lady who had a kind of home for destitute children.'

The story goes on to explain, that little could be made of Felicie, but that another child, Annette, was musical, and was encouraged by the maiden lady to study at the Paris Conservatoire of Music.

This is what we want to see once again – dedicated people, with plenty of time and money, who will devote themselves to the future of disadvantaged children. Such was the culture of voluntary service – where individuals received the practical help that they needed to gain a foothold in the adult world. We do not want paid agents of the State, who fail them, so that they end up in adult mental health services.

Interestingly, our service user, Rosamund, who had spent her teenage years in a Salvation Army Approved School, did get this kind of help. When it was time for her to leave the school, their officer got her a job as a wardmaid at the Royal Berkshire Hospital.

By contrast, the people whom we know, who have left local authority 'care', usually end up, unemployed, in prison, or, as our notorious social worker confessed, in adult mental health services!

1998 - 1999: Sadie Minton: 'She ticks all the boxes'

I regard Sadie Minton as a success story. She has suffered from mental health problems for most of her adolescent and adult life, and I have been involved with Sadie and her family for virtually the entire thirty years that I have worked in voluntary mental health services in Berkshire.

Sadie, as an adolescent, started with a diagnosis of schizophrenia, then went on to acquire the label 'severe personality disorder'. In due course, they added 'with schizoid features', and finally, with Sadie now in her fifties, went back to the original diagnosis of schizophrenia.

Sadie has been very disturbed over all the years that I have known her, so why do I describe her as a success story? The answer is that she has achieved a good quality of life in all areas – albeit in a limited way – despite her severe mental health problems.

First, she has a very nice house in a pleasant part of Wokingham. True, a well-to-do relative bought the house for her, and it is held in trust to protect her from predators. No matter, she has a nice house in a good area, and she has proved herself capable of keeping the house in a good state – albeit with some help from her family.

Secondly, Sadie works. True, she only works for two hours a day, six days per week, in a little, unsupervised, cleaning job. No matter, she works, and her employer is satisfied with her work.

This success was prejudiced, some years ago, by the meddling of a local employment advice service. Observing that Sadie was well-spoken, well-educated, well-dressed, and well presented, and, obviously, from a good background, they thought that cleaning was not good enough for her, and sent her on an accountancy training course. The stress brought about a breakdown, and another admission to hospital.

What intrigued us about this intervention, was their failure to see that a person who is capable of training as an accountant, doesn't usually wait until the age of forty-five, to do so! On recovery, we advised Sadie to stick with cleaning, and she has done so, successfully, ever since!

Thirdly, Sadie has a partner in a long-term, stable, relationship. True, she suffered for many years at the hands of exploitative and short-term sexual partners. No matter. In her forties, Sadie met a good, sound, person. True, the relationship is limited. They live separately – meeting up when mutually convenient, but Sadie is capable of cooking very well, they go out to places of interest, and enjoy holidays together. Their relationship is good, if limited.

Fourthly, Sadie looks years younger than her fifty-three years, is invariably very well-dressed, and well presented, and looks remarkably glamorous for a woman of her age. True, due to her mental problems, Sadie is constantly dyeing her hair, and changing her make-up. She is also a shopaholic for clothes. No matter, the result is excellent.

Finally, Sadie has hobbies. True, though attending Art School when young, Sadie achieved only a Foundation Course Certificate. No matter, she has an eye for design and colour, and has proved herself capable in knitting and craft-work.

So – not just in my eyes - but in the eyes of society, Sadie is a success. If, in twenty-first century society, you have a nice house in a nice area, you work, you have a good, stable relationship, you enjoy good holidays, you are of slim and glamorous appearance, and you participate in skilled hobbies, then you tick all the boxes, you are a success. Sadie ticks them all. She is a crisis house success story.

1999 – 2000: Manfred Jameson: 'Whatever love is'

'Youth's the Season Made For Joys. Love is Then Our Duty'
John Gay

Manfred Jameson came to us in 1999 – having a diagnosis of depression. He came from a good family, was very well-educated, and had an excellent job as a chartered accountant. His depression stemmed from problems in his personal life – for which I had immediate sympathy – since what had happened was so understandable.

Manfred explained that he had been depressed while at college, but had, nevertheless, qualified, and entered the accountancy profession. He had had various girlfriends, but had met no-one to whom he felt strongly attracted. He reached the age of twenty-eight. In his profession, by that age, it was expected that one should be married. All his colleagues were.

He reached the conclusion that romance, love, and passion, were the stuff of films and novels. So Manfred decided to play safe, and do the conventional thing. His secretary, Carrie, was blonde and slim, averagely good-looking, and a reasonably nice person, so he married her. They were happy for ten years, had two sons, and lived the conventional life. Manfred was churchwarden at the church they attended. He was content because he knew nothing else.

Until the Christmas Party! At the Christmas Party, down the stairs walked the beautiful Emily, and Manfred fell hook, line, and sinker in love – much as Romeo did when first encountering Juliet!

Manfred's problem parallelled, exactly, that of Stephen Farraday in

Agatha Christie's novel, 'Sparkling Cyanide'. [Published: Collins: 1945.] She writes:

'Often looking across the table at his wife, he [Stephen Farraday] felt gladly what a perfect helpmate she was. . . . . Yes, he thought, Stephen Farraday, that little, disconsolate, boy, had done very well for himself. His life was shaping exactly as he had meant it to be. He was only a year or two over thirty and already, success lay in the hollow of his hand.

And in that mood of triumphant satisfaction, he went with his wife for a fortnight to St Moritz, and, looking across the Hotel lounge, saw Rosemary Barton. What happened to him at that moment he never understood.. . . Across a room he fell in love. Deeply, overwhelmingly, crazily, in love. It was the kind of desperate, headlong, adolescent calf love that he should have experienced years ago and got over.'

Agatha Christie went on to say, that Stephen Farraday, for all his fine intellect, and political astuteness, lacked the insight to see that his former unemotional planning of a conventional, controlled, successful, life, and then his meteoric infatuation for Rosemary, beyond his control, fitted together only too well.

Manfred and Emily's affair started immediately. In due course, Carrie found out, and sued for divorce. By the time he came to us, Manfred was in a complete state of despair. He had lost his wife, home and children, and, worse still, Emily – being younger and single – had ended the relationship – which she considered had run its natural course. Manfred was at rock bottom, with nothing.

There were no financial problems. Manfred could afford to buy another house for himself, and could also afford to pay for private psychotherapy. He needed our support for about a year. We encouraged him to get back into dating, and, eventually, he met somebody suitable – though he did not re-marry until some years later – this time, quite happily. Manfred also changed jobs – still in a top position in financial services, but in employment which he found more congenial.

Manfred's was an example of 'life crisis' - where the individual needs time, and sanctuary space, to repair his broken heart, and his broken life. This was precisely the service that the crisis house provided. Success story!

2000 – 2001: Martin Threw: 'Good enough for God'

Martin came to the crisis house from the mental hospital - where he had been admitted under the emergency Section Four of the Mental Health Act – having made a suicide attempt. He expressed terror, to the hospital social worker, at the prospect of being Sectioned for a longer period, and becoming like the demoralized and institutionalized patients whom he saw around him - so she enquired as to whether we had a vacancy, and accompanied him to the crisis house, when we agreed to accommodate him.

Martin had been depressed because of marital breakdown, and because his carpentry business had been going downhill. The crisis house proved to be a godsend. His business had been located in Wokingham, so, isolated in a mental hospital, out in rural Oxfordshire, he would have stood no chance, at all, of re-establishing his business.

We are right in the heart of Wokingham. He could park his van outside the house, and start re-establishing contacts immediately. The first order he got, was to make some coffins; he expressed doubts to me, because this seemed macabre. My advice was 'Money is money. All a coffin is, is a wooden box, like any other!'.

So it proved to be, and soon Martin's business was flourishing again. He also acquired a new girlfriend, who proved very supportive during his stay at the crisis house. It took Martin exactly one year to get himself completely re-established in all areas. He then, successful once more, moved out of the crisis house, into a flat with his girlfriend, and never looked back!

A point about recovery from depression. Even when things started to go well, Martin still expressed low self-esteem. He told me that he had gone into the carpentry business, because it was the only work that he could get. I never push religion down people's throats, but his comment made me think of the Carpenter of Nazareth. A job in a carpenter's shop – of low status - but it was good enough for God! A cheering thought!

Sometimes I reflect upon Martin's success story with a tinge of sadness. It is so much a case of 'It is better to light one candle than to curse the darkness!' Suppose the social worker had not been prepared to look at alternatives – even though the Mental Health Act required her to do so. Suppose we had no vacancy! Suppose, like National MIND, we feared the risk involved in accepting the suicidal! Would Martin have recovered? Would his business have flourished once more? Would he have met a suitable new partner?

All those sad, oppressed, institutionalized, mental patients, were once lovely babies! They were all bright young people, with potential! The kind of intervention one gets, when experiencing mental health problems, is the crucial factor in subsequent outcome.

Chapter 9

The Continuing Of The Same 2001 - 2006

2001 – 2002: Malcolm Chase: 'Manners makyth man'

Malcolm came to us in 2001 – he was suffering from depression – but with a diagnosis of bi-polar affective disorder. He had been sleeping in his car – his house having been repossessed because he had defaulted on the mortgage payments.

Malcolm explained that he was a Cambridge graduate, and that he had been very successful in business for years, had been married, with one daughter, and that they had owned a beautiful estate down by the river, at Wallingford. His illness, and manic episodes, had caused him to squander their money, and led to the breakup of the marriage. His parting shot to his wife was 'You can have it all! I have made a million before, and will do so again!' He then left, and moved into a tiny bedsitter in Reading.

He did not make another million, but he did well enough to buy a house at Spencers Wood – this being worth about five hundred thousand pounds - as compared with the two million pounds estate in Wallingford. He did well for a time, married again, but suffered further bouts of mania – leading him into the destitute state that he was in when he came to us.

Malcolm stayed in the crisis house for four months. He made some progress, and like so many of our guests, was a limited success. We found him quite a nice little council flat, but it was quite sad to see him hanging those beautiful, expensive, curtains from his former house, at those plebeian windows.

As we often discuss in the crisis house, how you feel about your circumstances, all depends upon where you are coming from.

If you have had a beautiful estate in rural Oxfordshire, a council flat in an urban complex, seems such a comedown, but if you have been living in cramped conditions, or, worse still, on the street, a council house, or flat, seems like paradise!

I recall a television programme on the subject of garden cities, the Quaker Sir Ebenezer Howard's, wonderful vision to improve life for inner city slum-dwellers. One of my college friends, lived in such a garden city, Letchworth, and was full of enthusiasm for the venture.

The television presenter interviewed some people who were the first to move from inner London into the London County Council's first council houses, at Downham, near Bromley, in Kent. 'What was it like?' he asked. 'Paradise,' was their answer.

For the first time in their lives, they had a bathroom, and a garden. What to others might be the mundane basics, to them, was perfect bliss!

Malcolm had found a girlfriend when living in Spencers Wood, and they continued with their relationship - though she did not wish actually to live with him. He tried to get back into work in the civil service. They did not have him back, but he did get a severance payment.

After leaving us, he also went for one-to-one psychotherapy – which he found to be beneficial. A limited success story, and as so often is the case in mental health, having to accept a lowering in social status - inevitable where there is severe mental illness.

Malcolm was so well-mannered, and our volunteers remarked that this was so refreshing - since courtesy is so rarely encountered in these days, but the old adage still applies – 'Manners makyth man'!

2002 – 2003: Daniel McLeod: 'It's the effort you put in'

Daniel came to the crisis house, suffering from post traumatic stress. He was a gay man, and had been the victim of an unprovoked attack in Reading. He had fled to his native Glasgow, but had been unable to settle there, so he returned to the comparatively small, and quiet, town of Wokingham.

Daniel was a worker. He worked hard on his problems, from day one - eventually regaining enough confidence to go back into Reading. His first attempt to get back into work failed, but his second attempt was a success. He found work running the cyber café in the station, opposite the crisis house, and this worked well.

Daniel had worked as a carer in statutory services, and he amused me, by constantly pointing out all the rules and procedures that the crisis house, should be, but was not, following. I don't think that Daniel ever really got it into his head, that we are a self-help group, and not a statutory service.

After some months, Daniel had recovered sufficiently to move into a rented flat in Reading. He found a new partner, and returned to working in care. He still keeps in touch with the crisis house. A success story!

2003 – 2004: Reg Gardiner: 'I prefer to work'

Reg was originally admitted to the crisis house – having been released from Section at the hospital. He had a diagnosis of schizophrenia. His sister came to us seeking accommodation, since the only alternative was the isolating Y.M.C.A. Hostel in Reading – some distance from his home town of Wokingham.

On his first admission, Reg stayed for two months – then returning to Germany, where he worked with a Dutch building firm, as a bricklayer. He became ill again, and returned to the crisis house. His second stay was longer, but when due to leave, we found him a nice council flat at Earley.

Reg continually fell foul of the Housing Benefit rules, when working. He did casual on-and-off work on building sites – sometimes working for weeks on end, and, at other times, being unemployed, for weeks on end. Every time he went back to work, his Housing Benefit was discontinued. Thus he sank deeper and deeper into rent arrears.

Reg was keen to work. He did not want to be idle, so in the end, he relinquished the tenancy on his flat – preferring to sleep in his car, and to drive around the country, getting any work on building sites, that he could. In the eyes of society, if you work, you are normal! So Reg qualifies as a success story.

When Reg came to us, I read his social worker's report. This was, the particularly useless, social worker who shouted 'For you! For you!' continually down the phone when we were refusing her an inappropriate, referral. She wrote 'Tends to isolate himself'. Hardly surprising, if you dump him out in a Y.M.C.A. in Tilehurst, when his family connection is in Wokingham!

Self help is the name of the game, and Reg Gardiner exemplifies this philosophy perfectly – as his latest venture illustrates. He has taken out a monthly subscription – costly, but still less than a monthly rent would be.

This is a subscription to a chain of health clubs. Provided that his membership is paid up, Reg can access their services anywhere in the UK. So he can use their restaurants, showers, laundry, swimming pools, gymnasia, libraries – in fact they offer everything, apart from a bed!

Reg has now up-graded his vehicle to a van – with a back seat, comfortable enough, to sleep on. So, as he tells me now, in 2015, he is using his wages to meet his actual needs, and not for renting a flat, which, much of the time, he would not occupy. A successful resolution of his living situation.

2004 - 2005: Ambrose Meyer and Sylvia Kann: 'I want my life back'

When in 2003, Ewan was admitted to the crisis house – suffering from schizophrenia and heroin addiction – I knew nothing of the latter. I soon found out! I could swear that heroin addicts reproduce asexually – by splitting! First, you have one, then two, then four, then eight!

So Ambrose and Sylvia came into the crisis house as friends of Ewan. Homeless, destitute, and heroin addicted, they presented themselves as being simply homeless, but I knew that they must be addicts, because all Ewan's friends were! They had been on the streets for some years, so, for the first three months, I simply let them settle – acquiring some stability and security with us – mixing in a non-drugs culture, and having a stable roof over their heads. During this time, I formed an amicable relationship with them – not intervening in their situation at all.

After three months, I explained that their life of crime, to fund their drugs habit, must stop, because, sooner or later, they would be arrested. I offered them the choice: 'You can either go through drugs detoxification with us – getting all our support, or, you can go the criminal justice way – under the Probation Service. Either way, it has to happen eventually.' They chose to go our way.

I was very lucky to get a local doctor – young, clued up, and with it – who was willing to supervise their treatment. Not all doctors are so willing. My role was to give support, and to get them interested in embracing a life free from drugs. They had some outstanding offences, so I had to accompany them to court, where they were placed on a Drugs Testing and Treatment Order.

I helped them to pick up the threads of a normal life – encouraging them to shop for new clothes, visit markets, take part in sports, visit places of interest, and, generally, get back into the community. In time, both got jobs.

Ambrose's family lived in Australia, and, once addiction-free, he contacted his mother and his sister. They were keen for him to return to them – which he did in September 2005. He went on to marry, and to have a family of his own, in Australia.

Sylvia stayed with us until January 2006. Then, addiction-free, she found a flat, and resumed care-work - eventually moving back to help run her mother's nursing home.

The relationship, between Ambrose and Sylvia, is what is known as co-dependency. It is sustained only by mutual addiction to drugs. Once addiction-free, the relationship evaporates. However, they stayed amicably in touch with each other, and with us - both – as a result of their stay in the crisis house, having achieved good quality lives. This achievement took us the full two years, but it was a success story.

Some of our members were not entirely sympathetic with our welcoming of heroin addicts into our ranks – even though addiction and mental health, are firmly wedded together. 'Let us return to mental health, pure and simple,' one declared. It is many things, but pure and simple, mental health will never be!

2005 - 2006: Cedric Billing: 'I'll settle down one day'

Cedric came to the crisis house suffering from depression. His nine-year relationship had broken down, and he was homeless – since his former partner had bought him out, and retained the property. So Cedric was obliged to live temporarily with his mother and her new partner – not altogether amicably.

Eventually, Cedric found accommodation in the private sector, and he returned to work. He remained depressed, and dropped into the crisis house regularly for support.

Over the years, Cedric worked his way through an incredible number of relationships – none of which worked out. Finally, after years of trying, he met a nursing sister, Katie. They came to the crisis house to tell us that they were getting married, and moving to live in her native Shropshire. Success story, at last!

Chapter 10

Continuing - Under Threat Of Closure 2006 - 2011

2006 – 2007: Maurice Santereau: 'What starts as disaster can end as triumph'

I think that I regard Maurice Santereau as our all-time, supreme, success story. Maurice came to us in February 2006 – referred by the local Citizens Advice Bureau. He had attempted suicide, by slashing his wrists. Maurice explained that his depression stemmed from a childhood of physical, emotional, and sexual abuse. This is the story!

Maurice's mother, who was mixed race African, came from the Reunion Island – a French-speaking province close to Africa. It was difficult for young women living on the island to find husbands - because most young men left, in order to find work. Maurice's mother worked as a secretary, and was probably already suffering from mental illness when, at the age of twenty-four, she put an advertisement in a 'Lonely Hearts' Column – in order to find a husband.

A man from Toulouse answered the advertisement, and she met, and married, him without further delay. He was seventeen years her senior, lived with his mother in Toulouse, worked as a refuse-collector, and had a history of violence.

Maria, Maurice's mother, wanted a child, but her new husband did not. Nevertheless, she went ahead, and had just one, Maurice. His parents lived in degrading filth, and treated Maurice with great cruelty. As a baby, he was slapped, and pushed off his potty by his father. No doubt the relationship between Maurice's parents had broken down after his birth, so Maurice became a substitute, and his mother sexually abused him. He suffered physical abuse from his father, sexual abuse from his mother, and severe emotional abuse from both.

At the age of eleven, Maurice ran away, but he was too terrified to expose his parents to the authorities, so he was returned to their abuse. At sixteen, having obtained his School Certificate, Maurice ran away to Paris, and never returned to his parents. He lived in hostels and worked in all sorts of jobs – offices, shoe shops, factories, restaurants. At the age of twenty-four, Maurice came to England, and worked as a waiter at Pizza Hut in London. Eventually, he moved from there to Pizza Hut in Bracknell – finding accommodation in a shared house. He then went into care work in Wokingham, and, after a wait of eleven years, obtained a council flat.

When he came to us, Maurice was off sick from care work at a local, Wokingham, nursing home. I advised Maurice, as I do everyone, that the sooner he got back into work, the better. Nothing is better than work for relieving depression, and for re-engaging with the normal world. Conversely, nothing is worse for depression than having too much time to sit around thinking about oneself, and mixing only with other people with mental problems.

Maurice returned to work promptly – firstly, as a cleaner. Having proved himself competent at this for six months, he was then reinstated as a care worker. Thereafter, it was literally a ladder from the bottom rung to the top!

Maurice climbed the career ladder with diligence, skill, determination, grit, and graft. He climbed from being a basic grade care worker [NVQ 1] to a senior care worker [NVQ2]. Then he took a post in the National Health Service – working for Consultants. Through a correspondence course, he obtained his International Baccalaureate. He also pursued an Open University Course in Child Development.

Due to his experience of child sexual abuse, Maurice, though extremely attractive, found great difficulty in relating to the opposite sex. Nevertheless, he eventually found a suitable partner, and married her in March 2012. They moved to a much better flat, at the college where she worked as an administrator, and, in due course, he started studying for a degree at the college – with a view to going into teaching.

In due course, they bought their own house, and Maurice started driving a car, once again.

The happy couple spend a lot of time travelling, and Maurice, who had never been able to face the prospect of returning to France, was even able to re-visit Paris with the encouragement of his wife. Supreme success story!

2007 – 2008: Nancy Shelton: 'Back in the rhythm of the dance'

'Let's face the music, and dance!'

Nancy came to us in 2007 – referred by her boyfriend – with whom the relationship was just ending. They had been living together, and he was concerned for her future welfare - since she had both mental health and physical health, problems.

Nancy was a very attractive redhead, who had been training as a dancer, until a back injury prohibited further involvement in this career. She suffered from Tourette's Syndrome as well as anxiety and depression, and she had a long history of instability – both in relationships, and in accommodation.

Once settled into the crisis house, Nancy quickly found a new boyfriend, and even got back into dancing, as much as was possible, with the limitations imposed by her back injury. Unfortunately, this caused the boyfriend to become jealous to a paranoid degree. He did not like Nancy, dancing, and thus having an opportunity to encounter other men. Eventually, he became violent, and since he knew that she was living in the crisis house, it was no longer a safe place for Nancy to be.

Nancy had a cousin who lived in Eastbourne, so she was able to stay there for a short while – giving Berkshire's 'Women's Aid' time to find her a place in an Eastbourne Refuge – well away from Berkshire, and the violent boyfriend.

From the refuge, Nancy graduated into an Eastbourne council flat, and then, on receiving a legacy from an old aunt, was able to buy a flat. In Eastbourne, she quickly found another boyfriend, but he also became jealous and violent, so she had to end the relationship, and to take out a Court Injunction – preventing him from contacting her.

We are still in touch with Nancy – now settled with a new partner and due to give birth to twins in April 2016. Nancy is a beautiful woman, and it is a fact of life, that beautiful women never go short of a partner. This may bring its own problems, but, being beautiful is, nevertheless, usually accounted a success!

2008 – 2009: Peter Black: 'Lonely no longer'

'Love's no thrill, by the water mill – all by yourself in the moonlight!'

In Agatha Christie's novel, 'Death in the Clouds', [Published: Collins: 1935.], one character, a Dr Bryant, makes a - most telling - pronouncement. He says,

'There comes to everyone a turning point in their lives, Monsieur Poirot. They stand at the crossroads, and have to decide. My profession [medicine] interests me enormously – it is a sorrow – a very great sorrow to abandon it. But there are other claims. . . There is, Monsieur Poirot, the happiness of a human being....'

The turning point, the time of decision. That is what I have always envisaged as the chief function of the crisis house. If a person can get support then, when they most need it, then whole lives can be turned around, for the better.

Peter came to us at the age of thirty – referred by his psychiatrist. He suffered from an anxiety neurosis, was unemployed, and was living with his elderly parents. Peter explained that he was homosexual, but that his parents found difficulty in accepting this fact. As a teenager, they had pressurized him into finding a nice girl, and marrying her.

He duly became engaged to a nice girl, and she gave birth to their daughter. Peter explained, that he could function with a woman, but didn't want to. Throughout the relationship, he was going off with boys all the time. Sadly, the girl was killed in a road accident, so her parents, who lived in the north of England, adopted the baby, and Peter, sad and desperate in his unhappy living situation, turned to alcohol. He had just finished successful alcohol detoxification, when he came to us.

Peter became very involved with our Association – serving on the executive committee, and acting as librarian. He was very pleasant, courteous, and mild-mannered – as homosexuals – in my experience – invariably are. He was also extremely efficient in all that he did. In 1996, Peter obtained Lottery Funding, to provide our Association with a holiday caravan by the seaside.

I think that it was a visit to this caravan in the summer of 1997, that brought Peter's crisis to a head. He saw all those young people, happy with their partners, enjoying themselves on the beach, and this brought home to him, just how intolerable his loneliness had become – hiding from the world, in a back bedroom, at his aged parents' house.

I had a friend who ran a gay socializing group in Reading, so I suggested that Peter contact him – with a view to finding a partner. He met a gay young man, Ken. They stayed very briefly in the crisis house, until I found them a council flat. Supreme success, this. Admittedly, it was located in the least desirable part of Wokingham, but I got that flat, for the couple, within three days! Oh, happy day!

We celebrated their wedding at the crisis house in June 1998. A local clergyman officiated at the ceremony – not yet enshrined in law, but, nevertheless, having the blessing of the church! This clergyman was able to reassure us, that church history indicates that the Christian Church was blessing same/sex marriage, as early as the fifth century A.D. In due course, they moved into a better flat, and took out a Civil Partnership - once these became available.

Nearly twenty years on, Peter and Ken are among the happiest couples that I know – partners in work as well as in love – running a successful internet business. Success story!

Homosexuality and mental health

Over the years, we have encountered quite a large number of homosexuals, who have experienced mental health problems – due to the stress of being in a minority. How they are regarded, it seems to me, depends, very much, upon where you are in history.

In ancient Greek and Roman times, homosexuality was celebrated – hence all the statues of splendid naked male athletes! By contrast, in Victorian times, and during the first half of the twentieth century, homosexuality was reviled – even being treated as a mental illness.

Thus you had the shocking maltreatment of Alan Turing, who cracked the Enigma Code – played so movingly, by the wonderful Benedict Cumberbatch, in 'The Imitation Game'.

How many lives did they estimate that the homosexual, and Asperger's sufferer, Turing, saved, by cracking the Enigma Code, and thus, shortening the Second World War? Fourteen million, wasn't it! They should have been down on their knees with gratitude to the man – not vilifying him!

After legalisation in 1967, homosexuality was tolerated, rather than celebrated. That is why you got sad characters, if Madame Ling Ling is to be believed, like the late, former Prime Minister, Edward Heath. In his position, in the 1960's and 1970's, he could not be openly gay.

Now, with gay marriage, we are moving towards a society in which homosexuality is celebrated, once again, but it is, of course, too late for many who have suffered, because of prejudice in the past.

2009 – 2010: Kurt Haddow: 'Good with computers'

Kurt Haddow was a latter-day friend of Ewan. [Chapter 9: 'I Want my life back'.]

When Ewan brought Kurt to the crisis house in 2009, he was, sad to say, practically dragging him by the ear, unable to cope with him any longer.

'Oh no, I thought, here we go again!' I would swear that heroin addicts reproduce asexually, by splitting! Ewan brought Kurt to the crisis house because he could no longer tolerate his behaviour – having Kurt living with him in the flat. Sure enough, once one heroin addict was with us, then they all began to congregate.

Kurt was homeless, destitute, freezing, and starving! His mother had been paying for bed-and breakfast accommodation for him, but he had spent the money on heroin, and so was back on the street. It was February, and freezing, so we agreed to put Kurt back into bed-and-breakfast accommodation, but supervised the payments, while we applied to the Council for Housing Benefit.

When Housing Benefit became payable, we asked the council to pay it into the charity's bank account, so that we could continue to pay Kurt's rent, and thus ensure a stable roof over his head. But they insisted upon paying the money directly to him – to 'encourage responsibility!' What nonsense! Addicts will always prioritise drugs above everything else!

Kurt spent all the money on drugs, and on paying off drugs' debts, and so was out on the street once more – albeit not in such a dire state, in what was now, the mild May weather. Bureaucracies are totally inflexible. You can't reason with them, so I have given up trying. I don't want to see them improved. I want to see them abolished!

I think that we despaired of Kurt, but he was highly intelligent, and, in particular, very good with computers. Through an internet contact, he found a job – setting up a computer system for London taxis. He got accommodation with the job, and did extremely well. We are still in contact, and Kurt has now completed a heroin detox and rehabilitation programme, and is looking towards a positive future. Success story!

2010 – 2011: Gavin Morton: 'Step by step to success'

As I state in 'This is Madness': [PCCS Books, Herefordshire: 1999.], 'There is no magic in mental health'. It must be rare indeed, after a severe breakdown, for an individual to resume a former successful life immediately. Indeed, I have NEVER encountered this. All my success stories were willing, to start back at the bottom, in a much humbler position, than their abilities merited, and then make the hard, strenuous, climb, back to normality. It is hard, it is gruelling, and don't I know it!

Gavin Morton made this climb. He suffered a severe breakdown, after one of his twin boys, died shortly after birth – the other twin being born, severely handicapped. The trauma also led to the breakdown of his marriage.

When I first met Gavin, he was trapped in the mental health system. He had a diagnosis of bi-polar affective disorder, and was very heavily medicated. He moved into mental health supported flats, close to the crisis house, and attended our drop-in centre. He suffered, a severe, manic episode, and was Sectioned under the Mental Health Act. He was still grieving about the loss of his child, and the breakdown of his marriage. More desperately than anything, he wanted a child, to compensate for his loss.

While in the mental hospital, Gavin formed a relationship with another patient, got her pregnant, and, once the baby was born, they moved into his flat together. Unfortunately, there was a terrifying incident at the flats – where a paranoid schizophrenic threatened to kill the baby. Gavin, wife and baby, fled to the crisis house, where they stayed for six months, until an ordinary flat, in an ordinary street, was made available to them – away from the mental health system.

Then Gavin started the slow, hard, climb back to normality. First, he started as a voluntary occupational therapy helper, at a local centre for learning disabilities. Then, he went on to be a low-paid, mental health support worker, with the local community mental health team. Note, as I state in chapter one, and as so many of these 'Success Stories' illustrate, most people who wish - having suffered mental health problems – to work in mental health – wish to go the professional route. I, in a minority, did not.

Prior to his breakdown, Gavin had already obtained a degree in Social Science, so it was not difficult for him to take the next step – that of qualifying as a mental health social worker. Once qualified, he took up a post with the local community mental health team

By now, his wife had relapsed into mental ill health, and the marriage broke down.

Gavin retained custody of their child. He did very well in his job – undertaking additional training as an 'Approved' Mental Health Professional – with the duty of applying for patients to be Sectioned, under the Mental Health Act. He was also given the task of setting up the local 'Personal Budgets' Scheme for mental health clients.

On his social work training course, Gavin met his third wife. In 2010, they emigrated to Australia, where she had relatives, and went on to have another child together. Gavin keeps in touch with the crisis house, and visits us whenever he is over in England, visiting family.

As I write this, Gavin is over in England, and has visited us at the crisis house – bringing photographs of his sons. I can hardly believe that his elder son is now eighteen, and is about to start music college. It doesn't seem long since he was in the crisis house, on my lap, with me singing 'Baby Face' to him.

'Baby face. You've got the cutest little baby face. No-one else could take your place. My poor heart is thumping. You sure have started something. Baby face. I'm up in heaven, when I'm in your warm embrace. I didn't need a shove, because I fell in love, with your pretty, baby face!'

On this most recent visit, Gavin explained that the Social Services, who employ him, in Australia, are just as bureaucratic, as ours are here. 'If you were under them, you would not be able to do what you do', he said. 'The managers are worried about keeping their jobs, and are obsessed with risk assessments!'

What is the answer? Get rid of them, of course! Establish a welfare set-up, where you have only volunteers, and do not have people in paid jobs, then there would be nobody to put those jobs before the welfare of the mentally ill.

I have always maintained, that the most valuable service that the crisis house provides – is asylum, and Gavin, looking back on his time here, confirms that, for him, that was indeed the most valuable feature of our service!

'IF you were under Social Services.' 'IF you allowed them to infiltrate.' 'IF you had 'professionals' on your committee.' 'IF', is the little word, with the big meaning! We are NOT under Social Services! We do not allow them to infiltrate. They are not coming on our committee.

Thus, as Gavin confirms, from personal experience, we are able to provide a service which actually meets the needs of the mentally ill, and that included him. A success story!

Chapter 11

Success Going Into The Future

2011 – 2012: Pamela McEllen: 'My heart is singing again'

When Pamela first came to the crisis house drop-in centre, she was extremely depressed, and alcohol dependent: she looked very ill. Pamela didn't return for some time, but when she came back in September 2011, she looked, and expressed herself as being, much better. She had freed herself of alcohol addiction, with the support of Alcoholics Anonymous, and of a local rehabilitation programme.

Pamela explained that she was getting her life back together, and was singing again. At the time, I was just preparing the programme for the Association's twenty-fifth anniversary – which was due to be celebrated in March 2012. I asked Pamela whether she would like to sing at this event, and she agreed to do so.

We arranged some singing lessons for her, and these went well. On the evening of the celebration, Pamela, tall and willowy, looked like a million dollars, and sang like an angel. It was a marvellous performance. Pamela, herself, chose most of the songs.

However, I did make the choice for the final item on the programme - mine. I chose Blake's 'Jerusalem'. Blake – the inspired Poet:

'And did those feet in ancient time, walk upon England's mountains green? And was the holy Lamb of God on England's pleasant pastures seen? And did the Countenance divine shine forth upon our clouded hills? And was Jerusalem builded here – among those dark satanic mills?

Bring me my bow of burning gold. Bring me my arrows of desire. Bring me my spear, oh, clouds unfold, bring me my chariot of fire.

I will not cease from mental fight, nor shall my sword sleep in my hand, till we have built Jerusalem in England's green and pleasant land.'

Why did I choose this hymn? The following questions give the answer!

'Was Jerusalem builded HERE – among the schizophrenics and the alcoholics? Was the Holy Lamb of God HERE among society's rejects? Is talent, and glamour, and beauty HERE – among the derelicts and the stigmatized?' What Pamela demonstrated, on that wonderful evening, was that indeed they were!

Pamela's mother was crying in the audience. For years, she had been with her daughter, through the dark, satanic mills of depression and alcoholism. Pamela had barely been able to get out of bed, and to get washed. Now she was standing in front of a hundred people – looking unbelievably glamorous, and singing like Callas! I think Pamela's mother concluded that we actually HAD built Jerusalem in England's green and pleasant land!

After her triumph, Pamela continued step-by-step, to rebuild her life. A supreme success story.

2012 – 2013: Petula Bateman: 'Free of abusive relationships'

'Don't need nobody. I can do without it'
Chas and Dave

Petula was the victim of a series of abusive relationships. She was very depressed, and was diagnosed with Bi-Polar Affective Disorder. We arranged for our befriender, Suzanne, to form a befriending relationship with her. Petula greatly appreciated this support. At this time, she was living in an isolated situation out in Shinfield, but, with our support, she obtained a council transfer to a house in central Wokingham, where she was much closer to her family.

Petula had been violently, physically, abused, and intimidated, by her father – who was a regimental sergeant major – unable to realise that a family, is not a regiment!

In order to escape, she chose the classic path of becoming pregnant at the age of fifteen. At sixteen, she married the father of her child, and so went out of the frying pan into the fire. In fact, this first husband, was not physically abusive, and Petula got some of the support that she needed at the time, by moving in with his parents. Nevertheless, inevitably, the marriage broke down.

In all, Petula gave birth to six children – all from abusive relationships. Her final relationship was so terrifyingly abusive, that Petula relinquished her home, and was admitted to a refuge for battered women. After this trauma, Petula decided to avoid all relationships – contenting herself with children and grandchildren.

In 2012, Petula entered a therapeutic community, and stayed the full course – completing the entire programme of therapy. She reported this to be very hard, and gruelling, but, ultimately, successful. A success story!

2013 – 2014: Lucy Farmer: 'Back to normality...'

When Lucy came to us, she was very unstable, – having just been discharged from hospital. She had just gone through divorce, and – although the split was amicable – this was still a major trauma - after thirty years of marriage. The last straw, which triggered the breakdown, was that, just as she was newly divorced, Lucy was made redundant from her job, and feared poverty, as a result.

Lucy had two sons – one living independently, and one, at that time, living with Lucy – not a very good arrangement, since he did not cope very well with her illness. The divorce settlement had ensured that the large marital home was sold, and that each partner then bought a smaller house. It also ensured that Lucy had a pension pot to provide for her old age.

Both of Lucy's aged parents were alive when she came to us, but, within a few years, both died – and Lucy inherited a lot of money, which she proceeded to squander at a manic pace!

She got involved with another of our former service users – an alcoholic, who also suffered from Bi-Polar Affective Disorder. Together, they romped through thousands and thousands of pounds – holidaying all over the world, staying in expensive hotels, dining in expensive restaurants, driving expensive cars, and generally having a wild time – until the money ran out!

Three years on, the alcoholic died of liver failure. Lucy then, tried living with a schizophrenic, but this did not work out as a relationship – since it was a double dose of mental illness! He moved out into shared accommodation, but they remained friends.

A remarkable degree of stability, and sensible behaviour, came to Lucy in the ensuing years. We put this down to the fact that she obtained a job, both sons married, and Lucy has been presented with three grandchildren!

Lucy had been office manager, and personal assistant to a businessman, prior to her breakdown. In 2012, she managed to get a little part-time office job, and – although she was made redundant after a year – this got her back onto the first rung of the ladder of working life, and restored her self-confidence.

With both sons now married, Lucy became the proud grandmother of a boy and two girls. She is a godsend to her daughters-in-law, and has a useful role in life – helping out with the grandchildren.

When I look at Lucy today, I am amazed. She has been discharged from the local statutory mental heath service. She is so stable, so sensible, and so happy. She goes for just one family holiday each year – a humble caravan holiday in Dorset. She thoroughly enjoys helping with the grandchildren, and even having the eldest, a boy of six, to stay overnight.

She has only a limited income, but manages well on that, and she is still able to socialize with, and support her schizophrenic friend – even though it did not work out as a relationship. Nor has the failure of former relationships, deterred her from participating courageously in internet dating – ever hopeful of finding a special friendship. In 2015 she found one. Lucy made the most strenuous efforts to get back into work, and was, finally, also in 2015, successful in getting temporary work. A, quite remarkable, success story!

2014 – 2015: Dan Kent: 'All the things that I have worked for'

Dan came to the crisis house in 1999 – having suffered a manic episode, and having, as a result, been dismissed from his job as an engineer. He was very depressed, and busied himself - doing a lot of voluntary work for the crisis house. He was not ready to go back into professional engineering, but was, nevertheless, keen to get back into work. With legal support, we had obtained for Dan, financial compensation for the loss of his job – since his inappropriate behaviour – which led to his dismissal – had been due to mental illness.

He took a job as a salesman with a local wine merchants. He also found a girlfriend. Eventually, he moved in with the girlfriend – renting his own house out, in order to bring in an income. In due course, Dan got back into professional engineering . He did very well in his job for the ensuing nine years – even travelling to China for the company. Then, at the age of fifty-five, he was made redundant.

Dan, through the local job centre, got a temporary work-placement which he enjoyed, but when he got back into a permanent position, things did not work out so well. He became very depressed – with suicidal ideation. We paid for him to go on a refresher course in order to brush up his skills. Armed with a bang up-to-date qualification, he was able to try himself out in two jobs, but neither worked out.

This is when Dan became morbidly depressed. When able to get out of bed, and into the drop-in centre, he would sit in a corner, hidden under a baseball cap – barely able to speak. We despaired. We thought that Dan would never recover, but he did!

Depressed no more, he became active, positive, and willing to look realistically at jobs available to older people, and with which he would be able to cope. Now, in 2015, he continues to contribute enthusiastically to local voluntary organizations. A success story!

Some mental illnesses – including schizophrenia, and bi-polar affective disorder, are life-long conditions. Sufferers will have periods of relative good health, and of relative ill health. Learning how to cope with this - is the art of gaining quality of life – despite the illness. Dan is a success story because he always lifts himself out of the depression eventually.

2015 – 2016: Tommy Warfield: 'Why not enjoy life?'

'Enjoy yourself, it's later than you think. Enjoy yourself, while you're still in the pink. The years go by, as quickly as a wink. Enjoy yourself, enjoy yourself, it's later than you think!'

Tommy first came to the crisis house early in 2002. He was very depressed – his wife having divorced him. He had been diagnosed with Bi-Polar Affective Disorder.

As a result of his manic illness, the couple had had to sell their beautiful house, in the centre of Wokingham. His wife had salvaged the remains of their public relations business, with difficulty. She, and their young daughter, moved to a much smaller property.

Tommy, himself, on discharge from hospital, was living in bed-and-breakfast accommodation – awaiting a move to a flat in the private sector.

Above all, Tommy is a social animal. He loves going out, going to the races, going to pubs. He had to leave his private sector flat, but we found him a super new flat, in a nice part of Wokingham. He managed there for some years – only having to go into staffed accommodation as his health deteriorated.

For years, he managed to get to the crisis house drop-in centre every day that we are open – partaking from our bar with relish! His favourite drink was Hendricks gin with tonic, thinly sliced cucumber, and a squirt of lemon, Very stylish!

Tommy's former wife remains very supportive, and his lovely daughter, Elizabeth, is obviously very fond of her father, and keeps in touch with him on a daily basis. I regard Tommy as a success story because, despite ill health, he keeps a grip on life.

Disabled by Bi-Polar Affective Disorder, living in NHS Staffed Accommodation, and having reached the age of seventy-three, he, nevertheless, enjoys life! Him they could not kill! A success story!

Ongoing success

Twenty-five years on, we are extremely fortunate that we continue to hold the Lease on the crisis house. In March 1991, when we obtained our first Lease, the deal was that we would continue to lease the building, until it was demolished to make way for the proposed link road. At the time, it could not be established whether this would be in a year's time, in several years' time, or whenever.

Acting on the firm belief that we are living now, this did not deter us from using our limited funds to improve the premises. As Judi Chamberlin describes so cogently in 'On Our Own' [Published by MIND – London,1988], the Vancouver Crisis Centre - which she attended, lasted for only eighteen months, but it was time enough for Judi to turn her life around, and success, even for just a few individuals, is always worth the investment.

Work on the link road finally commenced in 2012, and it had by then, been established, that the Crisis House, unlike a number of other local buildings, was not to be demolished, so we could continue.

Our situation was difficult. We were surrounded by work, noise, and rubble. At one point the house was totally surrounded by water – like the houses on stilts, that one sees in children's history books! We were barely visible, and what one could see, looked derelict. People thought that we had closed down, and the numbers attending fell.

But, the new road and station, were completed, eventually. We then became visible once more. We used some of our reserves of money to ensure that we looked as smart as our new surroundings, and the numbers attending started to soar. So in 2016, we are encouraging more people to become success stories like those whom I have described over the past twenty-five years.

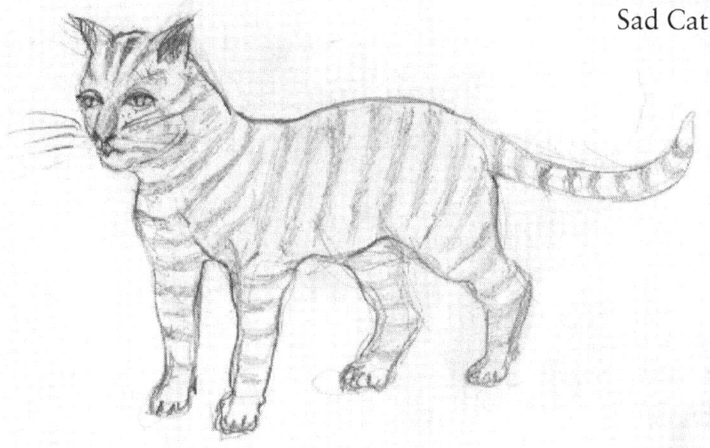

Sad Cat

Chapter 12

Twenty-Five Poignant Stories Triumph And Disaster

Duncan: 'Not so badly endowed'

'I want an old fashioned house, with an old fashioned fence, and an old fashioned millionaire!'

Duncan came to us – not as a service-user – but because he was courting one of our befrienders, Jane. Jane was an excellent befriender for female users. [We only allow same-sex befriending.] Nevertheless, Jane bore a grudge against men. She had married young, as a strict Roman Catholic, and had borne her husband four children - working hard to raise them. Then, in middle life, her husband left her for a younger woman – hence the bitterness. Jane – who was still attractive and well-dressed, in middle age – courted several men after the break-up of her marriage, and took out her fury on all of them. Duncan was one such victim.

He was a widower of sixty-eight, and his late wife, who had died of diabetes, had borne and successfully raised, their eight children! After a year of mourning, and of honouring his late wife's memory, Duncan started looking for a second wife, and found Jane. Their relationship continued for some time, but Jane was not serious about it, nor, for that matter, about any other such relationship.

Duncan lived near me, and used to give me lifts home in his car. It was then that he confided his problems. 'I have now been in love with Jane for a long time, he confided, but she tells me that I am no good in bed. and that I will never satisfy any woman, because I am not very well-endowed.' My private thoughts were 'You have successfully fathered, and raised, no fewer than eight children, so something, somewhere must be working OK'.

However, I replied, 'Duncan, I consider you to be very well-endowed indeed. You have three pensions – one from service in the Royal Air Force, one from working as an engineer at Sperry's, and one State Retirement Pension.

You own a lovely house - which you keep very well, because you got used to doing the domestic chores, when your late wife was ill. You can cook. You can drive, and own a good car. You can dance – the proper ballroom steps – not just galumphing, modern-style, around the dance-floor.

All this being the case, I should think that there would be a queue of widows, a mile long, who would jump at the chance of marrying you, and – were I in that situation – I would be first in the queue!'

Thus encouraged by me, Duncan put an advertisement in the local 'Lonely Hearts' Column. Almost immediately, he met a widow, Joanne. I attended their wedding, and Duncan confided further to me, that he had never been so happy in his life.

There was a bitter/sweet sequel to Jane's story. She had always complained, bitterly, that her former husband's new partner, would, unfairly, enjoy his company in old age, while she would be lonely, but he died of a heart attack at the age of sixty-eight. 'Well, I told Jane, she didn't get his company in old age. Life has a way of turning the coin!'

Louise and Patrick Henman: 'Playing fair…'

When Louise and Patrick first attended a National Schizophrenia Fellowship Support Group which I ran, I assumed them, erroneously, to be mother and son. Not so! They were man and wife, with a thirty-year age-gap between them!

They attended the group, because Louise's son, from her first marriage, had suffered a schizophrenic breakdown while in his first term at Cambridge. He was very seriously ill, and violent. Louise maintained that her first husband, the boy's father, who was a top psychoanalyst at the Tavistock Institute, had caused their son's illness, by his emotional abuse of him.

Louise was upper middle class, of very good family, had been a trained nurse, working at an exclusive private hospital, and had money. When Patrick met Louise, he was an engineer working for the British Government. He was then aged twenty-nine, and Louise was aged fifty-nine. Patrick needed money to study for a PhD, so he agreed to marry Louise in return for this money. Patrick was very good looking, and they had a high class wedding at the British Embassy, with Louise looking extremely elegant, in cream lace.

Patrick wasn't a chancer, he was a nice man, and he wanted to play fair. He probably thought that he would only have to stick by Louise, for ten to fifteen years. Then she would pass away, and he, having discharged his debt honourably, would still be young enough to marry a younger woman, and have a family of his own.

It was not to be. When Louise turned up at the crisis house, in a state of extreme crisis, in the year two thousand, she had reached the age of eighty-nine, and Patrick the age of fifty-nine. Patrick, now panicking, that if he waited any longer, it would be too late, had divorced Louise, and married a woman of forty-four.

Louise had stubbornly refused to accept the situation, and had baulked at the prospect of the marital home being sold, and the assets being divided, so, eventually, it was sold over her head.

Homeless, she had gone to her mentally ill son, but, after a violent incident, she escaped through a window, and arrived at the crisis house. After a short stay with us, we found Louise accommodation, in a local sheltered home for the elderly - where she continued, for a further twelve years – finally passing away at the ripe old age of one hundred and one!

Joyce and Bob: 'Till all my money was spent'

'She was a dear little dickie-bird, 'Cheep, cheep, cheep,' she went.
Sweetly, she sang to me – till all my money was spent! Then,
she went off song. We parted on fighting terms. She was one
of the early birds, and I was one of the worms!'

It is painful to have to stand by and watch a life being wrecked, but there are times, when that is all that one can do.

Joyce came to the crisis house, having been physically assaulted by her long-term lover. She was under the local Mental Health Team, for depression, but, no doubt, suffered from a personality disorder as well. Joyce had a long history of failed relationships.

She was thirty-eight when she came to us. At the age of nineteen, she had married Terry. They had one daughter, Philippa, who, sadly, died of infantile liver disease, at eighteen months. This tragedy caused the marriage to break down.

Joyce then married Mark Lane. He was a successful businessman, and they had a good standard of living, with a nice, big house overlooking the river. Joyce was very good on the domestic front, and made an excellent social wife and hostess. Not so good, though, in other aspects of marriage.

Unfortunately, Joyce started an affair with Andrew, a serving soldier in the army, who was stationed at our local garrison. Mark Lane found out about the affair, and divorced Joyce, so she moved into a council flat, near to the garrison, and her lover. Then Joyce met a partially-sighted man, Cliff; she married him, and they moved to her native Devonshire. This marriage lasted for eighteen months.

Then Joyce moved back to Wokingham - in order to resume the relationship with her soldier lover. Then, she met Robert, and, within weeks, married him. Joyce had assumed that Robert had money, but he turned out to be a conman, with huge debts. She divorced him, returned to her lover, and, some months after this, came to us in a battered state.

Life can be very unfair. Bob, a local plumber, just happened to be doing some work for us, at the time that Joyce was admitted to the crisis house. Bob was a forty-three year old bachelor – living with his parents. They, not unreasonably, had thought – once he turned forty – that he was unlikely to marry precipitately. So they suggested that he take over paying the mortgage on their house, that they, being retired, could live there for the rest of their days, and that Bob would then inherit.

Within weeks, Joyce had married him. We knew her history, but he did not. Furthermore, we could not interfere; to do so would have been futile, because we would not have been listened to, and heeded!

To begin with, the couple moved into the council flat near to the garrison, and, standing by helplessly, we predicted, accurately, each, subsequent, move in the game.

Joyce protested that Bob's parents [though only in their seventies, and able bodied], could no longer cope in the house – which she, of course, now jointly owned. No doubt Bob and his parents resented the situation, but a weak will inevitably bows before a strong will! Within weeks, Bob's parents were shunted off to an old folks' home, and Joyce and Bob relinquished the council flat, and moved into what was now, undeniably, their property!

But not for long. Property, in Wokingham, is amongst the most highly priced in the UK. Joyce decided that they should sell up, and move to the West Midlands, where the cost of an equivalent property is only half of that in Wokingham. I could not remonstrate – only to be told to mind my own business! My one intervention was gentle. I asked Bob if he was happy with Joyce, and he said that he was. Then I pointed out that in areas where property prices are low, work was not usually so readily available.

Agatha Christie, in her autobiography, admonishes her readers never to interfere in other people's affairs, pointing to a case where a woman, who appeared to be a gold-digger, made an excellent wife for her alleged 'victim'. Agatha had never seen a happier marriage. I take her advice, but this was not to be the case with Bob and Joyce!

They moved to the West Midlands. For the first eighteen months – using the thousands of poundsworth of profits made on the sale of Bob's parents' house - Joyce whirled Bob around the world in a flurry of extravagant holidays. When the money ran out, she divorced him, and claimed her half-share from the sale of the West Midlands property. Then, work ran out. Stuck on his own in the West Midlands, virtually bankrupt, Bob had to take a job as a postman.

The last I heard of him, many years later, Bob was back in Wokingham, and had a girlfriend – hopefully a wiser choice this time, but he had still been stripped of his property, and of all his assets.

I heard nothing further of Joyce. In the intervening years, she could have married a further six times. It is very sad when a situation renders one helpless.

I always advise our service-users not to get romantically involved with people at the crisis house, and not to seek partners there. True, there is no guarantee of success anywhere. One could meet someone with problems at a sports club, or at a camera club, or in amateur dramatics. The difference is that - at the crisis house - meeting people with problems is GUARANTEED!

People with mental health problems naturally gravitate towards other people with mental health problems, because it feels safe, and so far as ordinary fellowship, and mutual support, are concerned, this is fine. But as a way of finding a partner, it is a recipe for disaster, because one compounds the problem – resulting in a double dose!

Like everything else that leads to success, finding a suitable partner requires effort. One must look good, develop interests, get out there, and be prepared to meet people in the normal, competitive world. It is easier, infinitely easier, just to grab the depressed person sitting next to you in the drop-in centre, and sad to relate, many a time, I have seen it happen.

Joy: 'The dinosaur'

'Why did the pterodactyl become extinct?
Because it was not adaptable to social change!'

Joy used our services for a good twenty years – having suffered a breakdown after the death of one of her sons in a medical accident. She left us, because one of our service users, in all innocence, destroyed the fantasy, which had become the mainstay of her existence.

After the death of her elder son, Joy had nothing further to do with his widow and her children. The rift appeared to have been caused by a disagreement over the financial compensation which Joy's daughter-in-law received as a result of his death. This money, quite rightly, was awarded, so that the widow would have the wherewithal to bring up her two teenage children, and was not to be distributed to the wider family, but money – particularly, large sums – invariably causes family rifts, and Joy's bitter resentment caused a permanent fracture!

This left Joy, with only her husband, her one surviving son, her daughter-in-law, [never very close], and one grand-daughter, Raquel. Joy existed in a 1950's timewarp, and nothing could bring her into modern times.

'Put them all in the army!' was her answer to the problem of unruly youth. We pointed out, in vain, that service in the modern army, is a highly skilled, technical, career, and that the armed forces are no longer willing to sweep up society's riff-raff!

The next time that the subject of unruly youth was raised, Joy would declare, 'Put them all in the army!' You might as well have spoken to the wall!

Joy's granddaughter, like virtually all young people in the twenty-first century, obtained the usual clutch of GCSE'S, 'A' Levels, and then a degree in criminology – which is a social science.

Even in my young days, fifty years ago, degrees were becoming much more commonly held, and nowadays, virtually everybody has one. But, in Joy's eyes, Raquel was some kind of genius – a latter day version of Sir Bernard Spilsbury, and would be renowned in forensic science! But a genius Racquel was not. She was just a nice, ordinary, girl - of the twenty-first century!

We pointed out, in vain, that Raquel – with 'A' Levels in Art, Spanish, and Social Studies, and with a Social Science degree, could not possibly become a forensic scientist – because forensic science is about blood, and semen, tissues, and fibres. It is Biology and Chemistry.

My neighbour, Dr Christopher Groombridge, is a forensic scientist, working for the Home Office, and he, most certainly, has a degree in chemistry, and a Doctorate in Forensic Science!

Joy stuck to her guns! Sadly, this delusion was shattered – albeit unintentionally – by one of our number, Gerry.

Gerry, a somewhat rough-edged character, was known to us, affectionately, as 'Delboy'.

We were helping 'Delboy', to get back into work, by preparing a good CV for him. He typed this up himself, on our computer. "You have done very well with the CV, we said, you have put down all your GCSE'S and 'A' Levels, and all your work experience. It is a good record, and should enable you to get back into work?"

Joy's jaw dropped. She could not hide her astonished anger. Impervious to Jerry's feelings, she cried 'GCSE'S, 'A' Levels, him?' 'Yes, we replied, everybody has them, these days.' There was a good three minutes' silence. Then Joy cried out, 'I won't have anything said against Raquel. She has done very well!'

Nobody had said anything against Raquel. She had done well enough, but so had Jerry, and I think that he was, yours truly, bewildered! Nevertheless, the fantasy was shattered, and, after twenty years, Joy ceased to come to the drop-in centre. I call these stories poignant. Are they funny, or are they tragic, or are they both?

Dr Anna Higgett: 'Embroidered on silk!'

When Dr Anna Higgett, Government Mental Health Policy Adviser to the Department of Health, visited the crisis house in 1999, I showed her around – explaining that I thought it very important that the mentally ill had beautiful things around them. 'And talking of beautiful things, I said, look at those flowers! They are...' 'Embroidered on silk' – she finished for me.

It was all there in her voice. The poignancy. The sadness. If only one could have this in the statutory services! But you won't. You can't. That kind of commitment, and devotion, belongs firmly to the voluntary sector – whose services come from the heart – freed from the chains of bureaucracy.

I recall a 'Songs of Praise' programme, in which a participant asserted, that she bought all her clothes in charity shops – so that she would always have money spare – to give - in cases of genuine need.

That was exactly my thinking – when I gave up a well-paid professional job – in order to do voluntary work in mental health, full-time. Don't buy your clothes in expensive, London shops. Do without luxuries. Purchase essentials in charity shops. Then, you can do without a professional salary, and devote your life, full-time, to voluntary mental health work.

A second consideration was, there are plenty of good teachers, and plenty of good schools, but mental health services, are, generally, so awful, that mental health desperately needs the talent!

The hymn chosen by this lady was: 'When I Survey the Wondrous Cross', and when it came to singing the line, 'All the vain things that charm me most, I sacrifice them to His blood.' - they trained the camera on her face.

One might add, 'Love so amazing, so divine, demands my soul, my life, my all.' It is dedication that is needed in our mental health services, not money!

There are good people working in the National Health Service mental health services – I don't deny it. But the voluntary sector, working in partnership with them, would achieve nothing, and lose everything. You would be sucked into their bureaucracy. Instead of embroidering flowers on silk, you would be sitting in meetings – going around in circles!

My visits to NHS and Social Services mental health facilities, have been very limited indeed, because I am a separatist, I prefer to have nothing to do with them. But I do recall one visit to the old mental asylum in Oxfordshire.

In all innocence, I walked onto a ward. Half a dozen patients were sitting in identical 'granny' chairs, not grouped together to encourage interaction, but placed wide apart - so that each patient was isolated – staring at the completely blank wall. I could see no staff on duty at all. Then, I noticed at the far end of the ward, a wooden and glass structure, in which all the staff were sitting – drinking coffee, and talking to each other.

Eventually, it was feeding-time at the zoo. Out the staff came, to give the patients their medication, and food, and then they retreated back into their lair! The sad thing is, that therapeutic interaction with mental patients, if you are interested in them as human beings, doesn't even have to be hard work! A nurse could sit down with a group of patients, do the day's crossword with them, drink coffee with them, and so aid their recovery. Quite an enjoyable little activity – not hard work at all!

In the crisis house, we have fixed things, so that a group of people, relatively well, who might consider themselves to be volunteers, rather than service users, can't sit together in the office – talking to each other, and ignoring the more ill – because, deliberately, we don't have an office!

Although we have several rooms, all are used, equally, by everyone.

Our chairs and tables are placed like those in a normal, family, sitting room – in order to encourage social interaction. We all use the same toilets, and they are all kept spotlessly clean, because, in our stage of civilisation, everybody should have clean toilets to use!

'Oh, it's nice to have a home of your own, and sit by your own fireside. If you've only got a table and a chair, it's all yours, and you're welcome there. You're as good as anybody in the land, as happy as a king on his throne. What more do you want? You've got the wife and kids, and a nice little home of your own!'

The sentiments, expressed in this old music hall song, are what, we hope, service users feel about the crisis house!

Chapter 13

Brenda O'Malley: 'The cherry orchard'

'I love you, but we're strangers when we meet!'

Brenda O'Malley came to the Crisis House, to seek help with coping with her daughter-in-law, who suffered from bi-polar affective disorder, but her own story makes poignant reading.

When Brenda came to us at the age of sixty-five, she was still a beautiful woman, and one could imagine that, when young, she had been an absolute stunner. She confirmed that this had indeed been the case. Able to have her pick of any husband, Brenda chose a dashing RAF pilot. She married him at the age of nineteen – with only a small amount of secretarial work experience behind her. That was, indeed, the convention in those days. A woman's destiny was marriage, and, middle class women, in particular, were not expected to work. As Agatha Christie explains, in her Autobiography, the young woman's destiny was marriage. If, for instance, you were to marry a draper, then you took on HIS way of life.

Both partners were strict Roman Catholics, and, for the wedding, had the full works – including a Nuptial Mass. Brenda bore her husband four children. After leaving the Air Force, he went into business – which – in those days – involved a lot of travelling. We were not in the era of mobile phones.

The couple had plenty of money, a beautiful house, four beautiful children, and, what Brenda thought, was a perfect marriage. On Sunday evenings, after dinner, the whole family would sit together, and select a book. It might be something like 'Great Expectations'. Then each family member would read a chapter aloud, and then hand it to the next person. On one such evening, Brenda's husband was helping himself to a drink from the sideboard, and observing this idyllic family scene. 'In my own way, I love you all', he said. A somewhat cryptic pronouncement, but Brenda only realised its true significance, in the light of future revelations.

It was the husband's sister who spilled the beans. On a visit to Brenda, she said, 'If you knew what he is getting up to when away from home, you could not bear to be under the same roof as him, never mind in the same bed!' All was then revealed. Brenda's husband had, not one, but a number of mistresses – scattered the length and breadth of the United Kingdom. He had a son, by one, who was based in Scotland, yet another down in Cornwall, another on the South Coast, and so on. His travelling on business, enabled him to keep all these affairs going, and none of the mistresses knew about each other.

Once his secret was revealed, of course, it meant divorce – a very serious step for Roman Catholics to take. It meant the tearing apart of that lovely family. It meant poverty for Brenda. She only received a tiny amount of alimony, and the cheque for this was signed by the Cornish mistress, one of those who survived the revelations! Insult was thus added to injury.

Brenda, without proper training to fall back on, and having lost the marital home, had to take residential work as a chambermaid – getting up at the crack of dawn, and slaving away for a pittance. Fortunately, later on in life, she did meet a new partner, a former naval officer, and they did have a happy relationship for seven years until he died.

So it is better not to cut the cherry orchard down. Ignorance is bliss. If the sister had kept her mouth shut, Brenda would have gone on being happy, and would have continued to lead a contented life - with plenty of money, and security with the family.

The poignant aspect is, that when her husband said, that, in his own way, he loved them all, he was speaking the truth. He wanted the beautiful, pure, wife, the lovely children, the nice house, and the respectable, contented, lifestyle of a successful businessman. However, he also wanted lots of extra-marital affairs – probably never intending that they should ever be anything other than that. What is truth? Too often it is the thing that upsets the applecart!

Bonnie Perry: 'Pack up your troubles'

*'Pack up your troubles in your old kit bag, and smile,
smile, smile! Don't let your joy and laughter hear the snag,
smile boys, that's the style. What's the use of worrying,
it never was worthwhile. So pack up your Troubles in
your old kit bag, and smile, smile, smile!'*

Bonnie came to us because she was having problems with a psychopath, who was living with her, and who was refusing to move out. Bonnie had married very young. She had been content to be a housewife and mother, but her husband had done brilliantly in his career as a TV sports journalist, and, moving in different directions, their relationship faded away. He found a new partner, and divorce became inevitable.

Bonnie was vulnerable. She had a son of twenty-one, but also a son of twelve – conceived in the [forlorn] hope that another child would save the marriage! Instead, he tied her down. The psychopath worked with Bonnie's elder son, and, lonely, she got involved with him.

On Bonnie's behalf, I think that we must have approached practically every authority that there is – from the Citizen's Advice Bureau, to the Mental Health Act Commission, to the Maudsley Hospital, to a local Consultant Psychiatrist – all in our endeavours to free her from this man's clutches – all in vain. Bonnie stayed with us for a full year, and, incidentally, during this time, ran an excellent Montessori Mother and Toddler Group at the crisis house. She was such a capable woman. This is what made us despair!

Finally, she moved to Cornwall. We all heaved a sigh of relief – thinking that she had freed herself at last. Not a bit of it! She had packed up her troubles in her suitcase – taking the psychopath with her, and it was only much later, by means of legal intervention, that Bonnie finally got out of his clutches. Poignant indeed – that an attractive, and capable, woman, could have become so vulnerable and beholden!

Jeannie Barnett: 'The glutton for punishment'

The lengths to which individuals will go to worsen their situation in life, know no bounds. They are a common phenomenon in depressive illness, but they are, nevertheless, fascinating in their awfulness.

One such example, was Jeannie. Jeannie came to stay in the crisis house, with her new, mentally and physically, ill, partner. She had four children by a previous partner, and they all suffered from learning disabilities. However, when she came to us, they were aged twenty-one, nineteen, seventeen, and fourteen – so they were progressing towards adult years. Jeannie was then in her forties.

Jeannie explained that she had suffered from uterine cancer, and so had undergone a hysterectomy. 'But, she explained, I can have a womb transplant – so that I can give birth to a child by Mick.'

Mick, at this time, was in his mid-fifties, suffered from very severe mental illness, and was also unable to return to work due to severe chest trouble!

I am fascinated, bemused. With four offspring with learning disabilities, one would have thought it enough of a burden for anyone to bear. It is poignant, if not tragic, that anyone could be such a glutton for punishment – disregarding the fate of the unfortunate child to be born into such unpromising circumstances!

When it seems to me that people are indulging in the most extreme of self-destructive foolishness, I turn to Agatha Christie in order to comprehend the psychology.

For instance, in the short story, 'The Cornish Mystery', from Agatha Christie: 'Poirot's Early Cases.': [Published: Collins: 1974.], Hercule Poirot explains to Captain Hastings. 'If you read the papers carefully, you will find that often a nice respectable woman leaves a husband she has lived with for twenty years, and sometimes a whole family of children as well, in order to link her life with that of a young man. . . . In the Autumn of a woman's life, there comes always one mad moment when she longs for romance, for adventure, before it is too late.'

In Jeannie's case, she willingly relinquished the tenancy of a four bedroom council house, [now gold dust to obtain], in order, in middle age, to set up home, in a flat, with her new lover, and to endeavour, by extreme means, to give birth to a child, by him. Agatha Christie was right. The mad moment had come for Jeannie!

Jim South: 'When the devil drives!'

Some cases are hopeless, and Jim's was. I got to know Jim over a period of time – though he only stayed in the crisis house briefly. He was a confirmed, and inveterate, heroin addict. At one stage, he had been caught importing heroin into Spain, was arrested, tried, and had to spend three years in a Spanish prison. As a result, he spoke fluent Spanish. Needs must, when the devil drives!

It appeared that Jim's troubles started when his mother died, very suddenly, of a heart attack, when Jim was just ten years old. His brother got over this tragedy, and went on to become a successful adult, but Jim got involved with drugs, and has been involved with them ever since.

I have stated elsewhere, that addicts will not recover from addiction, unless there is a worthwhile life awaiting for them at the end of the dark tunnel.

I had no hope whatsoever, for Jim, because he simply was not interested in anything other than drugs. If drugs were being discussed, his eyes would light up. You could not interest him in football, or motor racing, or current events, or anything outside the twilight world imposed by heroin addiction. More than a decade after I first encountered Jim, I still see him occasionally, and nothing has changed – not one iota! A poignant story!

Annie Hirst: 'If everybody's somebody nobody's anybody'

In the human individual, there exists a strong, and an entirely understandable, desire to be somebody in life. Who can blame people? Who would want to be a dispensable, and replaceable, cog in a wheel? In old-style, village communities, the need to be somebody, was largely satisfied naturally. You WERE the local butcher, baker, candle-stick maker, etc. The Industrial Revolution put paid to that. Then, people became replaceable cogs in machines, and, from that time on, life for many people, has become increasingly anonymous, and isolating.

I am convinced that the reason, that so many sad and disaffected adults, jump onto the current, and hopefully short-lived, abuse bandwagon, is that – never having been anything in life – this gives them their one chance to be a star. They are centre-stage, being looked at, being listened to. Was it not Andy Warhol who said, 'Everyone should be famous for five minutes!'? I like Cliff Richard, and Jim Davidson, so it is sad that genuine stars have to be the victims in this witch hunt, and there are better ways for ordinary people to acquire self-esteem without destroying our national treasures.

Furthermore, one would think that, after the appalling miscarriage of justice that occurred with the Wimbledon Common murder, Police would insist upon, and only act upon, hard forensic evidence – DNA samples, where no mistake is possible. Hearsay is not evidence, and even if hundreds of complainants assert that a rich celebrity is guilty, this is still not evidence. Hundreds of people may, easily, be attracted by the prospect of ready money!

In the crisis house, we have encountered many such individuals, who have never, before, been anything in life. Because we are user run, some, at last, achieve a position – small, but important to them – with us. One such early example was Paddy Rooney [Chapter 22: 'Have you seen my childhood?'] His paintings, and our appreciation of them, gave him genuine self-esteem – unfortunately, in his case, short-lived!

In other instances, if people have, at least, been something early in life – a school sports star - for instance, then they are able to settle into humdrum, adult life, relatively happily. One such – amongst our ranks – is Glyn – who, when young, was junior boxing champion for the County.

Adult life, for him, has been far from successful. But he does not appear to crave to be somebody, in the way that many others do. Instead, he still talks, with pride, of his earlier sporting achievements. Furthermore, as I write this, after a wait of more than five years, Glyn has finally been offered the tenancy of a council flat. No longer homeless, this may be his first step in getting his current life, successful once again.

When the drop-in centre is open, I sit in my chair – sipping coffee or sherry – and [deliberately], create the impression that I have infinite leisure, in which to focus upon people's problems. It looks such an easy, pleasant, role, and numerous service-users, over the years, have wished to take it over for themselves.

Gabriela Rani tried to do so in an aggressive manner. [Chapter 34: 'Outright Battle'.] If such people realised the amount of work [some of it, extremely mundane], that has to be put in – in order to keep the crisis house the way it is, they would not want my chair! But they are seeing the created illusion, not the reality!

One such individual was Annie. She came to us in 1997 – explaining that she had mental health problems, and had been a Sectioned patient in a mental hospital for some considerable time. Of experiences there, she related the poignant, and awful, story, of the psychiatric nurse who used to rattle her keys – threateningly, and triumphantly – as she wielded her indubitable power over the Sectioned patients. I wish, in my narrative, that I could relate some good stories about the behaviour of mental health professionals, but, alas, I cannot.

Annie's husband, in her enforced absence, had an affair with her sister. In due course, he married the sister, and, because he was awarded custody, of Annie's and his, two daughters, he also obtained possession of the marital home. On discharge from hospital, Annie was abandoned, alone, and homeless. Eventually, in order to secure a roof over her head, she married somebody who, according to the lease, was only allowed to share his accommodation with a wife. So it was a marriage of convenience.

Annie, understandably, had a strong desire to be somebody, and she tried, strenuously, to take over my role in running the crisis house. She attended the drop-in centre regularly for some considerable time. Then one day, abruptly, she just ceased to come. Our befrienders visited her, but she never came back, and no real reason for her departure was ever given.

I think that Annie had finally realised that she was not going to take over the crisis house, and, if she were to attain a position in life, it was not going to be that one. Interestingly, Annie's second [empty] marriage was to someone with a position of importance in a small village. This gave her status vicariously, and so, partially, satisfied her need to be somebody in life!

The irony in this story, is that there is absolutely no need for anybody to feel useless in life. There is voluntary work of all kinds – available galore – and finding such a useful role for oneself, is often an important element in recovering from mental ill health. A poignant story!

Chapter 14

Val and Jean Burgess: 'We'll build a sweet little nest - Somewhere out in the west'

'With someone like you, a pal good and true, I'd like to leave it all behind, and go and find a place that's known to God alone – just a spot we could call our own.

We'll find some perfect peace, where joys never cease, somewhere beneath the starry skies. We'll build a sweet little nest, somewhere out in the West, and let the rest of the world go by!'

At just about the time that I was moving over to Berkshire, I had some friends in the National Schizophrenia Fellowship, who were doing exactly the same thing. Like me, they had got their mentally ill relative settled into care, and having just retired, from working hard all their lives in the grocery trade, in London, Val and Jean, Burgess, decided to move to a nice, quiet, little market town, in the West of Berkshire.

'After a lifetime in the hustle and bustle of London, we want some peace and quiet in our old age,' they said. So they moved to the charming little town of Hungerford – to the extreme West of Berkshire.

Only a few weeks after moving there, they were in the town's supermarket, doing their weekly shopping, when the manager came running in, and called for everybody to get down, flat on the floor. Then Val and Jean heard the gunshots – close by.

Michael Ryan, in a severe state of psychosis, had gone berserk on the street! Sixteen people died in the Hungerford massacre. My friends were among the lucky ones. They survived with their lives! This is a poignant story, but so telling! Mental ill health occurs everywhere, not just in inner cities. It touches all sections of society, and all communities.

Gilbert, and the director of Bracknell Mind: 'You saucy little perisher'

Readers may wonder why the crisis house, which, realistically, can only serve Wokingham, operates under the auspices of the Wokingham and WEST BERKSHIRE Mental Health Association. The reason is historic.

Some years ago, the Director of the, then, Bracknell MIND, paid us a visit. Reading MIND had closed down some time before, Windsor, Slough and Maidenhead had only small, local, mental health associations, and the towns to the West of us, had nothing.

So he saw an opportunity for empire building. He wanted to take over the whole county – as Director of Berkshire MIND. We were the only fly in the ointment. He promised not to interfere with us, if we agreed that this plan could go ahead.

My refusal was measured. I simply explained that, with the formation of a county-wide Berkshire MIND, we would become redundant overnight, and thus cease to get any funding! I also disagreed with the idea, as a good way of delivering mental health. I think it better, for the diverse county of Berkshire, to have local mental health associations – based in each of its towns – in order to meet their very diverse needs.

Our wonderful, late, Vice-President, Gilbert, was less measured in his response. 'You saucy little perisher, he said, that bloody thing [Bracknell MIND] has folded up three times.' It was quite true. It folded up in the early eighties, and, then again, in the late eighties, and then again, and then again! Losing its contract to Rethink in 2007, it staggered on for a while – with just an office base. Then the organization closed down completely in 2011.

At the time, I simply suggested, that, if the Director of Bracknell MIND wished to expand, he should form East Berkshire MIND, and that we, in order to protect our territory, could become Wokingham and West Berkshire MIND. This was done – with disastrous results for the East of the county.

When we formed, in 1987, there most certainly was, a Windsor and Maidenhead Mental Health Association – independent of MIND. There was also a Slough Mental Health Association. He took these under the umbrella of East Berkshire MIND, so that, when that folded up, they folded up with it. Then Rethink, in Bracknell, closed down as well, so East Berkshire is now, effectively, without a voluntary mental health service. A poignant story!

Fenella Bewley: 'Everybody's problems but her own'

Fenella Bewley came to the crisis house with the familiar problem of having a mentally ill son, who was still living with her, and this was inhibiting her, from having a life of her own.

This is her story. Fenella was married, and had raised five children. Her husband had a good job as an engineer, and they lived in a lovely, big house in a good area. Her two girls were married, and her eldest boy was established, and living independently, when Fenella's husband died, very suddenly, of a heart attack, at the age of only fifty-three.

Fenella still had her two younger boys at home – Jan, who was twenty-one, and Dean, who was eighteen. All the family were traumatised, but Dean, who was training in an apprenticeship, got a lot of support from his boss, who acted as a surrogate father, so he came through the ordeal. Jan did not.

It is terrifying how money trickles away, if you are not careful with it. Fenella decided to sell the big house, which, at today's prices, would be worth more than a million pounds, and buy a smaller one. She did this, and then, in an attempt to get Jan living independently, sold the second house, put money into building a granny annexe, at her daughter's house, and bought a mobile home for Jan. She moved to the annexe, so that she would be on hand to help with the grandchildren.

The mobile home did not work out for Jan, so Fenella sold it, and bought him another one, in a quieter, more rural area. That didn't work out either, so he sold it, and used the money to go to the motor racing in South America.

On his return, Jan had nowhere to live, so he went to his mother in the granny annexe.

Then her son-in-law lost his job, and could only get a similar one, if he agreed to move to Paris. So the house and granny annexe were sold. Daughter, son-in-law, and children, moved to Paris, and there was only enough money left in the kitty, for Fenella to move into a little one bedroom house – with Jan. This was her living situation, when she came to us for help.

I gave the standard advice – which I have given hundreds of times. 'Get the mentally ill son or daughter settled independently, before you become too old to cope. They will then be used to living independently, so it will be less of a trauma, when you do become infirm, or pass away.'

I thought, that, at the age of sixty-seven, Fenella was still a little young to think of going into sheltered accommodation for the elderly. She suggested this, because she had a friend, already settled, in a local scheme. I nevertheless, concurred, because Jan could not go there with her, and so would have to move into independent accommodation – or so I, in my naivete, thought!

All this was arranged. The little house was sold, Fenella moved into sheltered accommodation – for which she paid a rent, and Jan moved into a rented flat in the private sector. This didn't work out, so he moved into another private sector flat, and that did not work out either. He lasted for five years in his third flat, but having disputes all the time with the landlord and neighbours. Then the owners decided to sell up.

Fenella then found Jan a tiny cottage in a pretty little Oxfordshire village. He seemed to be very happy there. Then, unfortunately, after only six months, the owners decided to sell up, so we were back to square one.

After this, Jan failed to settle anywhere independently, and went to live, illegally, in his mother's sheltered flat. So, Fenella had gone - from owning a house worth more than a million pounds, down to a house worth half of that, down to a granny annexe, and then, down to a little one bedroom house – probably worth about an eighth of her first house, and, finally, down to a scruffy, little, rented, flat in a sheltered complex – where you couldn't swing a cat round – and now owning nothing. What a poignant descent! This was a classic case of a person who was very good at solving other people's problems, but she could not solve her own!

Once I knew that Fenella was terminally ill with cancer, I was determined to salvage some good from the situation, and I also knew that Jan would not be able to stay in the sheltered flat, because this would be given to another elderly person.

I therefore worked with a housing officer, to obtain a secure tenancy for Jan. This was also for a cottage, but under the auspices of a Housing Association. This arrangement worked well.

The very day before I wrote this narrative, at the end of August, 2015, I encountered Jan – doing his shopping in Bracknell, and evidently coping well. His mother died nearly three years ago, but he has coped, living alone, in the cottage.

In October 2015, I encountered Jan, once again, doing his shopping. He was looking very well. He confirmed that things were going O.K., and I noticed, amongst his shopping, a fresh chicken. So evidently, Jan is cooking for himself, and eating, properly. So I did salvage something from a very poignant situation.

A poignant story – indicating that one can lose a million pounds, and end up with nothing, if one is not careful with money.

Such a poignant story, also stimulates one to look carefully, at the policy of extending 'Right to Buy' to Housing Association tenants, as well as to Council tenants. We need to be sure that there will be enough secure tenancies available for people who will never be able to afford to buy property, and for whom the insecurity of private sector rentals has adverse mental health effects.

Alexander Hopkins: 'The highest in the land'

Alexander came to stay in the crisis house – having suffered a psychotic episode. He had been playing the drums with a band in France, when he became ill, so his fellow musicians thought that he should return to England.

This is his story. He said that he was bi-lingual – having started his life in the South of France. His grandfather had been an English aristocrat, who, early in the twentieth century, had made pregnant a young waitress in the South of France. Against all the conventions of the day, he married her.

Alexander's mother was the twelfth child of this union – thus bringing us into the mid twentieth century. In due course, she also married a well-to-do Englishman, and had three boys – of whom Alexander was the youngest. When he was only three, his father died, so his mother moved from the South of France to England, remarried, and went on to have a girl, and a boy, by her second husband. Her cousin, educated at Eton, retained the family Title.

Alexander suffered from depression, and Asperger's syndrome – which included obsessive/compulsive symptoms. He had reversed the biological clock, so members of our drop-in centre, did not see much of him.

I used to spend the early evenings with him – knocking back a bottle of Chablis together. He maintained, that to appreciate this vintage properly, you had to be on the French Riviera. Nevertheless, I thought that we two coped quite well! Alexander stayed in the crisis house for almost two years – largely due to the failure of the mental health team, to intervene on his behalf.

When he had been with us for just over a year, a new social worker, on the mental health team, came to see the crisis house. I explained that Alexander's pressing need, was now for move-on accommodation, so the social worker promised to appoint a community support worker – to arrange suitable housing for him.

Eight months passed, and nothing had been done, so I called them to the crisis house. The social worker asserted that Alexander wasn't mentally ill, and so did not qualify for a service from the team, and the community support worker asserted that it was up to Alexander to find accommodation for himself, and not up to her to do so!

I complained to their employer, the local authority, and, pointed out that – if the mentally ill person has to fend for himself – why are we, the tax payers, paying Social Services' employees – to do nothing? Days later, a council flat dropped from heaven.

Alexander went on to have severe problems, but he was one of my success stories, in that I did succeed in winning an appeal for him to continue to receive Employment Support Allowance. With his complex mental health problems, Alexander would never have coped in open market employment. A poignant story, and a stark example of the fact that mental health affects all strata of society – the aristocratic as well as those of more humble origin!

Stephen Miller, and Jenny: 'She danced with the Royal Ballet'

As I point out in the chapters on the Battle for the Crisis House, at times, over the years, I have wondered whether all my efforts to make the crisis house, the way it is, are properly appreciated. My fears were further allayed by this story.

I saw a beautiful, original, oil painting of a ballerina, in a pink tutu, that I would have liked for the crisis house. But it was huge, and heavy, and in a charity shop in Bracknell, so I doubted whether I would be able to carry it all the way over to Wokingham. You will have read of my brief encounter with driving!

I debated with myself, and then I decided to have a go. I staggered across with the picture – and very beautiful it looks, hanging in our main lounge.

Stephen suffers from very severe schizophrenia, and has, at times, to be Sectioned. He comes into the drop-in, and says, 'I have come here, because I want to sit and look at that beautiful picture of the ballet dancer. My sister, who danced with the Royal Ballet, died of leukaemia at the age of only thirty-two, and that picture reminds me of her – in her dancing heyday.'

A poignant story, and so telling. It just shows how important effort is, and how such simple endeavours, can be so important for the individual's mental health.

Chapter 15

Patrick and Jude Johnson: 'Tell me the old, old story'

Patrick Johnson, simply could not accept that his son, Jude, suffered from a severe mental illness, schizophrenia. Patrick was a trained Freudian Therapist, and had worked in the local youth service. Jude was diagnosed, when a teenager, and it seemed possible that the heavy use of cannabis had contributed to his illness.

Jude had been tried out in various unsupported, ordinary, accommodations, and none had worked out. Fellow residents voted him out of one, a therapeutic community. In one bed-sitter flat, he proved so disruptive, that his immediate neighbours drove their car to Virginia Water, and slept there – rather than putting up with the noise – that went on all night. It seemed that the options for Jude were running out.

I raised the subject with his father. 'Why, I enquired, is Jude not in the high support hostel, on the London Road?' 'I'll tell you why, his father responded, with fury, because the Social Services are crap, and I am not having my son living with a bunch of raving lunatics!'

What is so poignant about this story, is that – had Jude been accepted for the high support hostel – he probably would have been the most severely mentally ill resident, there!

Patrick worked in the local services, so it was the old, old, story – that they were good enough for other people's sons and daughters, but not good enough for his. This is the acid test, is it not?

I recall working in a top private school in North London. One of my colleagues said to me, 'This is the only school that I have ever worked in, to which I wouldn't mind sending my own children.' By contrast, I worked in, yet another I.L.E.A. school, which was not actually, one of their worst, because it was a Roman Catholic school, and so, retained some standards.

But the staff said that they would not be willing to send their children there. They wanted something better for them – a nice, private, convent school. Don't want your own services? What an indictment of them! By contrast, I can put my hand on my heart, and say, that were I to need a mental health service, the only place that I would go to, willingly, is the Wokingham Crisis House!

It is actually quite nice when individuals who have set up an excellent service, benefit from it themselves, at a later stage in life. Thus, Dame Cicely Saunders, received excellent palliative care, when dying of cancer, in St Christopher's Hospice, the pioneering hospice, in Sydenham, South

London, which she had founded in the early nineteen-seventies. I have only ever heard one word used to describe this hospice – 'Marvellous!'

By contrast, if one were not personally affected, one might even find service-providers' rejection of their own services, funny! As Groucho Marx would have it, 'I would never join a club that wanted me as a member!'

Patrick was also in denial that his son had limitations. Because, as a schoolboy, Jude had participated in making an amateur video film, for television, Patrick still saw a future career as a film director, as being a realistic option for him!

This poignant story has a, relatively, happy ending. Many years after my conversation with his father, I encountered Jude, by chance. By this time, he was living in supported mental health accommodation, and, since he was receiving the care appropriate to his condition, seemed to be in relative good health, and to have achieved some measure of stability.

Arthur Blake, and Elizabeth Strange: 'Like something from the third world'

Arthur was a schoolmaster – who had suffered a breakdown – as a result of the stress inherent in teaching. His story is most poignant. He was suicidal, and so had to be admitted to a mental hospital – under a Section of the Mental Health Act.

On his first admission, there was no bed available at the county mental hospital, so a bed was bought for him at an exclusive, private, hospital in London. With no previous experience of mental health facilities, at all, Arthur assumed that this hospital, at the beginning of the twenty-first century, was just as you would expect modern, mental health care, to be.

All patients had an individual, private room, with an en-suite bathroom, and colour television. The food was very good, and there was plenty of choice – from a well-planned, and varied, menu.

Each day, there was a proper programme of activities – which included line-dancing, [to get patients interacting], art, individual counselling, and a full range of therapies. Arthur recovered fully, and returned to work.

After a time, Arthur became ill again, but, on this occasion, there was a bed in the county mental hospital! A Victorian lunatic asylum! Dormitories, and shared toilets and showers. Awful food, and no programme of therapies.

Arthur's sister, and husband, came to visit the crisis house, when he stayed with us briefly. She had visited him in the mental hospital, and could hardly believe that such places still existed in the twenty-first century. 'What you would expect of Romania!' was her comment.

Another school teacher, who had a similar experience of the mental hospital, left, because it was so awful. 'There wasn't even a bedside lamp, so that I could read', she complained. If you didn't laugh, you would cry.

The crisis house, in addition to having a thousand pictures, has twenty lamps! The provision of softer lights is so important in a therapeutic environment. Main, fluorescent, lights, can be experienced as being harsh – especially by depressed people, who, frequently, suffer from hyperacuity.

The sad truth is, that the basic, human, necessities, can be supplied at practically no cost at all. What is needed is caring staff, and the abolition of bureaucracy. If the crisis house can equip itself from charity shops, at minimal cost, so could other mental health facilities. You need to get rid of bone-idleness, and find voluntary staff who will make the effort to provide good environments.

Bella Hutchins: 'I am qualified. Therefore, I am normal!'

I found Bella's situation to be very poignant. When she came to stay in the crisis house, she had practically no possessions. Nevertheless, she did bring with her a bookcase, and this contained all the textbooks on learning disabilities, which she had studied when training for work in this field. The tacit statement was, 'I am normal, I am normal. Look, I qualified!'

Bella had indeed, qualified, and worked, in learning disabilities, but she was suffering from a mental illness – which necessitated anti-psychotic medication, and she had become too ill to continue with her job.

I still see Bella occasionally. She did not return to her job, but lives, independently in a flat, has a partner, and attends a mental health drop-in centre.

So often, people with mental health problems, see a certificate in mental health, as a kind of protection from their illness – an immunisation! Alas, there is no inoculation against mental ill health. Knick-Knack made the same mistake. [Chapter 17: Give a dog a bone.'] I find this misconception to be poignant, and funny, and tragic, as well!

Tom Stafford: 'The diamond sorter'

It is poignant to reflect that Tom Stafford may never have suffered a mental breakdown at all – had not the unendurable stress of doing two people's jobs, caused him to become ill.

Tom, on leaving school, went to work as a sorter with a big Diamonds Company. When a colleague left, he was not replaced, and Tom had to shoulder both jobs. One day, at his bench, the stress overwhelmed him, and he flipped.

Tom attended our drop-in centre, regularly, for some time. He had a lovely, supportive, family. He had been living with his mother and father in a big house in Surrey. First, his mother died. Then, his father died, and left the house to Tom, but he could not cope with living there alone, so he came to live with his sister and her husband, in Wokingham.

I used to reflect, with rueful poignancy, how wonderful it would be for mental health, if all families were like Tom's. Tom's sister and husband were living in high-cost, rented, accommodation in Wokingham – having lost the property that they owned, when a former business partner had defected, with all the money – leaving them bankrupt!

So the whole family sat down together, to find a living solution which would work out to the optimum benefit for everybody! How rare! Look at Sonia, and her awful sister, Joan! [Chapter 47: page 260.]

They decided to build an annexe to Tom's house. This would be for Tom's exclusive use. His sister and husband would occupy the main body of the house. They would have some meals together, and some, separately. So it worked out, that Tom had a good balance of support, and independence. It all worked out very well, and I am in touch with Tom to this day.

A funny, and poignant, addendum to Tom's story. After moving back to Surrey, he, nevertheless, continued to attend our Christmas parties. But he was now attending, regularly, the local MIND drop-in centre, in Surrey. And yes, he confirmed, ruefully, it had plastic chairs, and bare walls!

Brian Gittings: 'Ability and disability'

Although we had not seen Brian for some years, when we heard of his suicide, we were still shocked. He had been such an excellent volunteer with us. He was so able, so intelligent, so caring. Brian was also an excellent problem-solver.

At the Inquest into his suicide, Brian's wife explained that he had held a very high position in working life, and had never adjusted to retirement. He had seemed, to us, to be well adjusted.

When he first came to us, Brian explained, that his offer of voluntary work with the Citizens' Advice Bureau, had been declined, on grounds of age. They did not have volunteers beyond the age of seventy – and since he was approaching this, the resources put into his training, would not be justified.

Quite sensibly, Brian then came to us, instead. He was, obviously, quite capable of seeing alternatives, and of finding a useful role for himself.

After two years with us, as an excellent befriender, he had gone off, first, to visit New Zealand, and then to go climbing in the Himalaya Mountains!

Brian was well into his seventies, when the tragedy occurred. He threw himself from a high building, and death was instantaneous.

I find it very poignant that, with all his abilities, he could not solve the problem. I would have sworn that Brian was capable of solving such a problem.

His story has some features resonant of the tragedy from, [Chapter 24: 'You can't be on page three forever'].

Chapter 16

Johnnie and Charles Hewitt: 'The reversal of fortunes'

Johnnie Hewitt was one of our early crisis house service users. He used to come to us for sanctuary and asylum – away from a very difficult living situation.

Johnnie was very intelligent, and had qualified in law. His problem was that he had been bullied, and abused, by his father, and, in his younger years, stood in abject terror of the man.

Latterly, his father had suffered a stroke, and was very incapacitated – needing a lot of care – which Johnnie had to deliver. He did this - with such a complex mixture of emotions. He couldn't decide whether he hated his father, whether he still feared him, or whether, now that he was the stronger in the relationship, that he pitied him. It was a most poignant situation.

Johnnie was an example of a person, for whom the standard services simply don't cater. What he was looking for, was respite, somewhere to come and relax, and try to sort out all his, conflicting, emotions.

Janey and Ellen Rainer 'Can you beat it?'

The failure and inadequacy of the social services, is ever my song! Janey, and her daughter, Ellen's story, provides a particularly annoying example.

When we had guests in the crisis house, we always tried to give proper preparation for their eventual moving on – in order to maximise their chance of success in their future accommodation.

For this reason, we had a well thought out schedule – to cover the longer stays in the crisis house.

Stage one, was the coming in, and settling in – and, during this period, we suggested that the person – just rest - and recover from their emotional trauma.

Stage two, after some recovery had been made by the guest, was to sit down with them, and discuss together – just what the problems, solutions, and future goals, were.

Stage three, was active working on the problems, and solutions, and working to achieve the goals.

Stage four, was the smooth process of moving out of the crisis house, and on with one's life.

It is credit to our Association, that having followed such a schedule, the great majority of our guests, over twenty years, used their experience with us, to achieve resolution of problems, and success in their future lives.

Janey and Ellen had been with us for some months, and had achieved all that they were going to achieve, so I spoke to Ellen's social worker – giving her a full month's notice – so that she could sort out appropriate, long-term, accommodation, for them.

On the day that the month was up, I contacted her – expecting, in my naivete, that all the arrangements would be in place. Not a bit of it. She had done nothing. 'No, Ellen was not going to be allowed to stay any longer', so I suggested that the social worker got her skates on!

She flapped around – trying to find something – and came up only with, completely unsuitable, bed-and–breakfast accommodation.

Fortunately, Janey persisted with the authorities, in her determination to get proper, long-term, care, for Ellen, so, eventually, she was admitted to a high-support nursing home. But why the wait? Why was this not arranged during the full month's period of notice? Can you beat it?

This social worker was very critical of Ellen's mother – accusing her of instilling 'learned helplessness' in her daughter. Whatever is learned helplessness? It sounds like a lot of social workerese rubbish, to me! In fact, Ellen had very high support needs, and the nursing home, which her mother found, was the right place for her to be.

Caterina and Sandra: 'She is a lovely girl'

One of our helpers, Caterina, had two daughters – Alice and Sandra. Alice married while very young. She was only just twenty. Caterina confided that her second daughter, Sandra, had never had a boyfriend, and had never been asked on a date by anybody. When her mother broached the subject with her, Sandra burst into tears. She wanted a boyfriend, but it never happened. 'I can't understand it, Caterina said, she is a lovely girl.'

I was able to concur that this was, indeed, the case. I had seen the photographs of Alice's wedding – at which Sandra was a bridesmaid. Naturally, she would look at her very best on such a day, but, even so, she was slim, and extremely pretty. She was an intelligent girl, a maths teacher, and had a pleasant personality, so neither of us could understand why nobody wanted her.

Caterina then confided, further, that she had experienced exactly the same problem, herself. As a young woman, she could not get a boyfriend, and so, in desperation, had ended up marrying her boss – rather than remaining a spinster, and was extremely unhappy with him. Again, I was puzzled. Now middle-aged, Caterina was slim, and, still pretty. Odd, isn't it.

Agatha Christie always comes up with the answers to these puzzles. In 'The Moving Finger' [Published: Collins: 1942.], Joanna Burton, remarked to her brother, Jerry. 'It's funny, isn't it? Some people have lots of looks and absolutely no sex appeal. That girl [Elsie Holland] has. It seems such a pity.' Her brother remarked that the reverse was also true. He said 'I have seen a little sad monkey-faced woman whom no-one would turn to look at twice. Then she opened her mouth and suddenly enchantment had lived and bloomed and Cleopatra had cast her spell anew.'

This is the Eartha Kitt of 'Old Fashioned Girl' fame. In her seventies, she still had IT. Nobody knows what IT is, but they recognise it, when they see it!

Sandra's was a poignant story, and many years later, I learned that she was still a spinster school teacher. I wish that I had a happy ending to all my stories, but I haven't! However, teaching is a useful occupation, so it doesn't have to be seen as a waste of a life, if one remains an unmarried school-teacher.

Furthermore, when you come to read of the timid, blonde, lady, in my chapter, 'Early Crisis House Experiences', you will, no doubt, concur, that there are far worse fates, in life, than spinsterhood!

Agatha Christie's opposite phenomenon, observed by Jerry Burton, is so poignant, as well. When Joy [Chapter 12: 'Till all my Money was spent'.], was about to embark upon her fifth marriage, [not counting the soldier lover], I actually asked my husband, who had met her at a dinner party at the crisis house, what was it that she had, that attracted all the men. I could see no attraction at all. He replied that she had 'IT'. Blessed if I could see it. But then, I am not a man!

Violet: 'I wish you wanted my love, baby'

I have written of Violet's situation in my chapter on 'Advocacy', and I was delighted to hear the latest news – that Violet has successfully completed her parenthood training courses, and is keeping her latest baby.

We found her situation, most poignant. Violet had, herself, been sexually abused as a child, and had been in care. She had all these lovely children, all taken away from her. We were most involved with Tommy and Ellie – and bought baby things for both children.

I can see Violet, sitting in the drop-in lounge, and saying 'They will take her [Ellie] away from me'. She was so sad, so helpless. Thank God that her situation is now resolved!

Anita White: 'You can't go back'

Anita White came to stay in the crisis house because her current partner was violent and abusive. Anita appeared to be well bred and well educated. The partner was neither, so we wondered about her story.

It transpired that, at twenty-three, Anita had married her first cousin. Unfortunately, he was then involved in a car accident, and his injury necessitated amputation. Anita had trouble coping.

Her current partner was younger, could drive a car, and so, appeared to be a more attractive proposition. She met him at work, and the affair commenced. She left her husband, and moved in with the new partner, but the relationship was disastrous. The new partner turned out to be, uncouth, and violent.

When she came to us, Anita was hopeful that her former husband, to whom she was, fundamentally, much more suited, would have her back. He declined. He didn't mind her visiting him, on a friendly basis, but the trust had gone, and he did not want her back.

The great poignancy of life is that you can't go back. Anita left the crisis house to see whether she could patch things up with her second partner, but this did not work out either, and they split up. A poignant story.

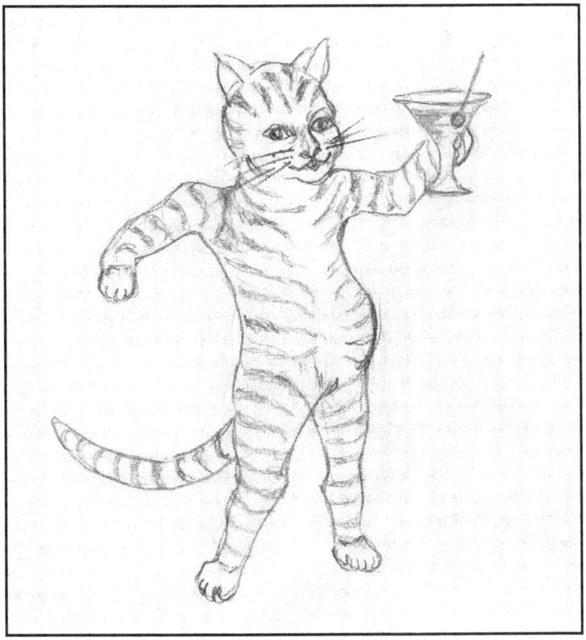

Chapter 17

Twenty-five Funny Stories

Ted: 'The emissary of the Queen!'

We ran a drop-in centre at the Wokingham British Red Cross HQ in Denmark Street, from June 1989 until March 1991 – when we took over the Crisis House. The hall was bare and clinical – with hospital beds there, for Red Cross first aid lessons, but their volunteers were very kind, and we had the use of a kitchen, and toilets, during our drop-in sessions. Our two years' experience there formed an excellent foundation for our subsequent work at the crisis house, so we were grateful, and kept in touch with the British Red Cross ladies, after we moved into the crisis house.

The Queen instituted 'The Queen's Award for Voluntary Service' at the time of her Golden Jubilee in 2002 – and the first of the awards were to be given to voluntary groups in July 2003. At Christmas 2002, the ladies from the British Red Cross – invited, as always – came to our Christmas Party.

One volunteer, Joyce, arrived, and asked if it would be all right if she brought Ted in with her, to see the crisis house. Assuming Ted to be either a mental health service user – looking for a drop-in, or a relative looking for somewhere suitable for a patient, I replied 'Of course! Come in Ted, sit your old self down, and have a glass of sherry, and a mince pie!' We then settled down to all our usual jokes about the awfulness of the mental health system, and our contempt for Social Services!

Joyce showed Ted over the crisis house. Some time later, Ted telephoned – asking whether we would like invitations to the Buckingham Palace Garden Party. Ted – in addition to holding a very high-ranking position in the British Red Cross - was an emissary of the Queen! Our association was one of the first to receive the Queen's Award for Voluntary Service in July 2003.

Ackbar Ahmad: 'I'm a Chinaman'

Ackbar, an Asian man, came to stay in the crisis house just after Christmas in 2001. After a stay of six months, we found him a flat. Our usual practice, then, was to get the flat a nice, new, fitted carpet, and furniture, so that the person could feel that they were setting out on a good basis. The former guest would choose their carpet from a local carpet supplier, and then we would arrange the fitting, and pay.

There were protests from other service-users, when Ackbar's carpet turned out to cost twice as much as those of other former guests. I had given Ackbar instructions as to how much we could pay per square metre – wanting the former guests to have good quality, but not the luxury end of the market. Ackbar had complied, but, of course, his flat happened to be twice the size of that of other former guests, so he needed twice as many square metres!

Other service users were convinced that I had treated him preferentially, because he was Asian, but I had not. The rooms were bigger, and if that was racism, then I'm a Chinaman!

Peter Black: 'Bully for you!'

I liked Peter's story about the way he dealt with attempted bullying at school. Peter – homosexual, mild-mannered and courteous – as I have invariably found them to be – and quite ruthlessly efficient!

A gang of school bullies targeted him, so he challenged them to a fight, on some local common ground, after school. Laughing aloud, they turned up – expecting to find Peter cowering in terror.

Peter, himself, may be affable and courteous, but he sure did have some rough friends and acquaintances! The bullies found themselves confronted by two hundred skinheads – armed with bicycle chains – all organized by the efficient Peter. The bullies ran for their lives!

Janey and Mick: 'Sauce for the gander'

Janey and Mick stayed in the crisis house in 1998. Both had mental health problems, and I thought it unlikely that their relationship would stand the test of time. That being the case, when I found them a Housing Association flat to move onto, I insisted that they took out a Joint Tenancy – so that rights to accommodation would be protected for both of them if, [or rather, when], the relationship broke down!

Of the two, Mick was the more severely mentally ill, with physical problems as well, and so he was under the aegis of the local community mental health team. Janey had used local, statutory, mental health services, but did not come within their ambit of 'severe and enduring', and, therefore, qualifying for an ongoing service.

The relationship lasted for about another eighteen months, and then Janey came to the crisis house to explain that she had been locked out of the flat, and was homeless, and roofless. I was staggered that, in a democracy, a doctor, a social worker, and one tenant in a joint tenancy, could hold keys to a flat, but that the other lawful tenant, could be locked out. The whole point of a joint tenancy, is to protect the rights of all concerned, and any individual can only be evicted by a court order – due process having been adhered to.

It was a Friday afternoon. Mick had gone to stay with his brother for the weekend. I hastened to engage a locksmith. The locks were changed, and Janey, no doubt, with a considerable feeling of empowerment, was then able to re-occupy her flat.

Prior to changing the locks, I had broached the subject with their social worker. I told her that Mick and Janey's relationship – good or bad – was not her business, and she replied that it was not mine! I then told her that I would raise the subject with the Housing Association – to see what they thought about having their tenancies interfered with illegally.

I did this, and they complained to the social worker's employer, the local Council. The Council wanted us to accept that the professionals knew best! We did not. We took up the matter with the Local Authority Ombudsman – who upheld our complaint, and, cheeky little monkeys, said that they had another client with similar problems, and would we act for him as well?

The couple's solicitor thought it very funny that we had changed the locks, but what is sauce for the goose, is sauce for the gander. How would it be if everybody, for convenience, took the law into their own hands? Furthermore, it demonstrates, just how important it is, to have genuinely separatist mental health organizations, to safeguard the rights of the vulnerable mentally ill.

Knick-Knack Paddy Whack 'Give a dog a bone'

'Knick-Knack, paddy whack, give a dog a bone,
this old man came rolling home!'

Our Association has been very lucky with the students, whom we have had on placement with us, over the years. We are very keen to invest in the young, and I have devoted an entire chapter of this book to our experience with students, but there has been the occasional exception!

Pam approached us in the summer of 2009. She explained that she was undertaking a Counselling Training Course, and needed an informal placement, as well as the formal placement which she already had. Could she come to us?

Pam explained that she was homeless. She had been living with an alcoholic who had died. Due to his abuse of alcohol, they had defaulted on their mortgage payments, so their flat had been repossessed.

She was currently staying, unhappily, with some acquaintances. Their house was very dirty, but, for the time being, she was trapped there. She had been working as a carer, but could not cope, so she was currently working as a cleaner. She was having difficulty in coping with this as well: the boss was always telling her off.

We began to wonder who would be counselling whom! But training for counselling was, in her fantasy world, evidently to be her escape route from the problems of daily life. Give a dog a bone!

We gave Pam the affectionate soubriquet of 'Knick-Knack'. She actually fitted in quite well with us - because she was, obviously, a mental health client herself. The fantasy was the piece of paper – the Counselling Certificate that would enable her to escape from her situation. As I explained to our members, she probably would get the bit of paper, and she did!

'Once I qualify, said Knick-Knack, I can get fees of forty-five pounds per hour – counselling people.' It is fascinating to observe how people can fail to think things through thoroughly! Where did Knick Knack intend to do her counselling, if she set up as a private practitioner? – in the squalid house of her acquaintances? Or in the scruffy little council bedsitter, that she went on to occupy?

If she hired suitable premises, there would be to pay – rent, business rates, public liability insurance, cleaners, electricity, gas, telephone, internet, refuse collection, etc, etc, and don't we know it! These costs would not leave much out of the forty-five pounds per hour, that she was not going to earn - from clients who were not going to come forward.

There are employment opportunities for counsellors, but, as with psychologists, not as many as the number of people qualifying for such work. It follows that one has to be tip-top. GP's surgeries sometimes employ counsellors, but these usually like people who have some medical background in addition – a trained nurse with a post graduate counselling certificate, for instance.

Poor, old Knick-Knack. I still meet her occasionally. She is still hanging on, by her teeth, to her cleaning job, and still fantasizing that, one day, she will be in business as a counsellor!

I never like to concede that anything is a total disaster, and sure enough, on the last occasion that I bumped into Knick-Knack, there she was in a nurse's uniform – with a 'Care Assistant' badge proudly displayed. 'Back to nursing, then?' I enquired. She had managed to find a small amount of care work, to augment her cleaning, but Knick-Knack was not entirely enthusiastic about her new situation. I thought that it was, at least, a step up, an improvement, and that is always to be applauded, but, no doubt, Knick-Knack will go on fantasising that, one day, the counselling job will fall from heaven!

People who have suffered from mental health problems, commonly wish then, to work in this field, and, unlike myself, prefer a professional position. I have always preferred an informal, voluntary one. Some can be successful, but – as with all professional positions – one has to have the ability to think things through realistically, and to behave with objectivity.

The client has problems enough of his own. He does not want to spend the session listening to yours! A common complaint that we get about social workers in the mental health team, is that they spend their session with the client, talking about their own problems!

That is the difference between genuine, and pseudo, professionals. Doctors, for instance, are used to making objective judgements. When they are examining your legs – to see whether your veins are varicose – they are not thinking about whether or not they like you, or whether you can sort out their marital difficulties – which might be more severe than yours! This idea that 'professional' equals 'magic' is a falsity. Genuine professionals are, indeed, skilled in their particular field, but it does not follow that they have the answer to all life's multifaceted problems!

Chapter 18

Lord Baron Peter James Strathan Ellis Hythe: 'Good Lord!'

'Everyone knows me, from Smith to Lord Roseby,
I'm Burlington Bertie from Bow'

One morning at the crisis house, I received an urgent telephone call from the Wokingham Town Mayor's secretary. 'Pam, she said. A man has marched into the Town Hall – calling himself - Lord Baron Peter James Strathan Ellis Hythe! He is demanding to see the Mayor, and won't go. The problem is that I have already spent half an hour with him, and I have a big civic event to organize today. Pam, I'm desperate – I think that he is one of yours! Could I send him down to the crisis house?'

'Yes, send him down, I replied. I'll make a cup of tea, and see what I can do to help him.' Lord Baron arrived. He explained that he had a grievance about the way that he had been treated by the National Health Service. Then he went on to explain his background.

Lord Baron explained that he was the illegitimate son of a girl who had been seduced by a soldier from a local barracks. Her parents had been unwilling to take in their daughter and baby, so – in those days – 1961 – he had been put up for adoption. His adoptive parents were good, but very strict. He had to eat up all his greens, and his adoptive father, an army sergeant, believed in corporal punishment if a child misbehaved.

His biological mother had given him the name 'Peter': his adoptive parents called him 'James': his mother's surname was Strathan, his father's was 'Ellis', and his adoptive parents' surname was 'Hythe'. Through internet research, he discovered that there were lords and barons in Scotland whose family name was 'Strathan'. So, by Deed Poll, he changed his name to Lord Baron Peter James Strathan Ellis Hythe!

As a keen Agatha Christie fan, all this reminded me of the young man, Edgar Lawson, in her novel – 'They do it with Mirrors'. First, this young man claimed that his father was Sir Winston Churchill. Then, he claimed that his father was Viscount Montgomery. 'That Edgar guy', Walter Hudd asked of Miss Marple – 'what do you make of him? Says his father's really Lord Montgomery. . . . He told Gina something quite different. Some bunk about really being the heir to the Russian throne.

Hell, doesn't the chap know who his father really was?' 'I should imagine not, said Miss Marple, that is probably just the trouble!'

I took all Lord Baron's problems seriously – because they were serious to him, and we had his papers spread the length and breadth of the carpet. He claimed to be a qualified engineer, but, among all his papers, the only evidence of any qualifications that I could find, was one for attending a one-day course in kitchen hygiene!

I referred Lord Baron to PALS – the patients' liaison advocacy service - which deals with complaints about the Health Service.

Lord Baron started attending the drop-in centre regularly, and valued our support. He had a history of violence, but we never experienced any of it. He was always affable, and grateful, and, I would suggest, that this was because we always treated him with respect and courtesy.

At the age of forty-one, Lord Baron explained that he had never had a girlfriend, because he did not have the confidence to approach anyone, and ask them for a date. However, he finally met a woman at a pub, and he brought her to the drop-in centre. This led to one of the very rare occasions when I thought that we might have had a violent incident, but, with careful handling, we averted it.

Lola: 'Nearer, my God, to thee!'

'There let the way appear, steps unto heaven.
All that Thou sendest me in mercy given.
Angels to beckon me nearer my God to Thee. Nearer to Thee.'

The girlfriend, Lola, was an alcoholic. She explained that she and her siblings had been separated when they were young, and had all been placed in 'care'. In due course, she had married, but her husband was very violent. 'So, I dun 'im, I dun 'im', she said. 'You divorced him? I enquired.' 'No, I killed him!' she replied. Lola served eleven years in Holloway prison, but had recently been released – having completed her sentence.

As colourful characters, Lord Baron and Lola attracted a lot of attention in the drop-in centre, and this was much resented by the notorious Gabriela Rani. One day, she started provoking Lola – who – don't forget – had already killed! I feared a violent incident.

I sweet-talked Lola – explaining that she was extremely pretty – and that was why Gabriela was so jealous. All the time that I was sugar-talking her, I was edging her nearer and nearer to the door! It was 'nearer my God, to Thee' – metaphorically, but, thankfully, not literally.

Through she went to safety. Sweet relief!

Lord Baron had a history of violence, and prior to coming to us, he had attempted to murder a Police Officer – by stabbing him. His psychiatrist had made a diagnosis of paranoid personality disorder, and recommended this as his best defence – with a plea of 'diminished responsibility'. His plea was upheld, and, instead of going to prison, he was Sectioned into a secure unit. I always liked Lord Baron, and – although I have included him in my 'Funny Stories', his story could equally well be included with the poignant - or even with the tragic!

Angie Higginbottom: 'The secretary of the Politbureau'

When our Association formed, we had the conventional executive committee – composed of Chair, Vice-Chair, Secretary, Treasurer, and, then, ordinary committee members. We had to do a lot of paperwork – which we handed over to our secretary.

'Oh, no, I don't do paperwork, she protested. You have a very old-fashioned idea of what a secretary does - if you think that she does paperwork. What I always say, is that the Secretary of the Politbureau [who was, at that time, Mikhail Gorbachev], doesn't type the letters!' My colleagues remonstrated with her. 'I don't suppose that the Secretary General of United Nations types the letters' – quipped our Chair of the time.

The committee's more prosaic concern was – if, in a tiny, local, voluntary organization – the secretary doesn't type the letters, then who DOES type the letters? The lady would not budge. We suggested that – instead of holding the office of secretary – she became Vice-Chair instead – a role with very few executive functions. 'No, that is a trumped-up position. I am staying as secretary, but I am not doing the mundane paperwork.'

The problem remained. Who would do the paperwork? How did we resolve it? We were with MIND at the time, so I consulted one of their officers about the problem. 'There are training courses for committee secretaries' was her advice! A fat lot of good, this advice – lack of training wasn't the problem! This officer also annoyed me by suggesting that I put the problem in writing, and send it to her. I was not the Association's secretary. It was not my job to send out the letters. That was precisely the problem!

We had with us at that time, a volunteer, who had been a secretary in working life, and who was willing to take on, both the position, and the work. But how could we get her voted into office? The Association's annual general meeting was approaching, so we decided that we should

ALL resign, all stand again for re-election, and, of course, the Secretary of the Politbureau failed to be re-elected. Problem solved, and our new secretary then went on to do an excellent job for us for the next five years.

I have included this as a funny story, and, without a sense of humour, one would not survive in mental health at all! At the same time, that IS mental health. Delusions of grandeur go with the diagnosis of bi-polar affective disorder – from which this lady suffered. When one is adamant, as I have always been, that ours is a USER-run organization – from which mental health professionals are excluded, then one must take the rough with the smooth.

Yet another MIND Officer, on yet another occasion when they were assessing us, laughed at me, because I had raised the subject of an unwise decision made by some of the service-users. Her stance was, 'If you are stupid enough to be user-run – without professional support, then you have to put up with their stupidity!' This is what led me to the conclusion that, despite its rhetoric, MIND was not what it said on the tin. MIND did not believe in user-run services.

User-run organizations can do marvellous work, but it is not professional work, and it will always be limited by the disabilities which its members suffer, so one must always accept that reality. A useful comparison is with the Olympic Games – and, then, the Paralympics!

Bryan Hanrahan: 'A can of biscuits'

As I explain in 'This is Madness', [PCCS Books: Herefordshire:1999.], not everyone in the crisis house is in sweet and harmonious agreement about everything. When it comes to street drugs, I, personally, belong firmly, to the legalization lobby.

Heroin destroys lives. So does alcohol. Cannabis causes psychosis. So does alcohol. An expensive, cocaine habit ruins families. So does alcohol. People die from abusing ecstasy. They die from abusing alcohol. Not only do current laws defy logic, but prohibition doesn't work anyway. Legalisation of all mind-altering substances, would bring in very welcome tax revenue, and would also free up precious police resources to deal with other crime.

Some of my colleagues do not agree, and this has, on occasion, resulted in quite heated debate in the drop-in centre. Such a debate, about the use of cannabis, was being fiercely pursued one day, when one of our befrienders, Bryan, walked in. Unfortunately, he suffered from some hearing loss. 'What are they arguing about?' he inquired. 'Cannabis', I replied. 'A can of biscuits?' he inquired. We rolled around laughing. He repeated the story at a dinner party that evening, and brought the house down!

Rene Fancett: 'One person, one vote'

Rene was actually quite a good volunteer at the crisis house for a number of years, but she was yet another one who had held, for decades, a position of importance, as headmistress of a school, and could not adjust to retirement, and the consequent loss of status and power.

No longer having a school to dominate, I fear that she tried to dominate us. She disrupted committee meetings with her demand to have things her way, and it all ended in a dispute over a telephone bill.

When we set up the crisis house, twenty-five years ago, this was in the era before the proliferation of mobile phones. We always made a, free, landline, available to guests, so that they could contact people, in crisis, at any time of day or night. This was an, absolutely essential, part of our crisis service.

Furthermore, we always advised guests. 'If you need us to come out, in response to crisis, in the middle of the night, we will always come. You only have to telephone. But, if it is just that you can't sleep, and want to talk to someone, the telephone is there, freely, available, just get on to the Samaritans.'

Over the years, we had one or two cases of abuse of the telephone, but, very few, in the context of the fact that we accommodated one hundred and seventy-five individuals – in the crisis house – over a twenty year period.

Jack came to us in 1998 – referred by the local mental health team. He was eighteen years old. The first telephone bill that he ran up, was for about three hundred pounds, and we recouped this from his benefit money. The second one was for four hundred pounds – mainly run up through contacting sex chat lines in South America. We could not recoup this money, because Jack had then been taken to prison – having stolen seventy cars! The funny thing was that, apart from abuse of the telephone, Jack was well-behaved in the crisis house, and stayed with us for six months.

We sent the telephone bill to Social Services – on the grounds that Jack was not so much a mental health client, as a juvenile delinquent, and that the crisis house, with its philosophy of freedom and responsibility, was not a suitable place for people who needed external controls!

One of their social workers reckoned, that he knew a way in which the abuse of the telephone, could have been avoided. I am intrigued as to how. You can't leave vulnerable people, overnight in a crisis house, and not provide them with a free telephone.

They refused to pay. We refused to pay! Then, Rene, said, that because she had been a local headmistress, she knew the people in Social Services, and would sort it out. She came cheerfully to the committee meeting – she had sorted it out – and had agreed that we would pay! At this juncture, I believed it necessary that we put the matter to the vote. Rene said that if we did not vote to pay, she would resign. We voted, by a large majority, not to pay. She resigned.

We were still, early in 1999, a MIND Local Affiliated Association. The way that MIND worked then – was that one could, if one wished, join national MIND as a member, and pay a membership fee directly to them, but, if one preferred, one could join one's local association, and obtain MIND membership through the annual affiliation fee that the association paid to MIND.

I confess that I never enquired of our service users, whether they were direct MIND members, or not. Some may have been, but they were all MIND members through membership of our local, paid up, affiliated, association, and all, most certainly, had a vote.

Rene contacted MIND HQ – complaining about our decision, and also claiming that, because she was a member of national MIND, she was the only one entitled to vote! Only ONE person in an organization with a vote – it gives a whole new meaning to the word – dictatorship! Even the National MIND Officer saw the problem – or the joke – whichever way you looked at it! If only one person votes, why bother to have voting at all?

On a less hilarious, and more serious, note, this woman was actually a professional – though not a mental health professional, and we could not help coming to the conclusion that she did not really regard our votes as valid. We were all either mentally ill, or carers of the mentally ill, and so, in her mindset, occupied an inferior position, where her, professional vote, could overrule us. Funny, yes, but also serious, because this is the crux of the whole power struggle in mental health, which we have battled so hard to win.

NOTE: Social Services caved in. They paid!

Sandie Sacareau: 'Beer money'

'I'm only here for the beer!'

We have long argued that a lot of the statutory services are a compete waste of the tax-payers' money – because those who receive them are in no way furthered. They are box-ticking bureaucracies.

There can be no better illustration of this fact, than that provided by the local drug and alcohol rehabilitation service. The people involved, may be well-meaning enough, but, in the absence of commitment by the addicts involved, all their efforts are useless. And we don't need such statutory addiction services anyway, because where there is commitment, Alcoholics Anonymous, and Narcotics Anonymous, suffice – and they, like us – are independent and self-funding.

Lack of commitment, is illustrated perfectly by Sandie. I can see her sitting in the crisis house lounge – counting out her money – and she doesn't have much, because she is addicted both to alcohol, and to heroin and cocaine. 'I have just two pounds left', she tells us. 'I have to go across the road to see my alcohol adviser, and then I have just enough money, to get two cans of lager to relax with, after I have seen him.' We sit there speechless – not sure whether to laugh or cry.

Even funnier, was a second occasion on which Sandie sat in the crisis house – this time ringing someone impatiently on her mobile phone. 'I wish that he would reply, she said. I am desperate to get a line of crack [cheap cocaine], and I have to see my substance counsellor in a few minutes time!' Well, you can't deny it, at least the lady is conscientious about keeping her appointments!

What is so extraordinary, is that Sandie herself – who is not unintelligent – sees no irony. Society is requiring her to see the substance adviser. If she fails to turn up, her benefits will be axed. So she is going to do what is required of her – see the adviser – and then she deserves to relax - with a large amount of alcohol or cocaine – or both.

Sandie's story is not unique. When the twins, both heroin addicts, stayed in the crisis house, I was reliably informed, they used to work out when opiates would not show up on their statutory saliva tests – carried out by the Probation Service. They would inject heroin at exactly the right time – in order to avoid detection.

As I have explained elsewhere, I belong firmly to the legalization lobby. Apart from anything else, I know when I'm licked! So does one laugh or cry? Well, I have included 'Beer Money' in 'Funny Stories'.

Yet another of our service users, Pat, is an inveterate alcoholic. He uses drugs as well, but he is not addicted to them to the extent that he is addicted to alcohol. His party piece is as follows.

He attends the Alcoholics Anonymous meeting in the Methodist church, and then walks straight across the road into the pub. Pat is always bemoaning the fact that he can't get funding for residential rehab, and yet, at the same time, he has absolutely no intention of coming off alcohol.

My university psychology lecturers, who were behavioural psychologists, always used to say, 'Behaviour has a source'. So what is the source of Pat's irrational behaviour? We have reached the conclusion that, by getting money spent on him, he perceives that he is being valued – even if the money is being wasted - and, by seeing substance advisers, he is getting attention – albeit to no purpose. We can see it. Why can't they? It is not as though the public purse is brimming over with money, and has no legitimate demands being made upon it!

Chapter 19

Anonymous: 'The considerate burglar'

All local charities suffer burglaries, and we have had our share. There is nothing that they would want to take from the crisis house – except, perhaps, alcohol from our bar – and even then - most of the bottles are open. The expense to the charity, is in the repair work that we have to carry out after a burglary - replacing windows, mending broken locks, etc.

So I have a sneaking fondness for the considerate burglar. He forced a window, but did not break it, so we incurred no expense. He stole nothing – not even a bottle of whisky openly displayed in the bar. He left the bedroom, if anything, even cleaner and tidier than it was when he broke in, and he even made the bed!

The only reason I knew that we had been burgled, is that I always placed the duvet on the bed, broad stripes upward, and he made it with the narrow stripes upward. If I had known who he was, I might have felt inclined to ask him to come to see us, and receive our help legitimately!

Dora Leggette: 'Put me in the picture'

'It was only a beautiful picture – in a beautiful golden frame!'

You know that nice, yet weary, feeling, when you have completed a very good job – to everybody's satisfaction, 'you thought!' It is 6pm, it is

Friday night, and you are going off for a nice, long, holiday weekend. On just such an occasion, I was about to lock up the crisis house, when the telephone rang!

It was my former guest. She had stayed in the sanctuary, with her two young children, just for a short time, while the authorities were organising bed-and-breakfast accommodation. I thought they had settled there, and I could go home. Not a bit of it! 'Can we come back, she pleaded, there are no pictures on the walls here!'

Well, the crisis house must have close on a thousand pictures – displayed throughout. All the rooms are covered with them. I have put in an enormous amount of work – over decades – choosing, carrying, and putting up pictures in the crisis house, so it is something, to know that they are appreciated. But, I fear, no, we cannot accept guests back – just because their move-on accommodation is devoid of pictures!

Golf course: 'Holed it in one!'

I have included this story with the 'Funny Stories', because my wry, bitter/sweet sense of humour, never deserts me, but, on reflection, it could equally well have been included with the 'Poignant Stories', or even with the 'Tragic Stories'.

We get donations from time to time, and, on occasions, these are from the collection made at a funeral – where the family request donations for charity, rather than flowers.

Such was the donation to be made to us by an officer of the West Berkshire Golf Course. We were invited to go to the golf course – which is near Newbury – to collect the money.

I never wear trousers – always a dress or a costume. My lady colleague sometimes wore trousers, but was wearing a dress on this occasion, but our service user and driver, who had been a guest in the crisis house, was wearing jeans. The Golf Course wouldn't let us in! Jeans were banned!

In the end, we managed to explain that we had been invited to collect a cheque for our charity, and that the Golf Course Dress Code did not apply to us.

Eventually, they shunted us into a side room – well away from the Golf Course's august members, and, finally, the cheque was brought to us! Irony! They wanted to give money for mental health, but they also wanted to marginalise the mentally ill!

Josie Kidd and Ernest Pleydon: 'I can if I try'

I have always warned against romance between crisis house service-users, and some, including, Ernest, agreed with me. A service-user snuggled up to him on the sofa, and Ernest, who was, in any case, a confirmed bachelor, was having none of it!

It was a warm, summer's day, and the lady concerned looked most bizarre – in heavy winter clothes – including thick, woollen tights, and a woolly hat. She was eating an apple – spraying Ernest liberally with the juice. 'You should take me out, she said, I can look nice if I try.' 'Then why don't you?' he replied. Brutal, but so realistic. You will not get a suitable partner, by snuggling up to the mentally ill service user, sitting next to you. You have to try to look nice, and then go out to find one.

Ernest Pleydon: 'Drink to me!'

'The thirst that from the soul doth rise, doth ask a drink divine'
Ben Jonson

There is another funny story about Ernest - which dates back to the time when we were battling for the crisis house. At that awful time, we were receiving constant, harassing, letters from the Social Services, and constant visits from various Council officials – all looking, in vain, for reasons to close us down.

I was unfazed by it all. I was not moving out, and would, if necessary, have taken the matter to court – hiring a top barrister - to make mincemeat of them all! But our service users were very anxious, and Ernest, in particular, was worried that they would dislike our bar, so he dismantled it, and took all the drinks home!

Off he went – with all the bottles of whisky and brandy in his car. Eventually, we won the battle for the crisis house – so we were expecting Ernest to bring the bar back. Not a bit of it, he had drunk the lot!

Chapter 20

Edwin: 'The chance would be a fine thing!'

Despite being mentally ill, and having enormous problems in life, Edwin had a marvellous sense of humour.

Edwin stayed in the crisis house, when he was just nineteen years old. He came from a dysfunctional family. His father was a violent psychopath, and was also an alcoholic.

Edwin regaled us with the story of his time spent in the mental hospital. He was a very good looking young man – with blond hair.

One day, the Consultant Psychiatrist, said to him, 'Today, Edwin, I want to discuss sexuality. Are you heterosexual or homosexual?' Edwin, unsure as to how the psychiatrist, himself, would answer such a question, answered, politely, but, nevertheless, firmly, 'I am heterosexual'.

'How do you know?' – probed the psychiatrist. 'Because, when I see the girls going by, I am attracted, but when I see the boys, I am not' – further explained Edwin. 'But you are not seeing girls, now, said the psychiatrist, so is your only form of sexual satisfaction, at present, obtained through masturbation?' 'There's not much chance of anything else – stuck in this place', affirmed Edwin.

Edwin related the story – performing all the actions – and having us all in fits of laughter. What a thing it is to keep your sense of humour – even in the most dire circumstances!

Reg Gardiner: 'Just like a scene from a film'

In our earlier days at the crisis house, one of our service users made a video film of it, and, later, in 2007, a DVD was made – giving a complete tour of the house, which, to this day, can be seen on You Tube. Now, Lucy and Neville are making a bang up-to-date DVD – to go on sale with this book – in 2016!

But the incident that always reminded me of a scene from a film, was the occasion when Reg Gardiner returned from Germany – for a second stay at the house. It was December 1997, and a guest had just left. I went through the usual routine of cleaning the room, re-arranging furniture, putting up new pictures, placing flowers in water ready for the next guest, and, generally, making sure that everything was ship-shape.

I had literally just given the fresh duvet its final pat, when the doorbell rang. Down I went to answer it. It was Reg – complete with suitcase – just returned from Germany. 'Hello. I said. Have you come back to stay in the sanctuary?' He nodded, and followed me up the stairs – exactly as in a film sequence. I flung the door of the sanctuary open for him, and there it was – all gleaming and ready for him to occupy. What one may call, perfect, though totally unplanned, timing. Just like a scene from a film!

Anthony and Amy: '*Cui Bono?*' - 'Who Benefits?'

I have explained, elsewhere in this narrative, that the crisis house [deliberately] has no office, so the less ill can't congregate and talk with each other – neglecting the more ill.

Nevertheless, at the Christmas Party, Anthony spent the entire evening - conversing with our beautiful, blonde, psychology student – Amy. 'I consider that Capital Punishment is appropriate', I told him, as we tidied up, after the party.

Anthony was bewildered. 'She doesn't need you, I remonstrated. It is the schizophrenia sufferer who needs you to talk with him, not the beautiful, blonde psychologist.'

Yes, we laughed, but, all too often, mental health staff, spend time talking with each other – when it is their patients who need this social interaction. Again, the problem, is their ingrained, bone idleness.

Of course it is easier to converse with somebody normal, than it is to struggle to make conversation with someone who may be delusional – due to their schizophrenia, or, so depressed, that they can hardly articulate. I struggle, myself, to make conversation, when Dan Kent is at his most depressed. [Chapter11: 'All the things that I have worked for'.], and when Daniel Rendell is at his most ill, [Chapter 46: 'Bank Holiday Monday at the Crisis House: 31st August 2015.].

Nevertheless, the severely mentally ill, desperately need social interaction – in order to achieve recovery, and recovery, is what the mental health services should be about.

Hazel Raymonds: 'She's gone to Nirvana'

To appreciate the funny side of this story, you have to be a Wokingham local – which the Consultant Psychiatrist was not.

Hazel Raymonds was resident with us at the time, and her Consultant Psychiatrist telephoned us – in order to make an appointment for her to see him.

Busy at the time, I said to one of our service users, 'Tell him that she's gone to Nirvana'. My message was despatched, word for word, faithfully. Then the psychiatrist was very concerned. 'Whatever did we mean?'

'Nirvana' is a somewhat expensive, and exclusive, health club, in Sindlesham – which is local to Wokingham, but the psychiatrist, whose base was out at the hospital in rural Oxfordshire, did not know this.

We laughed. Perhaps he thought that we had all become Hindus, and had despatched his patient to the Hindu heaven!

Phil Heweth: 'Washington, here I come!'

When Phil Heweth stayed in the crisis house, he was on Section Seventeen Leave, from hospital, so he was still under the jurisdiction of the local mental health service.

He had explained to me that, prior to being Sectioned, he had booked a holiday in Washington DC. Crisis House guests were always supplied with their own set of keys, and came, and went, as they pleased – freedom, and responsibility being the essence of our philosophy.

Phil duly went off for his holiday in America – without saying a word to anyone. When I told his key worker that he had disappeared, she feared that he had gone off, and committed suicide, but I thought not, and sure enough, he duly returned from holiday, refreshed, and having enjoyed himself.

I have never had any desire to control the behaviour of other people, unlike many people who work in mental health. They think that they have power, but I doubt it. My experience is that, ninety-nine per cent of the time, people do what they want to do. Phil was determined to have his holiday, and he had it, Section, or no Section!

Chapter 21

Rickie Masurel: 'A bottle of vodka'

Occasionally, we would get a referral to the crisis house, which turned out to be inappropriate. Such was the case with Rickie – who had been referred by another service user. His abuse of alcohol was so extreme, that it frightened other guests. They feared that he would fall on a hot stove, and set fire to himself.

This was in September 2002, and was the first occasion when we placed a guest in bed-and-breakfast accommodation, because we thought the crisis house inappropriate. It was Friday afternoon, [it always is!], and the rain was coming down in sheets. In the light of the comments made by other guests, I telephoned the council's Homelessness Officer, assuming, poor fool that I was, that she would provide accommodation. She replied that alcoholism was self-induced, and that she would do nothing!

So what could I do? I could not throw him out on the street; I could not leave him in the crisis house – putting other guests at risk. Then I hit on the idea of bed-and-breakfast. I obtained a place for Rickie in a local one, and gave him strict instructions.

'I shall come with you, to pay, I said, and you let me do the talking. Keep your mouth firmly shut, because, if they realise that you are drunk, they won't accept you, and then we really will be up the creek without a paddle. As soon as I've paid, go into your bedroom, and sleep it off.' Fortunately, he did this, and all went according to plan!

I knew that Rickie was a chronic alcoholic, but even I was surprised, when tidying his room after he left the crisis house, to find a bottle of vodka – tied behind the cistern in his ensuite bathroom. I laughed, but it showed the hold that addiction has, and the lengths that addicts will go to – to make sure that their needs are met!

Abdul Sheikh: 'Madam you can pay!'

Being only a stone's throw from Wokingham Borough Council Offices, the crisis house was conveniently situated, if they wanted a crisis room for an individual.

One afternoon, the Chief Executive's Secretary telephoned. An Egyptian had entered her office, and was refusing to go – until the Council housed him. 'Could we help?'

Abdul arrived, sandwiched between two Police Officers. He stayed with us for one week, and then in short-term bed-and-breakfast accommodation – paid for, by us. I explained that he might be able to find accommodation in the private sector, but that he would have to arrange Housing Benefit with the Council.

He turned up at the crisis house drop-in – complete with a glossy folder – from a top class local estate agent. He had found a beautiful house to rent – in the private sector. 'But Housing Benefit will not cover that rent [thousands of pounds per month]', I remonstrated. 'No, madam, you pay!' replied Abdul.

Ernest, who was present at this conversation, loved this story, and would go around the crisis house, bowing, and saying, 'Madam, you pay!' and then, roaring with laughter.

Hattie: 'Half a bottle of Beaujolais'

Hattie was as mad as a hatter, but we all liked her. She was actually too ill to stay in the crisis house, and, after a trial period, had to return to hospital. Nevertheless, we had enjoyed having her.

Hattie was a vegan vegetarian, and would not use any animal products. Her stay with us was during the winter, and my first mistake, was to offer her a sheepskin rug – for extra warmth in bed.

Hattie used to cook vegetarian dishes of lentils – washed down with spring water. One evening, hospitably, she invited me to join her in this repast. I declined politely. 'I plan to have a steak, inches thick, and half a bottle of beaujolais', I explained. *Chacun à son gout!*

This story also reminds me of the funny occasions when we had to tolerate Council officials coming down to see us – for 'Grant Monitoring'. I always provided sandwiches for lunch – including a vegetarian choice, but they, of course, would not drink Chablis!

In desperation, I got some fresh orange juice – especially for them. I encouraged them to drink it. It was inconceivable that any of our service users would prefer orange juice to whisky or vodka, and I did not want the charity's money going to waste, throwing away fresh orange juice, that nobody would drink!

Patrick Woodhouse: 'Washing the walls'

Patrick was referred to us – specifically because the crisis house is clean. What an indictment of the statutory mental health services! It worked. Patrick was happy with us, but he, nevertheless, needed everything to be even cleaner.

Whenever I encountered him, his hair was wet from washing, and he had, recently, come out of the shower. One weekend, our befriender went into the crisis house, and there was Patrick – busily washing the walls! She made a joke of it. He intended repainting them as well, and she told him to make sure that the new paint matched!

It is so important, to have places like the crisis house, because behaviours that we can accept with equanimity, and humour, are so often, intolerable, to the service user's relatives. One reason that Patrick was referred to us, was that he was awaiting being accommodated in a council flat, but, while living with his mother and sister, drove them mad – because he spent all day, and all night – in their only bathroom!

It is so easy to see behaviours as funny, when you don't have to live with the person, and share facilities with them – or rather – be deprived of your share of the facilities! Our private house has three bathrooms – just for the two of us. Of course, in such fortunate circumstances, I am unfazed by Patrick's obsessional behaviour!

We were able to take the heat out of such situations – to the intense relief of the families concerned. This is why I am furious, to this day, that the Social Services, tried to get us closed down. Not a thought was given, by them, to the many people who needed our services, and would have been deprived of them – if the plot had succeeded.

Mark Runce: 'It's not my mind, it's my penis'

Mark was one of our few crisis house guests, who flatly refused to take his medication – even though he suffered from a psychotic illness. In the end, in desperation, I took him to see the doctor, myself.

'Doctor, it's not my mind, it's my penis.' He said. The doctor duly examined him, but could find nothing physically wrong. 'You need anti-psychotic medication', confirmed the doctor.

Having failed with the GP, I then took Mark to see a Consultant

Psychiatrist. Armed with medication, we returned to the crisis house. Would Mark take that medication? He would not.

We had to settle for the fact that Mark was convinced that it was his penis, not his mind, and laugh – always the better alternative to crying!

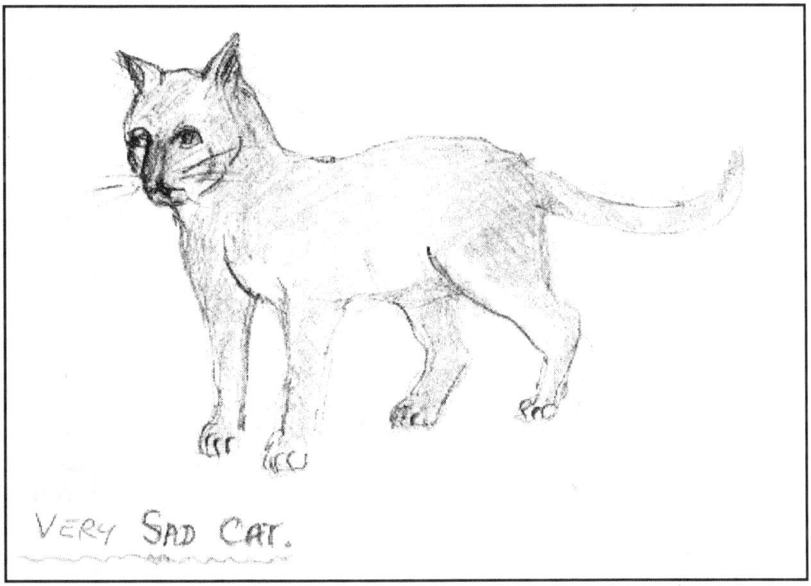

Chapter 22

Twenty-Five Tragic Stories

Our first suicide

You will not run a mental health crisis house, for twenty-five years, without having some suicides - hopefully, as few as possible. Similarly – in that time – you will also prevent numerous suicides. Suicide goes with the territory.

Just as a doctor, embarking upon his career, knows that he will cure most of his patients, but that some will die, in mental health, one accepts the rough with the smooth.

We barely knew Natalia. She was a twenty-three year old Polish girl – with a diagnosis of schizophrenia. She had attended our drop-in centre, only a couple of times – at just about the time that we were setting up the crisis house. My only memory of her is that she used to twirl around in a dance – to the music played in the drop-in centre.

Then one Friday evening, her distraught mother, telephoned to say that Natalia had taken an overdose of pills, and had died.

A tragic story! Had we had the time to get to know Natalia better, we may have been able to save her – as we have numerous others – with suicidal ideation – over the subsequent twenty-five years.

Paddy Rooney: 'Have you seen my childhood?'

'Have you seen my childhood? People say I'm not okay....
It's been my fate to compensate for the childhood I've never known.
Before you judge me, try hard to love me. Look within your heart and ask, 'Have you seen my childhood, the painful youth I've had.
Have you seen my childhood?'

Paddy Rooney was referred to the crisis house by his GP in April 1993. He suffered from psychopathic disorder, and had a history of violence, but his GP revealed nothing of this at the time – simply referring him for counselling and support. For two years, in the asylum ambience of the crisis house, Paddy did well, was happy, and stayed out of trouble.

When he came to us, he was forbidden, by a Court Injunction, to go into Bracknell, where his former girlfriend lived – in order to protect her, so he was living in temporary bed-and-breakfast accommodation in Wokingham. When this ceased, he stayed briefly in the crisis house, and then we found him a place in a newly opened mental health hostel. We also gave him a dog – Brucie – for company – when the drop-in centre was closed.

Paddy got back into his painting – he had learned to paint in prison! We even had an exhibition of his paintings, in aid of our charity. They sold very well, and a number still hang in the crisis house to this day.

But, inevitably, the time came for Paddy to re-engage with the normal world of stress and relationships. Paddy met Sheila, when both were out walking their dogs. She was twenty-nine, to his forty-nine years, and was very attractive. She was willing to be his friend, but not his sexual partner. Nevertheless, they spent a lot of time together, and Paddy formed a pathologically jealous attachment to her.

One Saturday in September 1995, Sheila explained to Paddy, that she had a male friend staying - not a boyfriend – just an old work colleague. This did not reassure Paddy. The paranoid jealousy stirred, and his violence was re-ignited.

He set off for Sheila's flat with a gun, and they were only able to save themselves when he fired, by barricading themselves behind a locked kitchen door. Thwarted, and then in a frenzy, Paddy tore through the night, back, from Sheila's flat in Finchampstead, to Wokingham – discarding the gun, en route, at California Crossroads. He rushed to the flat of one of our befrienders, and, Phaedippides style, dropped dead on her floor.

After weeks of deliberation, and no cause of death being found, the coroner brought a very distinguished pathologist out of retirement, to conduct a second Post Mortem. He found fatty tissue around the heart. So, the inquest jury brought in a verdict of 'Natural Causes' – death from a heart attack due to stress.

Due to his diagnosis of psychopathic disorder, Paddy had alienated all former family, and friends, so he had only us to arrange his funeral. A Roman Catholic priest had recently left us some money in his will, so this paid the funeral costs. What song do you choose to sing at a funeral - in such tragic circumstances? We plumped for Michael Jackson: 'Have You Seen My Childhood?'

In Victorian mental health services, people were 'put away' in asylums, and the sexes were separated. Reforms and modern community care, may have improved things for the mentally ill, but it does no harm to learn from history. Maybe, some of the Victorian ideas still have a place in mental health care today!

Had Paddy stayed in permanent sheltered conditions, he may well have been alive today!

Sophia: 'A tragic way to die'

Sophia was not a regular service user of ours, but visited our drop-in on a couple of occasions, because she had become friendly with one of our guests – while they were in hospital together. He explained that it was the usual story. Sophia had excellent 'A' Levels, and a glittering career ahead of her. Then, it had all ended in a schizophrenic breakdown. She had also suffered sexual abuse.

In due course, Sophia was re-admitted to hospital under a Section of the Mental Health Act. It was while she was on a supervised outing with a nurse, that the tragedy occurred. Sonia ran away from the nurse, and threw herself under a train that was coming into Cholsey Station. Her body was cut into pieces, and her head was never recovered. An awful, and tragic, death.

Sophia was sufficiently ill to need two nurses to accompany her on an outing from hospital, but no doubt, there were then, as now, staff shortages. Our Association firmly believes that mental health should be removed from the Social Services aegis completely, and that more resources should go into improving medical staff cover.

Gina: 'You were a beautiful woman'

Again, with Gina, she was not a service user, very well known to us. A hopeless alcoholic, who was already suffering from cirrhosis of the liver, she had been discharged from the alcohol detox programme at the mental hospital, because she was not co-operating with treatment.

She stayed, temporarily, with one of our former guests, Gary, but he only had a one-bedroom flat, so he asked if we would accommodate Gina until the Probation Service found her accommodation. Gina was under Probation, for drink/driving offences, and so qualified for such help.

Gina stayed with us for only three weeks. She then moved to a flat in Reading. Only three weeks after that, she was admitted to hospital, and died of liver-failure – at the age of only thirty! Gina was very ill when she came to us, so we never saw her at her best, but, I was assured, she had been a stunningly beautiful young woman! A tragic story!

Bill Hanrahan and Jeanette Aron: 'Don't leave me halfway to paradise'

'I want to be your lover, but your friend is what I stay.
Don't leave me halfway to paradise – so near, and yet so far away.'

Bill was one of the first to answer an advertisement for befrienders which we placed in the local paper when our Association started up in 1987. Bill explained that he had been a residential social worker in a children's home in Henley, but had suffered a breakdown when his homosexual lover was killed in a car crash. Bill was pleasant, courteous, and thus very popular, as I have found homosexuals invariably to be.

Jeanette started attending our drop-in centre some years later. She had been the victim of a series of very abusive relationships, and had, at one time, been resident in a women's refuge. Jeanette became very attached to Bill. He was gentle, kind, and gentlemanly – unlike all the other men with whom she had been involved.

They lived near to each other, and, although their ages were similar, Bill came to regard Jeanette as an auntie – giving her a key to his flat, so that she could pop in, and see that he was all right. But Jeanette saw Bill as a potential lover – inhibited from making any move, because he was a gentleman. She hoped, eventually, for marriage.

This is the phenomenon that one observes again and again. People simply cannot perceive, that relationships between men and women can be other than sexual! Bill was quite open about his homosexuality, but Jeanette simply did not believe it.

During the early part of 1996, Bill was in bed for a month with a chest infection. I started to have misgivings. That is an awfully long time, to be laid up, in these days of antibiotics. Then, in July 1996, I received a distressed telephone call from Jeanette. She had gone to his flat – only to find Bill dead – from a massive overdose of pills and alcohol.

The coroner confirmed that it was suicide. Bill had been dying of Aids, and had, presumably, chosen the quicker way out. Jeanette would not believe it. She was convinced that I had made it up – despite the coroner's report. 'Bill couldn't be homosexual. He was her partner, her future husband!' What was so tragic in the situation was that Bill HAD been genuinely fond of Jeanette, but not in the way that she perceived it.

Bill had been a devout Roman Catholic, and we had a Mass said for him, but Jeanette left our ranks, furious, and convinced that we had invented the whole story. Quite why? one fails to see!

We had had, on placement, a young volunteer, Myles, who was training to be a counsellor, and he still kept in touch with Jeanette. Some time after Bill's death, he called in – I think with a view to negotiating a path back into our ranks for Jeanette, but I did not broach the subject with him. His perspective was professional – where ours is one of freedom and responsibility.

We had not asked Jeannette to leave our service. She could, of her own volition, have returned at any time, but, no way were we going to solicit her return! Miss Bulstrode would not have run out of the boutique with the Balenciaga model dress – entreating the customer to buy it! [Please see: Agatha Christie: 'Cat Among the Pigeons.': Published: Collins: 1959.]

Overall, I liked, and respected, Myles, but I think that he was angry, when I did not broach the subject of a return, to our ranks, for Jeanette.

He made a parting shot. 'Next thing, you'll want to be paid for what you do.' 'No, I have never wanted to be paid for what I do. I want to do it voluntarily.' Then he said, 'All that voluntary organizations do, is pick up a few apples that fall.'

That is, indeed, all that individual, tiny, organizations, like ours, do. Have enough of them, though, and you could harvest all the orchards throughout the United Kingdom. You don't need bigger crisis houses.

You need more of them!

No, I liked Myles, but I stuck to the Association's philosophy. People have the freedom to choose, and then must take responsibility for what they have chosen. That is, after all, what happens in normal life, and we are all about getting people back into normal life - which means accepting its disadvantages as well as its advantages.

I come to Agatha Christie, once again. More than once, in her books, she quotes the old Spanish proverb, 'Take what you want, and pay', says God. My sentiments precisely!

In relating these stories, it occurs to me that a number of people have left the crisis house – angry, and intent upon our destruction – unfortunately thus playing into the hands of our enemies.

There was the irate ex-headmistress, the only one with a vote! There was the furious Gabriela Rani – so angry, when I declined to recommend her for a bungalow – on the grounds that – since her previous twenty accommodations had all ended in disaster – that one would as well, so there was no point in putting the effort in! There was Joan – angry because her sister was not going to be allowed to live, for free, in the crisis house, for the rest of her life!

Do these people hate the crisis house? No, they like it too much. They want it on their terms – even if – as with Jeanette – these terms are in the realms of fantasy!

I have also seen anger in service users, who, infantilised by conventional mental health services, actually perceive the crisis house as a threat. It is adult. It requires responsibility. It encourages a return to work. Though I perceive a lifetime trapped in the mental health system, as the worst fate that could befall anybody, nevertheless, some service-users choose this route – rather than putting in the effort that a return to normality requires.

One such was Elaine Whitely. She had come to the crisis house drop-in centre, in its very early days, and then we didn't see her for some months. It transpired that she had tried to kill herself, and to murder her two infant children, in the exhaust fumes of a car – shut up in a garage. Fortunately, the three-year-old escaped, and alerted a neighbour – so all three lives were saved.

Elaine was Sectioned in the mental hospital, and custody of the children was awarded to her former husband. Never reasonable in outlook, Elaine was most indignant. 'How dare they not let me have the children!' she complained. Well, she had tried to murder them!

We saw Elaine, from time to time, after that, but she never became a regular service user. We hadn't seen her for five years, when, one day, in October 2006, she turned up, out of the blue, to enquire about our services. She duly noted our adult ethos – including, of course, our bar.

Some days later, our regular service users were just about to sit down to lunch, when Elaine Whitely charged into the crisis house, like a bat out of hell. She was brandishing a copy of a letter that she had sent to Wokingham Borough Council. She had been allowed to type and print this letter at the local, statutory, mental health centre. This letter called for our funding to be withdrawn, and given, instead, to the local statutory service, which she used regularly, so that they could provide more of the same. She preferred their services to ours!

Why? Because no effort, nor responsibility, is required of their service-users. Once, in their services, one can sit for the rest of one's life – drawing childish pictures – like an infant in kindergarten. For people who choose to settle for this, our, adult, services, present a threat, so, instead of just not using them, and opting for the infantilising mainstream services, people like Elaine Whitely, actually set out to destroy the alternative. Needless to say, her attempt failed, and we banned her from the Association.

The employee who ran the statutory day centre which Elaine Whitely preferred, was laughing when I raised the problem with her. She would have liked to see us destroyed as well – but for different reasons.

This employee, and all her colleagues, eventually fell foul of a process known as 'Dismissal, and Re-engagement'. It is legal, but not considered to be good, employment practice. Its purpose is to enable employers to avoid paying redundancy money.

Thus the employer dismisses the employee, but offers another job, of lower status, with less pay, and inferior working conditions. Some employees will settle for this, but, for those who don't, redundancy payments do not apply, because they have not been made redundant.

In this instance, all the employees, but one, chose to leave, and this one left, eventually.

This day centre has ceased to exist. The building was demolished to make way for the new road, so the Elaine Whitelys of this world no longer have access to a day centre at all! When it existed, what threat did we present? The threat to the staff's livelihood, of course! Volunteers can easily provide the only drop-in service necessary, and now we do!

Chapter 23

Nigel Hills: 'A waste of a young life'

Nigel, and his twin, Stephen, were homeless, and roofless, heroin addicts. I accommodated them in the crisis house, only because they were friends of Ewan - who was resident at the time, so I knew that they would be there, morning, noon, and night, anyway.

Nigel was under the jurisdiction of the Probation Service, for drugs offences, and, during the time that he was staying with us, he was found to be in breach of his Drugs Testing and Treatment Order. This meant prison.

It was the Police who informed me that Nigel had been found dead. The coroner recorded an open verdict. Heroin could have contributed to the death: alcohol could have contributed, but although Nigel was found hanged, he could have been trying to get a vein in his neck, in order to inject heroin, and then slumped forward in a drunken state – so there was not the evidence of intentionality - needed to establish a verdict of suicide. It could have been an accident. Whatever, it was a tragic waste of a young life. Nigel was at the time aged only twenty-seven.

Throughout the entire twenty years that we ran the beds in the crisis house, I always took the same stance. If I thought that I was about to go out of the door - feeling uneasy about leaving someone there, I would not go. I would make other arrangements for them. As a result, we never had any suicides on the premises – nor any other significantly worrying incidents.

The problem with Nigel Hills, was that I had no such misgivings. He wasn't really a mental health client. He was a heroin addict – and always jolly, and cheerful. The coroner's verdict was open, so mine has to be, as well, but I think that the most likely verdict was 'accident – trying to find a vein in his neck to inject heroin, while drunk, and then, accidentally hanging himself in the shoelace – which he had tied around his neck'. A tragic story.

Steven: 'The tragic twin'

On the night that Nigel died, the entire crisis team came out to the crisis house. His surviving twin, Steven, was, naturally, very distraught. 'Why did he do that? I loved him!' he cried. At this juncture, we were regarding Nigel's death as suicide, but the coroner did not concur with this. He recorded an Open Verdict.

Perhaps his twin's death brought Steven to his senses. Whether he continued to use heroin or not, I am unsure, but he certainly settled down with a partner who had children, and went on to have his own child with her. The twins' mother established organizations for the support of the families of drug addicts. Like so many of us, she felt called, to use the rest of her life, in relieving the suffering of people, who were going through what she had been through.

Celia: '*Mens sana in corpore sano*'

Celia came to us – having dropped out of Birmingham University Law School. She explained that she had achieved five starred 'A' Grade 'A' Levels – which meant that you were expected to study either medicine, or law. Celia wanted neither, but, bowing to parental expectation, plumped for law. She hated it.

I asked Celia whether there was anything that she thought she might prefer, and she suggested journalism. I therefore encouraged her to study English. She started the course at Exeter, but dropped out again, and came back to volunteer at the crisis house.

She became friendly with Nigel Hills, who was resident with us at this time. As I observed them laughing together, Nigel, so young and handsome, Celia, so young and beautiful, I would never have dreamed in a million years that – less than eighteen months later - they would both be dead – both having hanged themselves!

Celia went back for a final, abortive, attempt to study English at Exeter, but telephoned me from there, to say that she was wandering around, out of her head, and not knowing what she was doing. 'Could she come back to us?' 'Yes, come back immediately', I replied. Alas, Celia came home, but to her parents' house. Her mother had died of cancer the previous summer, so there was now only her father.

Both of Celia's parents were chronic alcoholics, and Celia, an only child, had always been trapped – having to cope with their behaviour, once the front door was closed. Her mother had been a school-teacher, and her father, whom I actually met, presented a completely normal, and respectable, front to the world.

True, there are problems for families like my own, who have far more children than the parents can cope with, but there are also problems for families with an only child, like Celia.

If parents are mentally, or physically, ill, alcoholic, or drug addicted, but have a large number of children, then an elder sister might to be able to assume some of the functions of the inadequate mother. If a sick father is incapable of working, a number of brothers, together, may be able to bring in sufficient income for the family to survive.

Once the front door is closed, an only child is alone – sometimes coping with the most bizarre and damaging behaviour. Celia used to say to me, 'If only I had a brother – someone, at least to ratify, that I am indeed suffering what I am suffering!' Other members of our Association, who are only children, have confirmed that they felt what Celia felt – abandonment to their fate.

Celia left a note for her father to call the Police when he came home, and not to go upstairs. She then hanged herself in the loft.

When seeking my advice, Celia explained that her mother was never satisfied with less than starred 'A' Grades for everything. I tried to explain to her, the concept of being 'good enough', and even, something in which I firmly believe, the supreme satisfaction of scraping through by the skin of your teeth, and not giving the examiner one penny more than you have to!

I told Celia that, if she were my daughter, I would not want her to achieve five starred 'A' Grade 'A' Levels. Looking at her dropped jaw, I said that, I would prefer a daughter of mine, to have more balanced, all round, development. *Mens Sana in Corpore Sano* – a healthy mind in a healthy body!

We have had other service users who have solved the problem of not coping with university, and have still obtained their degree. An example is Jeremy March. [Chapter 49: 'Advocacy'.]

The art of coping with mental illness is to work one's way around the problems – so that one eliminates unnecessary stresses, but still achieves the things that matter in life. Jeremy's science degree from the Open University was every bit as good as a science degree from anywhere else. As my husband, who, as a Windsor Grammar School boy, used to play Eton College scholars, at sport, told them, (Tongue in cheek) 'Wherever you learn it, two and two always makes four!'

Angus McDonald: 'Defeating the object'

I liked Angus. He was highly intelligent, and with a very good sense of humour. He suffered from paranoid schizophrenia, and I first encountered him, when he sought a bed in the crisis house. We were full, but I was able to get him into a bed-and-breakfast hotel in Reading.

Angus explained that his parents were Polish immigrants, who had settled in Scotland. His father was a fully qualified lawyer, but, because of linguistic difficulties, he had been reduced to seeking work as a bus conductor. So, understandably, Angus's parents were desperate for him to be well-educated.

Angus achieved an undergraduate degree, and a Masters degree in chemistry. He was also studying for his PhD, whilst teaching science in a Roman Catholic boys' public school. He explained that his family were devout Roman Catholics, and that he was forbidden any sexual experience prior to marriage. It was while teaching at the public school, that Angus started experiencing paranoid symptoms – believing that the pupils were putting poison into his food.

Thus, Angus entered the mental health system – frequently under Section, and hating its demeaning facilities. He said that he had to share rooms with people who snored, and so, frequently, could not get to sleep.

Things seemed to be on the up when, one day, Angus called in at the drop-in centre – very smartly dressed – and, explaining that he had attended an interview for a job at Wokingham Library. Thereafter, I kept in touch – sending him a poem by Rae Unzicker: 'To be a Mental Patient'. Angus treasured this poem.

To be a mental patient

To be a mental patient is to:
* Be stigmatised, ostracised, socialised, patronised, psychiatrised.
* Have everyone controlling your life, but you. You're watched by your shrink, your social worker, your friends, your family, and then you're diagnosed as paranoid.
* Live with the constant threat and possibility of being locked up, at any time, for almost any reason.
* Live on £82 a month in food stamps, which won't let you buy the Kleenex to dry your tears, and to watch your shrink come back to his office from lunch – driving a Mercedes Benz.
* Take drugs that dull your mind, deaden your senses, make you jitter and drool, and then you take more drugs to lessen the 'side effects'.
* Apply for jobs, and lie about how you've spent the last few months or years, because you've been in the hospital, and then you don't get the job anyway, because you're a mental patient.
* Watch T.V. and see shows about how violent and dangerous and dumb and incompetent and crazy you are.
* Not to matter.
* Never to be taken seriously.
* Be a resident of a ghetto, surrounded by other mental patients who are as scared, and hungry, and bored, and broke, as you are.
* Be a statistic.
* Wear a label, and a label that never goes away, a label that says little

about what you are, and even less about who you are.
* Never say what you mean, but to sound like you mean what you say.
* Tell your psychiatrist he's helping you, even if he's not.
* Act glad when you're sad, and calm when you're mad, and to always be 'appropriate'.
* Participate in stupid groups that call themselves 'therapy'. Music isn't music, it's therapy: volleyball isn't a sport, it's therapy. Sewing is therapy. Washing dishes is therapy. Even the air you breath is therapy, and that's called 'the milieu'.
* Not to die – even if you want to – and not to cry, and not to hurt, and not be scared, and not be angry, and not be vulnerable, and not laugh too loud. If you do, you only prove that you are a mental patient – even if you are not.

And so you become a no-thing in a no-world, and you are not.

Rae Unzicker – 1984

As an ally of the radical mental health service users' movement, in the early 1990's, I invited both Judi Chamberlin, and Rae Unzicker, over from America - to speak at two of my conferences – and most successful they were!

The bitter irony, in these days, a quarter of a century later, is that you are lucky if you get any music, or volleyball, or any other activities deemed to be therapeutic! The former mental health services may have been infantilising and demeaning, but, at least, they did exist! Now, they are practically non-existent!

Sadly, in August 2006, I received a telephone call from Angus's sister – to say that he had died in a London hospital. She did not give full details, and may not, at that stage, even have known the full facts, but I presumed that it was suicide – since Angus was then only in his thirties.

It was so sad - because one can understand only too clearly why the parents pressurized Angus into such high educational achievements. We used to laugh together about this. Your education is to prepare you for life. If, at the end of it all, the one thing that you cannot cope with is life itself, then it defeats the object!

It was with the tragedies of Celia and of Angus in mind that I had the following letter published in the local Press in February 2014.

Letter published in local paper - Gove reforms will add to breakdown

"Michael Gove's education reforms will not result in a better educated society – only in a more neurotic one. Wokingham Mental Health Association sees many victims of undue academic pressure. His drive for

radical reform suggests that there was once a golden age in which everyone was a high academic achiever – lost in the last fifty years of lib - eralisation. Not true. Fifty or sixty years ago, only a small minority of children received an academic education in grammar schools. The great majority attended secondary modern schools, left at the age of fifteen, with no qualifications, and learned their occupations in the workplace.

That everyone needs to achieve basic literacy and numeracy, is undeniable, but most people will learn to read and write, and all the mathematics necessary to cope in life – in primary school. Foreign languages are also to be compulsory, but these are best mastered – by people who are actually interested – spending time in the countries where the people speak them. I don't despise the academic. One can learn things of value in the Classics which are relevant to this debate. 'Mens sana in corpore sano' – *'A healthy mind in a healthy body.': Juvenal.* 'Salus populi suprema lex esto' – *'Let the welfare of the people be the final law.':* Cicero.

That is what society needs in its education system – balance in all-round, healthy development – with social and emotional aspects receiving as much weight as the intellectual. China may well be surpassing us in academic achievement, but is China a happy, healthy, society? I think not. It is a ruthless, repressive, regime where individuals cannot flourish.

Education should be tailored to the individual. You cannot force mental growth. Do so, and what you get is mental breakdown. One of our service users, for instance, achieved five starred 'A' grade A-Levels, and then committed suicide. A tragic loss.

There is also a suggestion in the rhetoric around the reforms, that our comprehensive schools are bog standard. Wokingham schools are not. They are excellent, but, as St Crispin's School motto has it, we need 'Excellence for All', and that means catering for children of all abilities, and valuing equally all skills – both academic and practical."

As well as seeking high standards in our education system, in order to keep up, in a competitive world, Ministers should also read the wisdom, that is in Agatha Christie. She asserts that 'educating somebody' can be a cruelty, and she is right. We have experienced it!

Dirty books!

I remember one occasion in the crisis house, when a concerned parent took my advice on her daughter's education – with a successful outcome.

I always admire the mission statement, issued by the Abbey School in Reading. The Abbey is one of the UK's top independent schools, and parents vie to get their daughters in. But the mission statement says categorically:

'The Abbey School exists to educate academically able girls.'

So you know exactly where you stand. The Abbey School is what it says on the tin! It follows that, if one is not an academically able girl, one should not seek an education there.

This mother explained that her daughter had scraped through the entrance examination by the skin of her teeth, and was now not coping. She was exhibiting psychiatric symptoms – constantly washing everything, and, in particular, washing everything connected with the school – even school books.

'Symptoms, I advised, always tell you something, if you take note of them. The Abbey School is only for academic high fliers. Take your daughter out immediately, and send her to Luckley Oakfield.' Luckley is a local private school – which also has an excellent academic reputation, but it does not exist, solely, for high fliers.

The lady took my advice, and came back, six months later, to say that the move had worked beautifully, and that her daughter was happy, and free of all psychiatric symptoms.

Piers Matthew: 'I am heartbroken'

I never met Piers himself. It was his mother whom I had been supporting, throughout 2007. She explained that he had been discharged from the mental hospital with no support, and that she was worried that he would not be able to cope alone in his flat.

Then came the tragedy. Piers jumped from a railway bridge in Reading, and was cut into pieces by an incoming train. His mother said 'I am heartbroken. I tried to get care for him, but none was available.'

Piers's death occurred at the time that we were fighting for the crisis house, and his mother wrote to the Leader of the Council – begging him to allow our work to continue – so that others would not have to suffer as Piers, the rest of the family, and she herself, were suffering. It was then that, Leader of the Council, David Lee, wrote to her – saying that he was, indeed, going to support the continuance of the crisis house, and even to help enhance its ongoing success.

Chapter 24

Betty Hermitage: 'You can't be on page three forever'

'If we can't be young, and beautiful, let's be happy, and old'
Gracie Fields

I first met Betty in 1994, and she struck me as being a lost soul. She was then in her thirties, but spoke constantly of the time when she was young, and was a Page Three model. After this first meeting, I saw her occasionally. She explained that her parents were divorced, and that her mother was an actress – living in Eastbourne. Her father, whom I met, had been teaching English in Saudi Arabia, but had returned to England – suffering from chronic alcoholism.

At the crisis house, over twenty-five years, I have encountered numerous alcoholics, but Betty's father, was the only one I ever saw, who was visibly suffering from delirium tremens. Not just his hands, but his whole trunk, would judder and shake!

This was the route that Betty, also, went on to take. She moved into mental health supported accommodation, and, apparently, had, whole crates, of red wine, delivered there, on a daily basis. Betty died of alcoholism at the age of forty-nine.

Betty was an intelligent woman, and this is what intrigued us. However beautiful one may be when one is young, an intelligent girl knows that a career as a Page Three model, is short-lived, and would, presumably, make contingency plans.

There are various opportunities for ex-models – running dancing or fashion schools, modelling in fashion magazines for older customers, hostess work in cocktail bars, where attractive women of various ages are needed, but Betty did not consider any of these. All the time, she harked back to the past. A tragic story.

Aubrey Bennett: 'Work likes you'

You may not like work, but work likes you!

Aubrey came to us in 2003. He suffered from Bi-Polar Affective Disorder, and from alcoholism. During the time that he was staying in the crisis house, a young woman, Gina, who was already diagnosed with cirrhosis of the liver, came in for a brief stay. She was awaiting accommodation, which was to be provided by the Probation Service. She duly moved into this, but died three weeks later – at the age of only thirty.

'Let it be a lesson to you, I said to Aubrey, it kills you!' After a stay of five months in the crisis house, Aubrey also had to go into hospital for liver treatment. He did well, got back into employment, and rented a cottage which we found for him – locally.

Then he was made redundant. The Department of Work and Pensions wanted Aubrey to go on a course, to help him get back into work. We strongly encouraged this, but Aubrey demurred. 'They will make me stack shelves in Tesco's', he protested. 'Far better than being unemployed', we replied.

But Aubrey took the mental health ticket, which, fortunately, is not quite so readily available – these days. He persuaded his doctor to sign him off as sick, lost his flat, and took the only alternative – a place in supported mental health accommodation.

There, having nothing else useful to do, he continued to drink. He died of liver failure in October 2010 – aged fifty-two. If only he had taken the other path!

'You may not like work, I tell our service users regularly, but work likes you!' I have never known anyone, ever do other than benefit, from getting back into work – no matter how mundane and limited it may be. Work is society's ticket back to normality – providing, not just an occupation and an income, but the chance to mix with normal people, and to re-enter normal social life.

Pierre Bulstrom: 'You are a good-looking man'

I liked Pierre. He suffered from alcoholism, but I could tell that he had come from a good background. He told me that he had recently split up with his partner. She was a heroin addict – heavily involved in the drugs subculture, and her daughters were also heroin addicts. 'Pierre, I said, you are a good looking man. Surely you can do better for yourself.'

I advised to no avail. Almost immediately, he got involved with an extremely unstable woman, who was also dependent upon alcohol and drugs, and who had been working as a prostitute.

They were together for a year or two, and then she brought me the tragic news that Pierre was dead. Exact details were not available, but alcohol and heroin were involved, and the verdict was not one of 'Natural Causes'.

This is another of those 'If only'stories! If only Pierre had tried to find a more stable partner, and to lift himself out of that awful subculture, the outcome may have been happier. A tragic story.

Murial Carsons: 'Valiant 'gainst all disaster'

'He who would valiant be 'gainst all disaster,
let him in constancy, follow the Master.
There's no discouragement, shall make him once relent,
his first avowed intent to be a Pilgrim.

Whoso beset him round, with dismal stories, do but themselves
confound. His strength, the more is. No foe can stay his
might – though he with giants fight,
yet he will have the right to be a pilgrim.

No hobgoblin, nor foul fiend shall daunt his spirit.
He knows he at the end, shall life inherit.
Then fancies flee away. He'll fear not what men say.
He'll labour, night and day, to be a pilgrim.'

We first encountered Murial, a journalist on the *Wokingham Times* Newspaper, in June 1989. We had just set up our mental health drop-in centre at the British Red Cross in Denmark Street, and Murial was detailed to cover the story for the paper. Murial then stayed a friend, and an excellent journalist for the crisis house, for the next nine years – until her untimely death in February 1998.

Murial was a Cambridge graduate, and had, in her younger years, been a journalist on the *Guardian* Newspaper. But she suffered from ill health. She had to resign her post, sell the big London house – in order to raise money for a dialysis machine – and move to a council house in Wokingham. Murial had three children late in life, her husband had a good job with a local aeronautical engineering firm, but Murial, due to chronic ill health, was only able to work part-time on Wokingham's local newspaper.

As soon as one disaster was confronted, and resolved by, Murial, another one would hit the family. The trials of Job weren't in it! Murial had undergone a kidney transplant operation, and then developed cancer – due to a damaged immune system. 'I've had seventeen operations, she would say, it is my brain, my resilient mental attitude, which enables me to cope with it all.'

Then, Murial's husband lost his job, because the company was reducing staff, and moving out of the area. For a time, he was completely unemployed, but even when he got back into work, it was low paid and unskilled. He was never able to find another job with equivalent pay and status to the job that he had lost. So the family fell into poverty.

I remember Murial coming into the drop-in centre one Friday afternoon – to see whether I could cash a cheque for seven pounds – so that the family could have a Sunday dinner! My jaw dropped. I hadn't realised just how poor they were. It was Murial who enlightened me about the way life was, on basic benefits. 'It is no good them attempting to teach me budgeting skills, she said, there is nothing to budget!'

'Valiant 'gainst all disaster', Murial soldiered on. Her eldest child experienced problems in the school system, so Murial taught him at home. He was dyslexic, but went on, in adult life, to work, so far as I know, successfully, as a chef. Her second child went to university, but dropped out – the Christmas before she should have graduated. We thought this, an unnecessary, additional blow for the family. At that stage in the game, the final year, one may as well stick it out to the bitter end!

One day, hunting for bargains in the local supermarket – which was all that her meagre income could afford, Murial went blind – just like that! A shutter fell down over her eyes, and she could never see properly again. Nevertheless, Murial struggled on with her part-time journalist's job – using a gynaecological surgeon's lamp, to try to decypher the words.

She found the local sensory needs social worker, extremely patronising, but got back at her by sending her letters back, with their grammar and spelling corrected. Don't forget that Murial was a Cambridge English graduate!

That is the difference between my attitude, and the attitude of social workers. This social worker demeaned and patronised Murial, whilst I stood, in awe and admiration, for her fortitude. Murial died suddenly of a heart attack in February 1998, aged only sixty-one. She had a weak and broken body, but the heart of a lion.

In our Association's obituary notice in the *Wokingham Times*, we had John Bunyan's hymn published in her honour. 'No foe could stay her might. Tho' she with giants fight. Yet she will have the right to be a pilgrim.'

Maurice Santereau and I have a particular feeling of fellowship. [Chapter 10: 'What Starts as disaster can end in triumph'.]

This is because we both had an awful time, early in life, and a much better time, in adult years [touch wood!]. For many people, it is the opposite. They have idyllic childhoods, and then a terrible time later in life – just like Murial. It is, of course, true, that those with awful early years, are easily satisfied, and find adult life – which might be - if looked at objectively – only average in quality – idyllic - compared with what they have experienced in the past.

When Murial Carsons was in relative good health, I would sometimes accompany her to the theatre. We did not have to pay for the tickets, because we would be reviewing the performances for the newspaper.

One play always sticks in my memory. The scene was at a graveyard, and a group of family and friends were gathered around one, particular, grave.

'It is so well-kept, exclaimed one of the people, and all done for free, as well!'

'Oh no, it isn't! said another, somebody must be paying', and such proved to be the case. The grave was being kept up, and paid for, by another relative.

How true! Nothing is free. Whatever the service is, somebody, somewhere, is always paying, so we need to see that value for money is always delivered.

The Wokingham food banks

People find it difficult to believe that a place like Wokingham, which, in September 2015, was, yet again, deemed to be the best place in the UK to live, and to bring up a family, could experience food poverty.

But, as I said in my letter to the paper – regarding homelessness, the Bible's wisdom is timeless, and states: 'The poor you have with you always'.

Murial and her family, would not have had a Sunday dinner, if I had not cashed that cheque! We had no food banks in those days, but now, we have them, and they provide an excellent service – for which there is a big local demand.

I don't want to go on about it, ad nauseam, but again, you've guessed it. Is it the Social Services who man these food banks? Of course not. It is volunteers from the Salvation Army, the Methodist Church, the Lions Club. I say that society's welfare should be handed back to volunteers. It already has been! What we need now, is to abolish the Social Services' useless bureaucracy.

Of relevance here, is my story of the Lions' Club's Christmas parcels – which I relate in my chapter on 'Benefactors'. We ended up distributing the Christmas parcels because the Social Services were too bone idle to do so.

The truth of this came to me years ago – when the London Borough of Greenwich, in which I lived at the time, and which was under socialist control, decided to get rid of its 'Meals on Wheels', service - which had been run, with complete efficiency, for years – by the Women's Royal Voluntary Service. I had helped with this service, myself, as a sixteen year old schoolgirl.

The volunteers were replaced with paid people, who in theory, were to provide the delivery of meals, to local elderly, or handicapped, people. Next thing you know, Greenwich's workers had gone on strike, so no meals were delivered to the elderly and handicapped residents of the borough. Get rid of paid people, and give welfare work to the volunteers. Then, you will get the service needed!

Ackbar Ahmad: 'A living tragedy'

Most of my tragic stories, are about untimely death, but I wish to include some, which I regard as living tragedies.

Ackbar Ahmad came to the crisis house in December 2001. Christmas is a terrible time for mental health, because all the usual places of sanctuary are closed, and families, are crushed together – often inharmoniously! Such was the case with Ackbar. He arrived, with a volunteer from the Citizens Advice Bureau, on the day after Boxing Day. You've guessed it. All the statutory services were enjoying a prolonged holiday, and only the voluntary services were working!

Ackbar explained that his family, Kenyan Asians, had come to the UK when he was just nine years old. At sixteen, he started a successful motor mechanics apprenticeship, with Fords Motor Company in Dagenham, and had gone on to work for them for twenty-five years.

He had married, [a Hindu arranged marriage], and had a son and a daughter. The family lived in a council flat at Forest Gate, in the London Borough of Newham – overlooking West Ham Football Ground! This was conveniently situated for his work at Fords.

However, Newham, like all London Boroughs, had a lengthy list of people waiting for council houses, so they introduced a scheme - whereby families, willing to relocate to Luton in Bedfordshire, would receive ten thousand pounds as a deposit on a house there. Ackbar and family took this offer.

No doubt, the house in Luton was a success in itself, but Ackbar continued to commute to his job in Dagenham, and so spent practically the whole of his life – either working, or travelling. Inevitably, in his absence, the family started to function without him, and this led to marital breakdown.

Ackbar then moved to stay with an uncle in Ilford – which was also within easy travelling distance of Dagenham, but he started to suffer from depression. His brother, Mohammed, had obtained a job as an accountant at the Oracle in Reading, so he bought a house in Wokingham, and he, their parents, Mohammed's wife and children, and Ackbar, all moved in together.

There was a big, family row at Christmas, with some violence, so Mohammed went to the CAB, and that is how Ackbar came to us. I was so pleased that a bed was available. The relief on Mohammed's face was visible – when we explained that Ackbar would be able to stay with us, free of charge, until we found him a flat.

He stayed for six months, and then, in the glad old days, we got him a council flat. He was seen by the local mental health services – who did precisely nothing to rehabilitate him. They got him drawing stupid pictures of motor cars, when he could – with the right support – have actually got back into motor mechanics.

Ackbar had the HGV 1 and 2 driving qualifications, so work as a driver could have been another possibility for him. I have actually been driven by him – in our old minibus – and he was an excellent driver. Nobody could be more nervous of the roads than I am, but I always felt perfectly safe with Ackbar.

Ackbar got a good golden handshake from Fords, but squandered this in a Reading Casino. 'Pam, they are very kind, he would say. They bring you coffee and sandwiches to the gaming tables.' I bet they did! Anything to keep you there – spending money!

Due to the lack of local mental health rehabilitation services, once he had left the crisis house, Akbar descended into chronic alcoholism. We still see him rolling around Wokingham, his pockets stuffed with cans of lager, which he starts drinking in the early morning – a formerly skilled man, who is now lost, and purposeless, in life. A tragic story.

Chapter 25

Robert and Lilian: 'For everything there is a season and a time for every matter under heaven'

The Book of Ecclesiastes assures us that 'For everything there is a season and a time'. That has been my experience, and Robert and Lilian's story confirms me in this belief.

'Youth's the Season Made for Joys. Love is Then Our Duty'
John Gay

Robert and Lilian were teenage sweethearts – at school together – at the age of sixteen. At the age of nineteen, both went on to marry different partners – Robert and his wife having one son, and Lilian and her husband, having two daughters.

Robert's marriage broke down after a few years. Lilian's lasted for sixteen. Robert remarried, and Lilian found a new partner. When they met up on 'Friends Reunited', an internet site that puts old school friends in touch, Robert was divorced for a second time, and Lilian was bored stiff with her second partner - of twenty years.

It was a whirlwind romance! Sixteen years old again, in their minds, they whirled through six months of passion. Alas, they were sixteen in their minds, but not in their bodies! After six months, Robert suffered a heart attack, and was confined to a wheelchair. Lilian then had to nurse him, until he died eighteen months later. There is a time, and a place, and a season, for everything, and middle age is not the time for wild passion. A tragic story!

Further evidence that middle age is not the time for wild passion, is to be found in 'Three Act Tragedy': Agatha Christie: [Published: Collins: 1935.]. The plot revolves around the fact that a middle-aged man has fallen madly in love with a young girl. I won't spoil the story by revealing any more, but 'Tragedy' is in the title of the book!

Kate Sanderson: 'Searching for myself'

Kate was one of our earlier guests in the crisis house, and a tragic figure. She suffered from severe paranoid schizophrenia, and it was thought that she would, eventually, commit suicide.

Kate was one of our few guests, whose behaviour was obviously, bizarre. She would, for instance, place a mirror, on a stair. It looked so odd there. We wondered what she saw it as reflecting!

She was very distraught that her husband had abandoned her, and that she did not have custody of her daughter. She was constantly searching for herself, and for her lost life.

At Christmas, we always have a party, and we have a sack of presents, just little things, like foam bath, and calendars – placed under the Christmas tree. But Christmas is always a very sad time for the mentally ill – when their situation is brought home to them forcibly.

From the Christmas Sack of presents, a lucky dip, Kate got a soap dish. She then left the crisis house, and left the soap dish, with a note for us, saying that she needed the bathroom to go with it, because she was homeless. A tragic character!

Daniel Rendell: 'What a comedown'

Daniel was an equally tragic figure. He had a degree in maths, and a good job as an actuary with an insurance company. At the age of thirty-eight, he had a paranoid, schizophrenic, breakdown, and has never really recovered from this. Thereafter, his descent was tragic.

He owned a house – which he sold, and moved into a mental health hostel. When this closed, he bought a flat, but could not cope unsupported, and so had to be Sectioned into the mental hospital. We have known Daniel for over twenty years, and when he is out of hospital, he cuts a sad figure, sitting alone on a bench, and smoking.

The very day before I wrote this narrative – in August 2015, Daniel came to the drop-in – having been discharged from the mental hospital. He was very heavily medicated, with little to say.

So high was his dosage of medication, that Daniel, literally, fell asleep in the drop-in centre. I get the impression that, now that mental health beds are at a premium, patients are discharged before they are ready, and just doped up with extra medication – in order to make them acceptable in the community – in other words, not disruptive, and a nuisance.

All that bright youth, where did it go? A tragic story.

Sally and Allen: 'The tragic brother and sister'

Both Sally and Allen have been guests in the crisis house – and neither made a recovery. They had an extremely unstable background. Sally was a heroin addict, and their father supplied both of them with drugs. Prior to coming to us, Sally had been sleeping on a tombstone, in a local graveyard. How macabre!

Of the two, Allen was the more ill – so much so, that he needed nursing. With Sally, the main problem was heroin addiction, and when clean, she was capable of work. However, she quickly relapsed into heroin use – after a short period of being addiction free.

Sally's work led to an amusing, but, nevertheless, telling, incident in the crisis house. For a short time, Sally worked, quite successfully – catering in a local pub. One day, she brought home some lemon meringue pie, and cream, which had been left over from lunch. Gabriela Rani devoured a large helping. Then she declared, 'Sally should not be allowed to bring lemon meringue pie, and cream, here. It is not fair to us with a weight problem.'

I recall, when fighting for the crisis house, that an, anonymous, letter appeared in the local paper – criticising the fact that we had a bar – when people were 'battling' alcoholism. We have seen this 'battling'. Begrudge an old dear her weekly treat, a lunchtime small glass of sherry, and then go home – and down three bottles of neat vodka!

You may laugh, but it is this conception that SOMEBODY ELSE is going to sort out your problems. This is the same mentality exhibited by Sandie – with her alcohol and cocaine. [Chapter 18: 'Beer money'.] There is no magic in mental health. No one else is going to sort you out, or prevent you from suffering the results of your own actions. Self help is always, and invariably, the answer!

Although self-help is always essential, we also advise service users to seek medical advice, if this seems to be needed. Thus Maurice Santereau and I, advised Gabriela Rani.

She had just moved into a new flat, in a new area, in the [forlorn] hope that she would not have problems there. So, she registered with a new GP. 'Since you are starting afresh with a new GP, we advised, why not ask him to put you on a properly supervised doctor's diet – so that you can lose weight under medical supervision?' Sound advice.

Not to Gabriela Rani, it wasn't! She – have to go on a diet! She – have to lose weight! The plot to close down the crisis house, and to destroy us, was probably conceived at that very moment!

To return to the story, in addition to other problems, Allen suffered from bulimia, and was constantly vomiting. We quickly realised, that we would not be able to continue to have him as a guest in the crisis house – because he needed nursing, and this was not a service that we provided.

When yet another situation had broken down for him, Wokingham Borough Council's Housing Officer, asked whether we could accommodate Allen, once again, in the crisis house. We could not. We could not accommodate either tragic brother or sister again.

When Allen was living in the local mental health hostel, his sister reported that his room was in a state of the most unbelievable filth, and that there were live fleas hopping in his carpet! I never saw this room, but it must have been dire, because, when Sally, herself, was asked to leave the crisis house, I paid our cleaner to clean her room twice, it was so filthy. If Sally was distressed by her brother's room, it must, indeed, have been in a state!

This tragic story demonstrates just how great a need there is for high support facilities in the community. In the old mental hospitals, nurses saw that patients were washed, shaved, and dressed in clean clothes. Bedding was changed. Wards were cleaned, every day.

Severe mental illness has not gone away – just because the mental asylums have been closed! It exists to this day, and, having office based community psychiatric nurses, does not meet the need.

Nursing involves more than the administration of medication. Seeing that the patient has a bath, is, for instance, a basic nursing duty, and patients should be visited in their own homes, and how they are coping, should be observed, so that appropriate services, such as cleaning, and laundry, can be arranged, if necessary.

When we had the beds at the crisis house, we always gave guests the choice. They could clean their own rooms, if they so wished, but they could have room service, if they preferred, or if they were too ill to do their own cleaning.

We did not undertake personal laundry, but we would launder linen, if this was needed. As a result, with a handful of exceptions, we were able to keep the crisis house up to standard.

We love success, but we had to accept that this brother and sister were not to be among our success stories. A tragic outcome!

Peter O' Reilly: 'My mother was murdered'

I don't regard Peter, himself, as necessarily, tragic – although his background is extremely so. He was born with cerebral palsy, and spent his childhood in a wheelchair – though an operation has enabled him to walk – albeit with a stiff gait.

The tragedy of his life, occurred in 1996, when his mother was murdered by a paedophile – who had got involved with his thirteen year old sister. Peter then had to go into care.

The paedophile was sentenced to life in prison, and has committed further murders, since being gaoled!

Peter is a regular user of our crisis house – where we endeavour to give him the home, of which he was robbed, so tragically.

When Gavin Morton came to visit the crisis house, the day before I wrote this narrative, at the end of August 2015, [Chapter 10: 'Step by step to success'.] I was singing my eternal song, that it is the individual who gets his life back together, and not the mental health service.

Peter remonstrated with me. 'How can I? I was born, physically handicapped, and I have mental health problems, as well!'

Nobody is denying that Peter was unfortunately placed in life.

Nevertheless, he is not the only one, in our ranks, whose mother was murdered. A former guest in the crisis house, Tom, explained to us, that his father had strangled his mother, when he was still a baby. That, naturally, led to Tom having problems in life. [Chapter 29: 'Rhys and Tom'.]

The trauma, as we explain regularly, to Peter, stays with you for the rest of your life. There is no magic wand that will take it all away, so you have the two famous choices – you either sit down and moan for the rest of your life, or you get up and make the best of it!

The point is that, like Judi Chamberlin before him [Please see: 'On Our Own': Publisher: MIND: London: 1988], Peter is waiting for the mental health system to sort his life out, and it won't.

We have known Peter for about eight years. He reached his thirty-second birthday on 3rd September 2015. In the eight years, we have seen no progress in his situation at all. I did manage to obtain for him a 'Personal Budget', for help with domestic tasks, in order that he would not be living in the squalor inhabited by the tragic brother and sister, but, apart from this, no improvements have been made.

Incidentally, I mentioned to Peter, the remarks made by the social worker, in a former local MIND association: 'After we have messed them up, as children, in 'care', they then turn up in adult mental health services.' Since Peter had been in care, he was able to confirm that that is, indeed, what happens. Yes, but you don't expect the social workers to be boasting about it!

This would be the equivalent of a doctor saying, 'After I have infected my patients, deliberately, with bacteria, they then turn up in my hospital, for treatment for infection!' Doctors neither do, nor say this. Why? Because they are a genuine profession. Social workers are not.

Peter's situation is one, which I have observed, many times, in all my decades in mental health. He has already lost his teens, and his twenties. He is well on his way to losing his thirties.

I often advise service users, because I firmly believe it to be the case, that, up to the age of thirty, you can get away with practically anything. Your body is young, so it can withstand immoderate amounts of alcohol, and drugs. You can go back-packing around the world, and still get back in time to establish, for yourself, a career, a property, a partner, and a family.

After thirty, one by one, the doors start closing. You can still get into a career, for instance, but the likelihood is, by that time, that your colleagues will already be on their way up the ladder. It is absolutely the case that 'It's later than you think'.

As Sadie Minton's mother proclaimed, so cogently, all those years ago, 'Start going there, [to the local, statutory, mental health day centre], and you could still be going at fifty!' 'The years go by, as quickly as a wink!'

Peter is very intelligent, but it will be only when he ceases to expect the services to give him a good quality life, and establishes one for himself, that his situation will be resolved. Peter is skilled with computers, for instance, so there may be an opening for him in this area of work. At least, in October 2015, Peter took some temporary work in a pub. Any work is better than no work, and is always a step in the right direction.

Peter is also an example of the fact, that throwing money at problems, does not solve them. Because Peter has both physical, and mental, disabilities, he is in receipt of a maximum number of benefits, but his quality of life is poor, and will remain so, unless self help is brought into the equation. A tragic story!

I recall one incident, with Peter, that was both annoying, and amusing. It was an absolutely freezing winter's day, and, no doubt, all statutory services had failed to open.

I struggled in, to open the crisis house, but decided to close the drop-in promptly, at four o'clock. Peter went off to get his bus, and I hurried to tidy up. The snow was falling thickly. Then the door-bell rang. It was a lady with Peter, and, evidently, she knew him, from working in the local services. He had fallen over in the snow, and there were no buses. The roads were impassable for buses or cars. There was to be only one more train that day.

I looked up at the sky. 'It's not going to get any better', I said, 'Peter had better wait for the train'. The station was crowded with people, so, evidently, a train was expected shortly. Peter went across to the station.

Hoping to get the same train myself, which was to be the last that day, I hurried on with my tidying up. The door bell rang again. The woman was back – complaining that I had sent Peter to get a train. I gather that the stupid woman expected me to take Peter back into the crisis house, and make a fuss of him – thus ensuring that we would both miss the last train of the day!

I did not find out exactly what she expected me to do, because I slammed the door in her face, leaving her bleating, that she was going to write to someone. So far as I am aware, she never did! Having got rid of her, I rushed to get the train, and, fortunately, caught it. If there is one thing that I can't stand, in life, it is a busybody!

This incident illustrates cogently the difference between dealing with an idiot, and dealing with somebody intelligent. The only person left with me when I had got rid of the busybody, was my intelligent heroin addict friend, Kurt Haddow. [Chapter 10: 'Good with computers'.] At this time he was still living in the bed-and-breakfast establishment – a stone's thrown from the crisis house. 'You need to get home', he said.

They are very keen to pile their problems onto you. Miss that train, and we would both have been stranded in the crisis house for the night, snowed in. Of course, how I was to get home, never entered the stupid woman's head, nor did it occur to her that it was inappropriate for me to be stranded, alone all night, with a male service user.

Fortunately, I got rid of her, in time for both of us to get home. Peter lives near Bracknell Station, so he had no problem. I had to struggle for another mile through the snow, but because plenty of other people were doing this too, it was not too much of an ordeal.

Chapter 26

Cynthia Topping: 'Inhabiting a twilight world'

Cynthia finally passed away in 2013, at the age of seventy. She was a lifelong victim of minor tranquilliser addiction, and that is how we first met her, in 1989, when MIND was conducting a campaign, to prevent patients with anxiety, becoming addicted to benzodiazapines. Our late service user, Rob Jenkins, used to complain, crudely, but truthfully, 'That woman never talks about anything but her bleeding pills!'

This is her story. Cynthia 'had to get married' – as was the convention, then, because she was pregnant – with a baby girl. At the age of four, this child died, of tubercular meningitis. She had contracted the tuberculosis from her mother.

Cynthia had been prescribed vallium after her daughter died, and had been on it, for all the decades since. I actually remember the introduction of benzodiazepines, because, when I was a university student, in the 1960's, I worked, as a nursing auxiliary, in my college holidays.

In those days, patients with anxiety, were prescribed phenobarbitone, and this was considered to be very unsafe, because the therapeutic dose, was close to the fatal dose. So when benzodiazepines were brought in, in the late 1960's, doctors hailed them with delight, as being very safe. It was only much later, that it was realised, that they were extremely addictive.

After the death of her first child, Cynthia did go on to have two more, a boy, and a girl, and, because of her mental health, she was allocated a social worker. Cynthia did have one funny story to tell us, about her experience of this 'service'!

The baby had been screaming all night long, so at nine in the morning, Cynthia telephoned the social worker. 'Why are you ringing me at this time in the morning? the social worker demanded. I've only just got up.' 'Well, you are bloody lucky, Cynthia retorted, I've been up all night!'

It was the same story, then, as now. They want a cushy little job, with office hours. Unfortunately, mental health cannot be accommodated within office hours. It requires round-the-clock dedication.

This brings me to an article which I read, recently, in the *Daily Mail*. It was written by a psychiatrist, and it concerned the, recently adopted, requirement, that all nurses should hold degrees.

This has been the case since 2014, and I suspect that the reason is, that, now that practically every young person has a degree, the Royal College of Nursing believes that it is sensible, to introduce this rule – rather than allowing a situation where nursing is the only profession without such a requirement.

What the psychiatrist said, was, 'Who can blame nurses with degrees, if they prefer to sit in the office studying pie charts, rather than being out on the wards, dealing with disease and death?'

I was flabbergasted! If one wants to spend one's life – studying pie charts, why not train as a statistician? Nursing, I can assure him, is about dealing with disease, and, inevitably, about death, in some cases. If one does not wish to deal with these, why train to be a nurse, at all?

Thus, Cynthia inhabited a twilight world – having no energy to participate in life. She wouldn't get up until the afternoon. Eventually, we only saw her on Open Days – when the crisis house was open into the evening.

Her husband felt, after a time, that he couldn't do other, than get on with his own life. He used to go off on his bicycle, so Cynthia was left trapped in the half waking, half sleeping, state, of minor tranquilliser addiction. We provided Cynthia with a befriender, who did her best, and was appreciated, but Cynthia's life remained, very limited.

From time, to time, she made an effort to conquer the addiction, but never achieved this. A tragic waste of a life!

Jim Force: 'Driving to tragedy'

Jim stayed in the crisis house as a teenager. He came from a very tragic background. His mother had committed suicide as a 'human torch'.

Two of Jim's brothers were adopted. He, and two other brothers, went into care. Jim came to stay in the crisis house, when he returned to Wokingham, after coming out of care. His behaviour in the house was fine, but, after six months, he went to prison – having stolen seventy cars!

Cars, they were his problem, and his obsession. After his time in prison, we didn't see much of Jim – though he did stay with us briefly, with his infant son, after a quarrel with his partner.

Then the tragedy occurred. Jim stole a car, drove it while drunk, and crashed it. His injuries caused permanent paraplegia. Our befrienders went to visit him in Stoke Mandeville Hospital, but the doctors there, could not repair his fractured spine.

Jim is now a permanent invalid – so tragic – at the age of only thirty-six.

Catherina Lynham: 'I love having children'

Catherina was an early-day version of Violet. [Chapter 49: 'Advocacy'.] She was always having children, and they were all placed into care.

When she stayed with us, she had an eighteen year old son, two girls of twelve, a boy of six, and she had just given birth to another baby boy. Blood is thicker than water, because, though he had been in care, her eighteen year old son came to see her at the crisis house. Hang the Social Services, Catherina was his mother, and he wanted to see her!

Where you have human beings, things are never simple. However deficient one's biological parents may be, you have come from them, they are your flesh and blood, and the need, in adult life, to contact them, is strong.

One of our service users, who had been adopted as a baby, also traced her biological mother, and found her to be an old prostitute! No matter. Blood is thicker than water!

This particular service user, Fiona Brown, changed the history of the crisis house, albeit, unwittingly.

Shortly after MIND had sent its failed social worker, to assess us for quality, we received a letter from their Chief Executive – detailing her concerns. On the morning that this arrived, Fiona Brown, and another depressed lady, came into the drop-in for support. Who takes priority – MIND and their letter, or the depressed ladies? No contest, I threw MIND's letter in the bin, and turned my attention to the mentally ill people.

I mentioned the letter to Fiona, and said that I thought that we had a good reputation in the community. 'Not half! She replied. You have a marvellous reputation in the community. You should hear Tony's mother speak about you, for instance. Your services are marvellous!'

Tony Friar's mother had despaired of him. He stayed in the crisis house, and kept our rules. 'Why, pleaded his mother, will he keep your rules, but not mine?'

We come back to Agatha Christie. In 'The Clocks' [Published by Collins: 1963], Mrs Ramsay cannot understand why her teenage boys obey Detective Inspector Hardcastle, and not her.

'Out!' he said. 'It was only one word, quietly uttered, but it had behind it the quality of authority. Without more ado both boys got up, shuffled their feet and shuffled out of the room.' 'How wonderful, thought Mrs Ramsay appreciatively, Now why can't I be like that?' 'But then, she reflected, she was the boys' mother.'

Due to the intervention of our Association, Tony Friar ceased to be a difficult young man. He got a good job, married, had two children, and bought a house in Yateley.

I told Fiona that I was glad that we had such a marvellous track record, and remarked, with a laugh, that if Tony had bought a house in Yateley, which is a desirable, and expensive, area, just over the county border, in Hampshire, then he had done better than most of us!

So I consulted my fellow trustees and committee members, service users, and crisis house guests. 'Should we sever the connection with MIND?' They all agreed that we should, and a cheer went up when the MIND sign came down!

Guest at the time, Leona, was particularly pleased. 'Do you really mean that we can take down that awful board?' She said.

People living in the crisis house did not like being seen going in and out of a place that was, obviously, a mental health centre! We told MIND that we had a marvellous reputation in the community, and did not need them! End of era.

After she left us, Catherina went on to have yet another baby, and for all I know, she could have continued to give birth, throughout the rest of her child-bearing years. So tragic, both for her, and for the children.

Later in this narrative, I include a whole chapter on 'Children the Strains, and Stresses, for People with Mental Health Problems'.

What is the motivation, one wonders, for giving birth to child after child – especially if you know that they will be taken away from you? A perplexing mystery!

Life is full of bitter, and tragic, irony. Sometimes, I believe in the Greek Gods. They are up there, on Mount Olympus, laughing, and mischievous. They fix things, so that everything is the opposite of how it should be!

I recall two British Transport Police, visiting the crisis house. In conversation, I said to them, that life is so unfair. The mentally ill, and socially, inadequate, person, will give birth to child after child. By contrast, you get the nice couple, with good jobs, plenty of money, and a lovely big house. For year after year, they try, and no child comes. 'Tell me about it', said one Police Officer! One so often thinks that one's problem is unique. It is not, it is the common lot of humanity! A tragic situation.

James Jervis: 'Climb every mountain'

'Climb every mountain, search high and low.
Follow every byway, every path you know.'

I have written in detail about Jamie Jervis in my chapter on advocacy. I climbed every mountain to see justice done. Suffice here, then to say, that he was only twenty-two years old, when he committed suicide, and that is a very tragic waste of a young life!

Mark Tildesley: 'The loss of a child'

Mark Tildesley's abduction, and murder, by a paedophile ring, occurred in June 1984 – two years before I came to Berkshire.

However, in our early days, the crisis house did support his surviving relatives. His mother, Lavinia, her son, Christopher, and his wife, and their baby, attended our drop-in centre, regularly, for support. I also met Lavinia's daughter, Christina, and her husband, and daughters.

Mark's mother and father, both now deceased, never got over the tragedy. It did not help that – although there were conspiracy theories galore, his body was never found. Unable to achieve closure, Lavinia, Mark's mother, went into a time warp – keeping his bedroom in her cottage in Rose Street – as though he would, one day, come back. He never did. The tragic loss of a child.

NOTE: Because the murder of Mark Tildesley is already in the public domain, this is the only occasion when I have not changed the service users' names.

PART THREE

Our befriending Service

Chapter 27

Good Befrienders

'Glad to have a friend like you, fair, and fun, and skipping free.
Glad to have a friend like you,and glad to just be me!'

Two of the most distressing aspects of mental illness are that it isolates people, and that it results in loneliness. Befriending is such an essential service, because the befriender is able to re-engage the mentally ill person with the normal world.

Loneliness brings with it numerous hazards. Lonely people are so vulnerable, and there are always predators, galore, out there.

In Agatha Christie's Short Story Collection, 'The Labours of Hercules', [Published: Collins: 1947.], I particularly like the story, entitled, 'The Flock of Geryon'.

Mentally ill people, and lonely people, generally, are always particularly susceptible to the lure of cults. One can understand it perfectly. If you feel that nobody wants you, or that you have never been anything in life, how affecting it is, to be able to take on board the belief, that God has chosen YOU - to be one of his few disciples, a special legion!

One of the things that I, personally, like about the Church of England, is that it is not a little cult. You are one among thousands. The wording for its services and sacraments have been decided, by committee, hundreds of years ago. By participating in these, you feel that you are, at one, with humanity. Cults engender the opposite feeling!

As Miss Carnaby explains to Hercule Poirot, in 'The Flock of Geryon', 'The whole sect centres around the head of the movement, the Great Shepherd, he is called. A Doctor Andersen. A very handsome looking man, I believe with a presence'.

'Which is attractive to women, yes?'

'I'm afraid so', Miss Carnaby sighed. 'My father was a very handsome man. Sometimes, it was most awkward in the parish.'

Needless to say, the handsome Dr Andersen had more than a passing interest in these lonely women, his cult members', money!

I had a, not dissimilar, experience, in my schizophrenia fellowship group. Janine came to the group because she had a son who was a flamboyant, paranoid, schizophrenic. He used to lurk around the local churchyard in a cloak, and the children called him 'Jesus'.

Janine's husband, who was a psychologist, deserted the family, and moved to America. Her daughter, at the age of nineteen, joined the Moonies! She married within the Moonies, and had a baby, within the Moonies. There was nothing that Janine could do, and it was only because she did not try to rescue her daughter from their clutches, that Janine was able to have any contact at all.

What this girl was looking for was security, and certainty. Her brother was raving mad, her father had absconded, her mother was over-burdened with the worry of it all! It is such a Godsend if such individuals can be provided with a befriender, to relieve their loneliness, and to keep them in touch with the normal world.

Our Befriending Service was the first service that we set up when our Association formed in March 1987. At that stage we didn't even have our own base. We laid down firm ground rules for our Befriending Service, and, as a result, we have never had any serious problems with it.

First, it is run on a same-sex basis. As I point out to prospective befrienders, 'You may be stable, sensible, and not, currently, vulnerable, but people whom you befriend, will almost certainly be unstable and vulnerable'. One, therefore, eliminates almost all sexual risks by having same/sex befriending. If the person to be befriended is gay, then the befriender must be someone who can ensure that there will be no sexual attraction between the two.

We don't allocate befrienders cold. Now that we have had drop-in facilities for twenty-seven years, we expect prospective befrienders, first, to volunteer in the drop-in centre for six months.

During this time, it becomes apparent, if they have any particular prejudices, and it also emerges if they appear to get on particularly well with any individual. If that individual needs a befriender, the volunteer can then be matched – arranging the befriending on a mutually convenient basis. Some people only want telephone contact. Some like getting out and about. We do not encourage the befriender to take the person to their own home. The befriender may be happy with this, but other members of their family may not.

As I explain, we are working with vulnerable, lonely, people. How will you cope if they stay until midnight, or get involved inappropriately with other members of your family? Once they know where you live, what can prevent them from turning up at all hours of day and night?

When my husband, and I, were looking for a bigger house, some twenty years ago, we looked at some suitable ones, in Wokingham, as well as at those in Bracknell, where we had already lived, for the previous ten years.

'Too close for comfort!' was my conclusion. People would be popping round, at all times of day and night, saying, 'Sorry to disturb you, but!!!' So we plumped for where we are in Bracknell, just off the Wokingham Road. In emergency, I can get over to Wokingham, by taxi, in ten minutes, but we are not within 'popping' distance!

There is long-term befriending – which can go on for years, and then there is short-term befriending – which is actually more like crisis work – often highly intensive, and designed to support the person through a particularly difficult period. Our befrienders enrich the lives of those whom they befriend – getting them out to places of interest, and even, in some instances, taking them on holiday – both at home and abroad.

Chapter 28

Good Female Befrienders

Catriona and Benita

Catriona befriended Benita. Benita was referred to us by another local charity. They thought that she was suffering from mental health problems – and so it proved to be.

Benita had arrived from Australia – just turning up at the house of a distant cousin – whom she hoped would provide her with a home. Of course it didn't work. The cousin found her some ordinary, rented, accommodation, but Benita failed to cope.

Catriona was a very good befriender. We realized that Benita was quite seriously mentally ill, so we obtained a psychiatric assessment for her. The psychiatrist recommended sheltered accommodation, and this we secured for her – out-of-area.

While we were trying to resolve Benita's problems, a local journalist friend took her in temporarily. She stated that 'Of all the flotsam and jetsam of life, that has passed through my doors, Benita is the saddest.' Benita had been married, and had children, but had lost all contact with them. All that she now had, in life, was an inventory of tawdry possessions. A sad story, but we did, eventually, settle her into supported accommodation with caring staff. Her befriender, Catriona, visited and supported Benita throughout this entire period.

Pat and Rosie

It was our excellent, volunteer, Pat, who pointed out to us, that Rosie needed a befriender. She then went on to assume the role, herself, very successfully.

At first, she saw Rosie in the drop-in centre, but, once Rosie came into the crisis house, as a guest, Pat would visit her in the evenings – talking over all the problems, Rosie's dilemma, and her confused feelings about her situation.

Thus Rosie got all the help and support that she needed, to resolve her life crisis, and went on to make a success of her future life.

Gillian and Yvette

Gillian was one of our early volunteers – helping with our Association, when we were still at the British Red Cross Centre.

Yvette joined our drop-in at the crisis house in 1992. She had a very sad background – as a battered wife, was colossally overweight, and suffered, from very severe depression. Yvette exhibited a symptom which occurs commonly, in mental health. So overwhelming was her latent depression, that one only had to exchange a glance with her, and her eyes would fill up with tears.

Gillian made a very stalwart and committed befriender – taking a great interest in Yvette, and sympathising with her situation. The befriending relationship lasted for a solid, eight, years. Yvette died of a stroke, aged sixty-nine, in the year two thousand, and Gillian retired to Dorset, that same year. An excellent befriending partnership.

Una and Ruth

Una, who joined us in 1994, had her own sadnesses in life. Her first husband, who had always suffered bad health, died, when aged only fifty-four. Una was thus a widow at forty-nine, and was left to bring up their two boys on her own.

When she joined us, Una was very happy. Through a Christian Marriage Bureau, she had met a new partner, and they got married. But life was not fair to her. After a year of marriage, he also died , of a heart attack.

Una made an excellent befriender for Ruth. Ruth was extraordinarily neurotic. She was involved in a long-standing battle with the Health and Social Services authorities – over their alleged neglect of her, while she was both mentally ill, and pregnant – the stress causing her to miscarry the baby. Una supported her through it all – with patience and fortitude.

Una and I laughed together. When I suggested that she took on the befriending of Ruth, I said that she would be easy to befriend. By that, I meant that Ruth was neurotic, rather than psychotic, so one could have an intelligent conversation with her. She was in touch with reality, and she would understand what you were talking about.

The day after Una took over as befriender, Ruth made a suicide attempt! Was that what I meant by 'easy'? Nevertheless, Una went on to be a very good, and supportive, befriender for Ruth.

Martha and Cynthia

Cynthia was a minor tranquilliser addict, of decades' standing, and I never expected dramatic success, in her case.

Nevertheless, Martha was willing to take on Cynthia, as a befriender, and a very successful partnership, it was. Cynthia rarely got up before afternoon, so this was not to be a befriending in which outings to places of interest were to be on the agenda. However, Cynthia was most appreciative of the fact that Martha was always willing to be available on the telephone, so Cynthia always had available a friend who was willing to listen.

Cynthia's life was extremely limited, so having a good befriender, enhanced it considerably.

Sandra and Gabriela

Gabriela was extraordinarily difficult. Sandra was kind, and patient, and willing to take her on. My lasting memory, is of their trip to London to collect the 'Lady Balfour Pictures'.

Gabriela was obsessed with the aristocracy, and dreamed of marrying into it. The Mental Health Foundation had contacted us – explaining that Lady Balfour, who was an amateur artist, suffered severely from mental illness, and was having to go into permanent care. She did not want her paintings to rot away in an attic, so she had asked the Mental Health Foundation to distribute them to mental health associations throughout the UK. We were one of those chosen to receive the pictures.

We thought that Gabriela would enjoy the trip to London, and love meeting Lord Balfour, so Sandra travelled with her, and they had a most exciting day. Lord Balfour told them – with proper pride – that it was a member of the Balfour family, Robert Louis Stevenson, who had written 'Treasure Island', and so Gabriela had the longed-for brush with the aristocracy – albeit briefly! Lady Balfour's paintings are hanging in the crisis house to this very day.

Barbara and Frankie

It was our befriender, Barbara, who first brought Frankie to the crisis house, and she went on to be one of our most valued volunteers. Barbara explained that she had a neighbour, Frankie, whose mentally ill son was living with her, and causing problems. We encouraged Frankie to come to see us so that we could advise in her situation.

It is standard good advice – that, if one has a mentally or physically disabled son or daughter - living with one, that one should get them settled into independent accommodation – with the appropriate support – well before one becomes old, frail, or dies.

Then when the caring parent does eventually, sadly, pass away, the handicapped son or daughter will at least be used to shopping, cooking, laundry, housework, budgeting, and all the other necessities of daily life – with support for these, if necessary, so that – while the bereavement will still be traumatic for them, at least they will be used to coping with ordinary life.

On this basis, if I, over the years, have helped one parent with a mentally ill son or daughter, to settle them into independent accommodation, I must have helped at least one hundred! Barbara's befriending, in this instance, was the valuable contribution of getting for Frankie the advice that she needed.

Suzanne and Petula

Suzanne came to us on placement. She had experienced mental health problems herself, and was planning to train in psychoanalytic psychotherapy at the Tavistock Institute.

After some experience in the drop-in centre, I asked her to befriend Petula. Petula had experienced a lifetime of abusive relationships, and was awaiting a placement in a therapeutic community. In the intervening year, she found Suzanne's befriending invaluable.

Suzanne supported Petula during the period when she was waiting to move from her isolated accommodation out in Shinfield – back to Wokingham, and near to her family. A most successful befriending, and Petula went on to complete the programme in the therapeutic community – finding it most valuable.

Anna and Joy

Anna arrived just at the right time to befriend Joy. Anna had worked in the drop-in centre for some eight months, and so had got to know Joy and Frank. Then Frank died – very suddenly. Joy was devastated. She had been totally dependent upon Frank for sixty-five years, and could not contemplate life without him.

Anna befriended Joy, for the first full year of her bereavement – supporting her through her move from the maisonette that the couple had occupied – into sheltered accommodation for the elderly. Joy liked Anna, and greatly appreciated her befriending and home visits during this difficult time – a most successful befriending partnership.

Jane and Jean

Jane was an excellent befriender because she was naturally sociable. Among others, she befriended Jean – who was her neighbour, and a widow.

As a result of Jane's befriending, Jean attended our drop-in centre regularly, and they went away on holiday together.

Getting people out of their four walls, into the drop-in centre, and, thus, mixing with other people, may be a limited achievement, but it is, nevertheless, invaluable, as a first step back into normal life.

Shirley and Sadie

Shirley came to us because the local, statutory, mental health service were not interested in taking on volunteers. We welcomed her with open arms, and she served us well as a befriender, for a solid, eleven years!

Shirley befriended three chronically mentally ill ladies, who lived in local, supported accommodation. This was an occasion when the befriending led to concerns being raised about the quality of care that the ladies were receiving.

Shirley had concerns about the premises where they lived, their personal care, nutrition – in fact everything about their lives. One of the ladies had toenails which had grown so long that they bent over at the ends – like a tramp's. Extraordinary, since their paid carer could have accessed free chiropody services for her residents – through their GP. They didn't even have to pay.

I noticed that one of the ladies, who attended our drop-in centre, regularly, was inappropriately dressed, for the winter. It was December. She was wearing a thin black skirt, and a white blouse [no vest underneath]. She wore sandals, and no tights.

Shirley reported that the carer's family would all have a traditional roast Sunday dinner, but that the residents were not included in this. They would get something out of a tin.

This brings me to the whole point of my perspective on statutory, and, therefore, paid, Social Services.

If you are a volunteer, you want to do what you are doing.

Apparently, in the early days of the Victorian mental hospitals, for instance, local volunteers would have the patients to Sunday tea in their houses.

Were these ladies being looked after by volunteers, the table would be laid. Everybody would sit down to a proper roast dinner – followed by homemade apple pie, and custard. Everybody would enjoy it – mentally ill ladies, and carers!

Too frequently, if people are providing 'care' for a livelihood, the mentally ill people are a nuisance – to be given just the basics, and sometimes, not even those – resulting in the situation which Shirley discovered. I had a similar experience when I visited the old mental hospital

I told the Social Services Inspectorate, that it would not be difficult for the carer, when she went to have her own hair done, to take her residents with her, and get their hair styled, as well. They thought that I was expecting too high a standard. Was I?

We need to give our welfare services back to volunteers – who enjoy the work that they are doing. We need people for whom enhancing the lives of the mentally ill, and the vulnerable, is a joy, and not a burden. You will only get that if it is all done on a voluntary basis. Volunteers love their work!

In due course, Shirley went on to befriend Sadie – getting her involved in local, social activities.

Shirley was an excellent befriender, and most deserving of the Civic Award – for which we nominated her – and which she received from the Town Mayor in 2008.

Bev and Dolly

Dolly was one of those whom, we befriended, but rarely saw. She was isolated in her house, and only attended the drop-in centre, three times, over a period of years. Bev gave Dolly invaluable befriending – visiting her at home, and even, on occasions, managing to get her out to visit a local garden centre. This befriending is what I describe as our 'hidden' work – invisible, but still achieving great things behind the scenes.

Frances and Everybody

I would describe Frances, as our most popular, ever, volunteer. Throughout her seventeen years of service with us, she befriended anyone and everyone – helping them to re-establish themselves in the community, and to make a success of their lives.

She and Dave, together, went around in the minibus – collecting furniture, and helping mentally ill people to set up their flats in the community. She was the wonderful source of everything that was needed by them.

My most colourful, lasting, memory of Frances, is of the occasion when a crisis house guest asked if we had a sewing machine. I confessed that I hadn't seen one in decades. Not half-an-hour later, in walked Frances, with the needed sewing machine tucked under her arm – a vintage, 1950's Brother model – in perfect working condition, and still in its original case.

Sadly, Frances passed away – at the age of eighty-three.

Lucy and Theresa

In September 2015, I said to Lucy, 'You are no longer just Theresa's friend, you are her befriender!'

Theresa is Lucy's neighbour. Earlier this year, she experienced a tragedy. Her husband, aged in his fifties, committed suicide, by hanging himself, in their garage. Theresa had grown-up children, but, as she explained to Lucy, 'They have their own lives to lead'.

Lucy proved to be a most stalwart friend. She keeps Theresa company, goes out with her, for coffees, and meals, and, most important, gave her marvellous support, throughout all the trauma of the Post Mortem, and the Inquest.

In October 2015, Lucy brought Theresa to the crisis house drop-in centre. We filled in application forms for her – for Personal Independence Payment, and for Employment Support Allowance.

Theresa said that she loved the cosy little crisis house drop-in, and will attend regularly. People always do. She said that she hated the cold, uncomfortable, and bureaucratic, offices at which the local statutory mental health service is based, and that she would not be going back there. People always do!

'Glad to have a friend like you!' expresses Theresa's feelings about Lucy, exactly!

Chapter 29

Good Male Befrienders

'To a good man of most dear memory –
O, he was good, if e'er a good man lived'
William Wordsworth

Gilbert and Jay

Gilbert came to us, as a befriender, before we even set up the drop-in centre, at the British Red Cross. In January 1989, we held a coffee morning, at the house of one of our volunteers. Members of the local community were invited. Gilbert attended, and then went on to deliver stalwart service to our Association for the next seventeen years, and remained our life Vice President until he, sadly, passed away in June 2015 – at the age of eighty-nine and a half.

Jay was a particularly difficult service-user. He had a diagnosis of schizophrenia, but was reluctant to take his medication. Gilbert, nevertheless, befriended him, and saw that he got into hospital when this was necessary. Throughout his years of service, Gilbert would drive people to hospital, and even drove our minibus, when we were temporarily without a driver. We remain in touch with his widow, Joan, and were most honoured, and grateful, to be remembered with a legacy in Gilbert's Will.

Rob

Rob came to stay as a guest in the crisis house in January 1996 – introduced by another befriender. He had been turned out by his wife, was on the streets, and was practically starving – because – having always worked as a refrigeration engineer, since leaving the Navy, and, having been made redundant from this job, he was unaware of the existence of benefits.

We organized a benefits claim for him, and he did splendidly. He stayed for five months in the crisis house, and during this time, saved five hundred pounds from his Income Support. This enabled him to pay the deposit on a flat in the private sector – into which he moved in June 1996.

Rob then continued to drive our minibus, for the next five years – covering the entire, vast, Wokingham District, and thus enabling people who were isolated, and without transport, to get into our drop-in centre. Some were as far-flung as Remenham – which borders on Henley – but

Rob became the familiar face who picked them up, and delivered them home. The many who received this service, were most grateful for Rob's befriending.

Sadly, Rob passed away in October 2001 – after a battle with motor neurone disease. We were able to comfort ourselves with the fact, that his last six years with us, were much happier than the years that preceded them.

Brian and Cuthbert

Brian was an excellent befriender. He came to us at the age of seventy, because he had retired from a top directorship at a local company, but was considered too old to train for voluntary work at the Citizen's Advice Bureau. He had an interest in mental health, because one of his sons had suffered a breakdown while at university.

Cuthbert was mentally ill, a widower, and somewhat isolated and lonely, in a flat on his own. Brian befriended him – taking him out to places of interest, such as Maple Durham House. Such enriching activities, by a befriender, can make all the difference to a mentally ill person's life. In the end, Cuthbert, himself, had to go into a care home, but his two years of befriending, by Brian, had been happy ones.

After the two years, and with Cuthbert settled in care, Brian left us, to go climbing in the Himalaya Mountains! There is one sad, and one funny, sequel to the story of Brian.

Some six years after he left us, Brian committed suicide by jumping from a high tower. At the Inquest, his wife said that he had suffered from anxiety in old age, [he was seventy-four when he died], and that he had never really adjusted to retirement. There is no doubt that this adjustment is much more difficult if one has occupied a very high level position. Those retiring from humbler occupations make the transition more easily.

The funny sequel occurred, when a man who had also been made redundant, but from an ordinary job, came to the drop-in centre for support, and recognized Brian, with some awe, as the top director of his company.

I suggested to this man that he took up voluntary work. His reply was scathing. 'Voluntary work is the pits, and only idiots would consider it.' Since I consider voluntary work to be, by far the most valuable, the most important, and the most rewarding, work that there is, I, naturally, found this opinion amusing.

Martin and Alexander: 'When I needed a neighbour, you were there!'

Martin came to the crisis house, for support, while he was suffering from depression, and went on to be a good befriender.

He befriended Alexander – who was a guest at the time. Alexander's parents owned a flat at Grasse, on the French Riviera, and a successful venture, was, when befriender and befriended, spent a holiday there one summer. It is lovely to have a flat on the Riviera, but no fun visiting it alone!

Martin befriended Alexander until Alexander found a girlfriend. Martin then laughed. 'The love of a good woman works wonders', he declared. 'Alexander doesn't need me anymore.'

'Well, I said to Martin, it is in 'Genesis', is it not? that 'It is not good that man should be alone'. Having relationships can bring problems, but NOT having relationships, can also bring problems – emotional loneliness, being the most poignant!

What is so important in mental health, is having the person you need, there for you at the time of crisis. Some befriending partnerships go on for years, but others, like this one, are relatively short-term, but crucial in the person's recovery.

There is a funny sequel to the story of Alexander. He had, while staying in the crisis house, reversed the biological clock, so he would sleep throughout the day, and only come down in the early evening when the drop-in centre had closed.

Then we would share a bottle of Chablis together. 'To appreciate it to the full, he said, you need to drink it, in the sunny South of France!' Ideally, perhaps, but I always manage quite well in England's, unpredictable climate, but, nevertheless, green and pleasant land!

Malcolm and Reuban

Befriending an alcoholic, or a drug-addict, is a specialized task, and Malcolm was ideal for this role – because he was, himself, a successfully recovered alcoholic. He befriended, and visited, Reuban, who was a chronic alcoholic.

Reuban's relatives were extremely grateful – because Malcolm understood exactly what the problems were. In due course, Malcolm moved on, from befriending for our mental health Association, to specialized befriending with the local drugs and alcohol rehabilitation service, and he continues with this work to this day.

Tony and Byron

I have been working with our veteran befriender, Tony, for the past thirty-seven years, and among his many qualities, he has the ability to stick with the difficult cases. With Byron, he has succeeded where everyone else has failed.

I did not regard Byron as one of our success stories. He stayed in the crisis house, for almost two years, and appeared to make no progress whatsoever, but Tony persevered.

I think that Byron intended to stay in the crisis house for the rest of his life, but we were always, quite firm, about appropriate lengths of stay. Indeed, in the twenty years that we had the beds, one hundred and seventy-five guests stayed with us, and only seven of those, including Byron, stayed for more than a year. No-one stayed for the full two years, because, in our view, whatever the needs may be after that length of time, no way could they be described as crisis!

On leaving us, Byron went, first, into bed-and-breakfast accommodation, and, then, into a mental health supported hostel. With Tony's support and befriending, Byron did move on. From the hostel, he moved into a flat, and started to do charity work.

Byron was very intellectual – with an Oxford Degree, and fluency in German. Thus, he stood shoulders above other candidates, when he applied for a job with a German scientific company. They were able to conduct the interview in German, and Byron was offered the job, accepted, and moved to Germany to work. Tony remains in touch with him to this day – a most successful befriending partnership. Late in 2015, Byron was visiting England, and came, with his befriender, to visit us at the Crisis House. He has made a marvellous recovery, and it must be so rewarding for Tony to see this - the result of such stalwart befriending.

Phil and Keith, and Edwin

Phil and Keith are a stable, gay couple, and Edwin is as straight as a die. It was, therefore, quite appropriate for them to befriend him.

He came from an extremely dysfunctional family, and was in desperate need of befriending, and support. They would meet up, socially, and also be willing to talk on the telephone.

In latter years, Edwin has suffered from physical [heart] problems, as well as mental health problems, so he needs his befrienders' support even more acutely.

Phil and Kath

It was also, quite appropriate, for Phil to befriend Kath. She had been married, to an alcoholic, and suffered from very severe anxiety neurosis. Phil had suffered, from anxiety, himself, and so was able to empathise, with Kath. He supported her, with great patience, in many telephone conversations – a service which she appreciated, greatly.

Johnnie and Delpha

Johnnie is a gay man, who has been involved with the crisis house, for the past twenty-three years. He befriended Delpha, who was suffering from post traumatic stress disorder – due to her alleged abuse, by a psychologist.

Johnnie is actively anti-psychiatry, while I am not. It is the QUALITY of treatment that I look for, and we obtained this, for Delpha, at the Trauma Clinic, at the Maudsley Hospital. Johnnie supported Delpha all the way through her crisis – an excellent befriender.

Rhys and Tom

Rhys was an excellent befriender, for Tom. Tom had a tragic background. His father had murdered his mother – while Tom was still a baby.

Not surprisingly, Tom had emotional problems in adult life, and became homeless. Rhys would have accommodated Tom, in his own home, had his own health not been so precarious. Rhys suffered from kidney disease, and was on dialysis treatment.

Tom stayed in the crisis house for a short time, but then he found a girlfriend, who was moving to Devon, so he decided to move there, with her. After this move, Rhys continued, the successful, befriending relationship.

Dominic and Alexander

With some of our befriending partnerships, the relationship resembles more that of mother/daughter, or father/son. That is not always the case.

Due to his depression, and reversal of the biological clock, Alexander, had ceased to have the usual group of mates, that young men usually have. People to go out drinking with, and 'on the pull', as they so graphically described it!

Our befriender, Dominic, became one such mate for Alexander. He got him out, and about, and back into normal social life. A successful, befriending, partnership.

Neville and Norah [Hank]

Incredible to reflect that, after more than fifty-three years in mental health, and twenty-five – running the crisis house, I can still be shocked by the deficiencies of the statutory mental health services, but on Friday 16th October 2015, I was shocked, once again.

Norah has been feeling very depressed and suicidal, so, when she came into the drop-in centre, obviously in mental health crisis, I suggested that I telephoned the statutory crisis service – with a view to hospital admission.

I explained to the voice at the end of the line, that Norah should be visited by them, at home, that evening. It was Friday; the weekend stretched ahead, and I was worried about her being left there alone.

The voice wanted to know what method of suicide Norah had in mind. Does it matter? She said that they would risk assess her on the telephone. How can you? But she gave no assurance that Norah would be visited.

So I appointed a new befriender. Neville and Norah had been friendly for some months, and got on well together, so I asked Neville to stay with her for the weekend – providing some money for food, and thus ensuring that Norah was not to be left alone with suicidal thoughts.

So, with our most recently appointed befrienders, Lucy and Neville, our befriending service has entered a new phase. With them, it is much more like the intensive crisis work that we used to undertake in the crisis house, when we had the beds. Now, our crisis beds service is being replicated in the community, by excellent people, who, are willing to undertake this very intensive type of befriending.

Chapter 30

Benefactors

From the day that the first bed was carried into the crisis house in March 1991, through to the day that the last one was carried out in March 2011, the service was under-resourced

When we moved in – in 1991, a three thousand pounds, per annum, voluntary sector grant, from Wokingham Borough Council, was paid to us, to go with the lease on the house. But this budget was expected only to fund a day facility, and so was calculated accordingly.

By 1994, our beds were in constant occupation, so we asked the Authority for more money, and we were granted an additional two thousand pounds per year – specifically for the beds.

No sooner had the money been granted, than an inappropriate referral was made by Social Services. Their idea was 'Your beds are now funded, so we can start dumping people on you'. We nipped it in the bud – sending the person back to them, with a note – explaining that the proposed guest needed round-the-clock nursing, and that this was a service that we did not provide.

After this, few, inappropriate, referrals were made, because Social Services, then knew, that we would send them back – making work for them, and that would never do!

Now that the beds are closed, I reflect on things, with bitter/sweet amusement. I am fully convinced, that the authorities are miffed, that we no longer offer this service. Extraordinary – considering my twenty-year battle, to keep the beds available – only defeated, at last, by that all-powerful foe – money!

I come again, to Agatha Christie. Her endearing character, the little social snob, Mr. Satterthwaite, did not underestimate, nor despise, the power of money. In his long life, he had seen too many things fall before its might! You and me, both, Mr. Satterthwaite!

Gavin Morton, a former crisis house guest, who went on to train as a mental health social worker, and who recently visited us from Australia, is very wistful about the closure of our beds. 'They have cut off their nose despite their face!' he proclaimed. Quite!

I have, therefore, reached the conclusion, that what infuriated them over the years, was not the crisis house itself, but their powerlessness to control it. Because we had banned them in the Association's Constitution, WE decided who stayed and left. WE decided for whom the facility was suitable, and they had no say in the matter.

Wokingham's mental health services have never been well-resourced, so, in the context of these deficiencies, the Wokingham Crisis House represented quite a large slice of the local cake, and they could not control it – hence their fury.

As part of our campaign on behalf of the local homeless, I had the following letter published in the *Wokingham Times* on Thursday November 27th 2014:

Letter to the paper: 'I write further to your article 'Homelessness does exist in the town [the *Wokingham Times*: Thursday November 6th] and to subsequent correspondence.

"The answer to destitution is work. George Orwell came to that conclusion in his classic on the subject: 'Down and out in Paris and

London'.

Most mentally ill people can work. We have members whose schizophrenia is, at times, so severe that they have to be Sectioned under the Mental Health Act, but who, on recovery, work – doing cleaning or casual work on building sites – anything to avoid being a total burden on the tax-payer.

However, to be fit to present oneself to an employer, one needs first the four basics – a bed, a bath, clean clothes, and a hot meal. In fact, a hostel place.

That was precisely the function of the beds that we ran successfully at the crisis house for almost two decades.

Get a secure roof over the person's head, get some good food inside him, then get cracking on helping him to solve his problems, and get him back to work.

We had to close the beds because their funding of two thousand pounds, per year, from the local mental health budget was withdrawn in 2007. The community mental health team was still referring to the beds after the funding was withdrawn, but found, to their chagrin, that the beds, like the money, had ceased to be.

It is peanuts that charities get by on, and not fresh air. So, in the absence of beds, as John Ferguson [Director of the local CAB] points out in his letter: 'Town's need for a hostel is obvious' [the Wokingham Times*: Thursday 20th November 2014], we are thrown back on Wokingham bed-and-breakfast establishments.*

We had four beds, so these cost the tax-payer five hundred pounds a year each. By contrast, a bed in a local bed-and-breakfast establishment, can cost more than five hundred pounds a week. If I had put myself in the position of having to pay five hundred pounds a week for something that I could have had for five hundred pounds a year, your readers would think that I qualified for one of my former mental health beds, and I would agree with them."

I would not describe the attitude of the authorities towards us - as angry - nowadays. It is more wistful or rueful. Once we got our legacy, they probably saw no reason why we could not re-instate our beds – despite having no statutory funding. But running a residential facility is enormously costly – and we struggled the entire time. As I point out repeatedly to my colleagues, spending capital, and not getting a predictable income, is like having a large swimming pool. Pull the plug out, and, one day, you will find it empty!

Because we have always been under-resourced, we have always been reliant on, and most grateful to, our benefactors.

From the day that we walked into the crisis house, the Wokingham Lions' Club has supported us financially. They helped pay for the installation of a shower in our first crisis suite, and, later, for a shower in our downstairs emergency room.

They also supported individuals in need – paying for alcohol rehabilitation for one service user, and for carpets and a computer for another. Yet another donation from the Lions, helped towards our most recent refurbishment of the Crisis House.

We were saddened by the death of Sue Balchin in January 2015. Sue had been Chairman of the Lions Club, and a close friend of the crisis house. She was also active in our campaign to bring an end to local homelessness.

However, a former colleague of Sue, Sue Jackson, has now been in touch. She has formed an organization, 'Wokingham in Need', which wishes us to be involved in the continuing campaign, to end local homelessness.

Their inaugural meeting was on 23rd September 2015. I attended, with my colleagues, Lucy and Neville. The foundation of this new charity convinces me, even further, that Social Services are on their way out, and that welfare is already being restored to the voluntary sector.

The Lions had a tradition of raising money, for Christmas food parcels, for the needy. One Christmas, Sue was desperate. Social Services had failed to attend two meetings which the Lions had arranged – in order to get a list of needy families to whom they could deliver the parcels – so the Lions were lumbered with them. Could we help?

Thus was established, what is now our Christmas tradition, of accepting food parcels from the Lions, and distributing them to needy, mentally ill people. Christmas is always a terrible time for mental health, so a little extra cheer – like a festive parcel – can make the ordeal less unendurable.

On the subject of Social Services, my view differs from that of the majority. Most people find them woefully deficient, and want them to improve. I, by contrast, find them woefully deficient, and want to see them abolished – with society's welfare being restored to charities, and religious organizations – as it was traditionally, before the foundation of the welfare state.

We need to get back the dedicated volunteers - hospital almoners, prisoner help societies, and in fact, armies of volunteers, who will deliver to people, the practical welfare that they need – not pursuing their own careers. Such volunteers cost the tax-payer nothing.

An example supports my view. Just two days before I wrote this chapter, a lady, Ellie, visited the crisis house drop-in. She had been detoxifying from alcohol, and had then started to attend a therapeutic community. Its programme proved too intense at this stage in her rehabilitation, so she relapsed into alcohol abuse, and then took an overdose – which necessitated admission to hospital.

Once Ellie had received treatment for the overdose, she was discharged from hospital - late at night – with no arrangements, whatsoever, being made for her welfare. Where was the hospital social worker? Ellie was not even provided with transport home. Nobody checked to see whether there was food in the flat. Nobody informed family, or neighbours, of her discharge. Nobody arranged follow-up treatment. She was just slung out on her own.

In the good old days – before we had self-serving Social Services – hospitals had, in post, excellent volunteers – known as Lady Almoners. The Lady Almoner was totally practical. Before discharge from hospital, she checked that you had an address to go to, and somebody to look after you. She saw that the heating was on in your house, and that there was food in the cupboard. She arranged for you to get your medication, and that your GP knew that you were being discharged. Get rid of Social Services. Bring back the Lady Almoners, and you won't find people in the dire situation in which Ellie found herself.

Ellie, with whom we have been involved for many years, was another victim of educational pressure. She had been pressurised into taking a Fashion Degree at Kingston University, hated it, couldn't stand the cut-throat competition, and lasted there only for days.

When Ellie stayed in the crisis house, she maintained, nevertheless, that she must return to Kingston, and finish that Fashion Degree. 'Ellie, I advised, unless you are a latter-day Coco Chanel, or have vast amounts of money behind you, with a Fashion Degree, you will probably end up, as a window dresser, in a department store. Since you don't enjoy it, there is therefore no point in putting yourself through the agony!' Ellie then told me that she actually liked admin and secretarial work. She took a refresher course in this – opting, sensibly, for something with which she could cope!

The Berkshire Community Foundation, is another body which has supported us, over the years. They paid for an en-suite bathroom to be installed in one of our crisis suites. They also helped replace our holiday caravan, when the old one was on its last legs.

The Foundation also administers the local giving.com scheme – internet giving – which has also benefitted us financially.

Both the Allen Lane Foundation, and the Yapp Charitable Trust, have helped to support us, financially.

One Trustee, from the Yapp Charitable Trust, commented, on visiting the crisis house, that he wished a crisis house, such as ours, had existed in the area where a relative of his, had lived.

She was a brilliant medical student, but, through mental illness, had to go into what he described as 'An awful place', and committed suicide there.

The Yapp Trustee was overwhelmingly impressed, that the crisis house, was run, entirely, by volunteers. How to explain, to those not involved in psycho-politics, that it would not have existed, had it been otherwise? He went on to ensure that the Trust supported us, generously.

How to get crisis houses, for people like his relative? Get rid of statutory Social Services, and restore welfare, to the voluntary sector! What makes me sad, is that everybody says the same thing, but nobody grasps the nettle. There was no need for this brilliant medical student to go to an awful place. There should have been a crisis house, like ours, available to her, in her local area.

The Allen Lane Foundation [Penguin Books], also supported us generously. On the subject of Penguin Books, I note that, in 2015, a new film version of 'Lady Chatterley's Lover' has been produced. Its history never fails to amuse me.

I am convinced that, all those decades ago, the Penguin Books' Board of Directors, sat down and said, 'Profits are flagging. We need to make some money. Let's publish 'Lady Chatterley's Lover'!'

Annus Mirabilus

'Sexual intercourse began in nineteen sixty-three – between the trial of Lady Chatterley, and the Beatles first LP'
Philip Larkin

As a sixteen-year-old, I lapped up 'Lady Chatterley's Lover'. I thought that it was wonderful. But, I can't say that I go a bundle on D.H. Lawrence, nowadays. I must be getting old.

Nowadays, I prefer Agatha Christie. In 'The Clocks', Detective Inspector Hardcastle, in pursuing his murder investigation, makes a visit to the Cavendish Secretarial Bureau, which specialised in typing up manuscripts for authors.

'Sex was represented by a photograph of a timid-looking, balding man, Armand Levine.' His sales were plummeting – proving that nothing, as Agatha asserts, can be duller, than dull pornography!

In her autobiography, Agatha Christie, also says, of marriage, 'Passion you can take for granted, but I think that, respect, is very important.'

However, there is one characteristic of 'Lady Chatterley's Lover', which I hope that my book, though not steamy, will share. I hope that people will be curious about its contents, and so they will buy it!

It was a shrewd move on Penguin Books' part. Queues, miles long, formed, to buy the book. Profits soared. Gentlemen, as the Obscenity Trial, Judge, said, may not have wanted their wives, daughters, and servants, to read the book, but human beings always do what they want to do, and if something is forbidden, they want it even more.

This is where a successful business, scores over bodies like the, defunct, Inner London Education Authority, and the – hopefully to be defunct, Social Services. Successful businesses, have an accurate perception of human nature!

I.L.E.A. was abolished, because no competitive society can afford to neglect education. Mental health is usually regarded as being, less precious, and getting it right, is less urgent, but it is nevertheless, a fact, that things that don't work, do go, eventually.

A competitive, capitalist, society, needs a mental health system that gets people back to work, and to contributing, as soon as possible. It also needs facilities that enable the more severely disabled at least to function within their capabilities. Our current system does neither! Look at Akbar Ahmad! [Chapter 24: 'A living tragedy'.]

Local businesses have supported us with donations, and we were the proud recipient of a cheque from Waitrose, when their customers – through their token scheme – chose us as the most popular, and deserving, local charity.

Our patron, Lady Elizabeth Godsal, and her late husband, Alan, came to the rescue, with a large cheque, when we needed to install a new fire alarm system, in the crisis house. Lady Elizabeth also made a generous donation to the twenty-fifth anniversary celebration of our Association.

The local Masons, Inner Wheel, and Round Table, have all supported us over the years. Chair of the Masons, Ally Goodwin, has been a particularly stalwart supporter.

Then there have been the sporting events. Our member, David, ran a full marathon for us – raising one thousand pounds. Others completed a sponsored walk, and Chris and Hope completed a sponsored swim – all helping to swell the coffers. A second sponsored swim is planned for 2016.

Every year, on the last day of Royal Ascot, we collect for our charity, outside Wokingham Station. Those going to the races, find the parking in Ascot so difficult, that they park their cars in Wokingham, and then whisk through to nearby Ascot – by train.

Last year, Neville Sandford, and I, decided to go one step further, and join in the fun. We dressed up for the occasion – Neville in a topper, and me in the full, Ascot, regalia. The public liked it, and we did well with our collection.We plan to repeat the performance in June 2016!

We have a service user, Rosamund Rudd, who always makes a point of collecting for us, and makes a very good job of it. She is unfazed by the day allocated – that means nothing to Rosamund. She just collects when the spirit moves her, and turns up, at most unexpected times, with the collection box full to the brim!

When the crisis house was under threat of closure, Rosamund commented, 'We can't allow them to close it. This is the cosiest little house that I have ever been in!' She spoke for all the mentally ill, who use our service. We are their asylum, and that, no doubt, is why Rosamund is willing to spend time, and energy, collecting for our cause!

I have a funny story to relate – with regard to collecting for our charity. As well as collecting under our own name, for ten years, we also collected for the Alexandra Rose Charity – and we were allowed to keep ninety per cent of the proceeds!

It was on the occasion, that England thrashed Denmark – in the quarter finals of the World Cup. I was collecting outside Wokingham Station, and not doing very well, so I decided to take my tray of roses into the pub – which was jubilant with victory. There was quite a carnival atmosphere.

'Roses for England', I announced! 'Come over 'ere, darling!' was the response. Five pound notes, and ten pound notes went into my collecting box. I had never, before, done so well at a single collection!

We have a number of benefactors who make regular, monthly, payments into the charity account. These include Shirley, Hope, Dennis, Chris, Tony H., Tony W., and Doreen. Tony H. has also given extremely generous donations, over the years. In fact, dozens of individuals, and organizations, have supported us financially, and thus enabled us to continue with our valuable service, in the absence of what was inadequate, and is now, non existent, statutory funding.

Chapter 31

The Gillian Homer Legacy

I have always been blessed with a great sense of humour, so it never fails to amuse me, that the two most important letters, ever to arrive at the crisis house, were opened, with my authorization, by the cleaner!

I had asked the cleaner to open any mail that arrived in my absence, and to telephone me, if there was anything of importance. Thus did I learn, that we were to receive the Queen's Award for Voluntary Service!

On the second occasion, I received a telephone call – asking me whether I knew a Gillian Homer. I did not. 'Well here is a solicitor's letter – explaining that she has died, and left half of her estate, to the crisis house.' Since this legacy included both property and money, and since, for years, we had scraped by, on six thousand pounds a year, this news changed our circumstances completely.

It could not have been better timed. We received Gillian Homer's legacy in 2009 - at exactly the same time that the local authority axed funding, for all small, local voluntary organizations. So this money has enabled us to continue running our services, and also to carry out much needed refurbishment of the Crisis House.

Chapter 32

Investing In The Young Students At The Crisis House

'The Young Ones: 'Live, love, while the flame is strong – for we won't be the young ones very long!'

On 8th June 2015, we held an Open Day at the crisis house – to declare 'Open' our memorial garden – in memory of our late volunteer, Frances Rowley, and for people to see all our improvements and refurbishments.

One who attended the Open Day, was the Student Placement Officer, from Reading University. I explained to her that her students – who are second year psychology undergraduates – do our service users good, just by walking through the door!

All our service users have severe problems in life, and, many are, in addition, elderly, suffering from physical, as well as, mental, problems, and are battered, damaged, and disillusioned, by life.

For them to see twenty-year-olds – bright, beautiful, innocent, and unaware of what life might do to them – provides instant therapy, and warms their old bones!

Over the years, we have welcomed nursing, social care, counselling, psychology, and psychotherapy, students. Here, I shall mention a few of them.

Myles was a counselling student who was taking the same course as Knick-Knack. There could be no greater contrast between them. Myles was very together, and had an empathetic, and pleasant approach to our service users – with whom he was very popular.

He came to our rescue for a short time, because he was able to drive the minibus while we had a hiatus period, between our first driver dying suddenly, and Rob taking over long-term.

Unlike Knick-Knack, Myles moved on from us, to take up a counselling post with drug-addicts – at which he was successful. They had the same piece of paper, but Myles also had all the other qualities needed to make a successful counsellor – the supreme of which, is that you are there to listen to the client's problems, and not to burden him with your own!

I have long held the view that one either is, or, is not, a nurse, or a teacher. You can't create one through training. Training is certainly needed, but the basic ability must be innate. I suspect that the same holds true for counsellors.

In 2001, Amy Taylor joined us from Reading University. She was taking an undergraduate degree in psychology, and wanted to train as a clinical psychologist.

Amy fitted in very well, and was popular with our service users. One service user, Steven, became besotted with her. He suffered from learning disabilities, and schizophrenia, and had physical handicaps as well. Amy, by contrast, was blonde, bright, beautiful, and shining with health – Quasimodo and Esmeralda!

Despite her youth, Amy handled the situation well. She was kind and polite to Steven, accepting his gift of flowers, and not becoming fazed by the situation.

There is enormous competition for places in the NHS Clinical Psychology Training Programme – with only one in five hundred applicants being accepted. Amy was well aware of this.

I suggested, that, as a second string, if she was not accepted for clinical psychology training, she might take a Post Graduate Certificate in Special Education, and thus use her psychology – teaching emotionally, and behaviourally disordered, children in special schools.

My advice, though sound, wasn't needed. Amy obtained a first class honours degree in psychology, and was accepted for the NHS Clinical Training by a local health authority.

Hope Clayton came to us in the summer of 2011, and has been in touch with us ever since.

Never was anyone more appropriately named. Young, slim, blonde, beautiful, Hope radiates all that gives one hope in life. She spent the summer vacation volunteering in the crisis house – returning to Cardiff to complete her undergraduate degree in the Autumn.

Again, it was a case of 'What next?' Hope went on to complete a Masters Degree, but, by the summer of 2013, it was the same old story. 'You have an excellent CV, and there is nothing wrong with your application, but we have received five hundred applications for one post, so we are only considering people who already have some experience', a prospective employer would say. How to get that experience?

Finally, in the Autumn of 2013, Hope was offered a Health Psychology Training Place – in Aberdeen! She accepted, and has completed this training, but visits the crisis house whenever she is able to get down to Wokingham.

Dal was with us during 2015, and she is a post graduate psychotherapy student – already having five clients of her own - whilst completing her theoretical training.

Dal fitted in extremely well, and was very popular with our service users. Perhaps we have been lucky with our students. All have been pleasant. We have never experienced any problems with any of them, not even with Knick-Knack, and, unlike some placement organizations, we do not exploit them – using them as free labour.

Our value to them, is the opportunity that we provide for them, to get day-to-day experience of the full range of mental illnesses - by simply mixing, and talking with our service users.

Bearing in mind that I rarely hear anything but criticism of practising mental health professionals, I conclude that our students are in a state of grace. The harsh realities of life – its cruelty, its unfairness, its betrayal, have not yet touched them This being the case, I even point out to their

Placement Officer that the crisis house is the light end of mental health.

We are a self-help organization, so we are largely well-behaved, co-operative, and self-motivated. If a student goes from a placement with us, to a placement on a dementia ward, for instance, then they may be faced with some of the harsher realities of life, so they may as well enjoy the lighter side of mental health while they can! 'Live, love, while the flame is strong, for we won't be the young ones very long!'

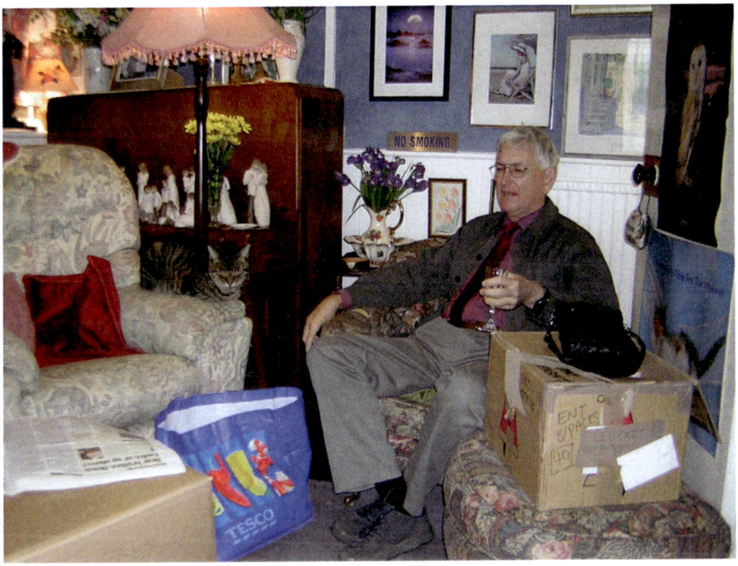

Good old Tony - Benefactor and supporter - for nearly forty years!

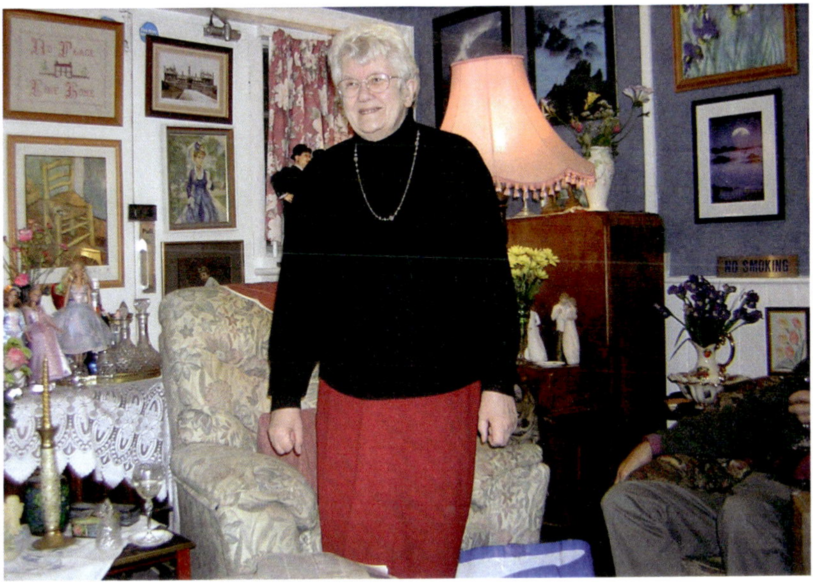

Frances - our all time most popular volunteer!

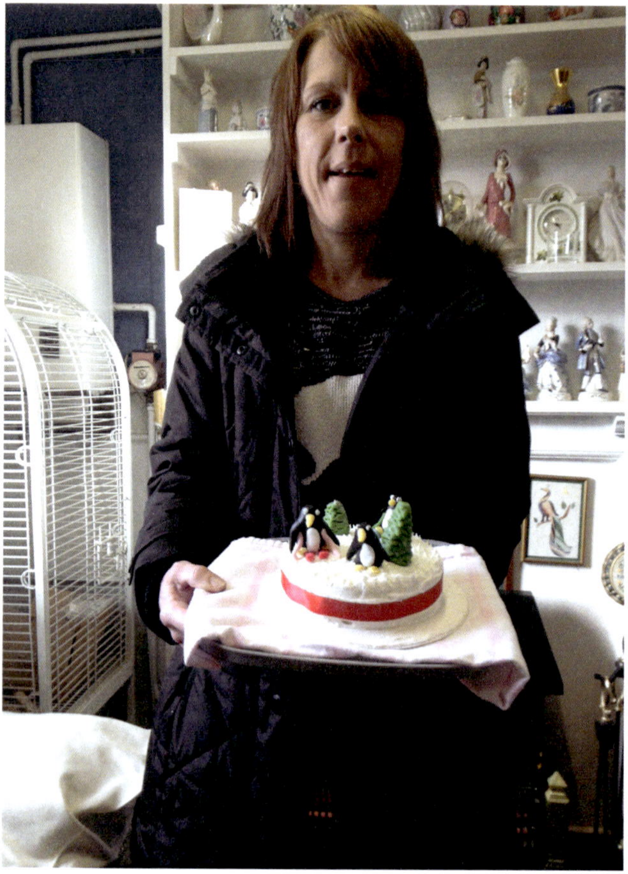

Kerry with her Christmas cake!

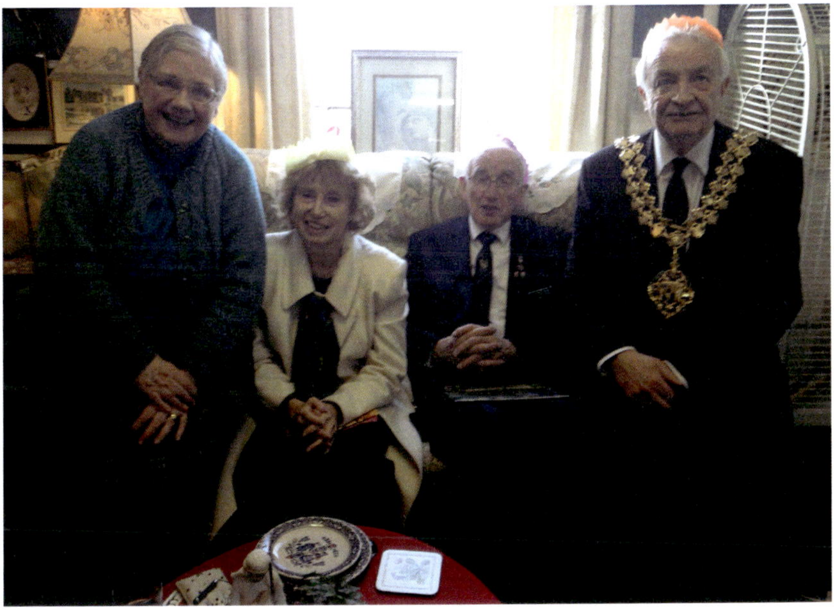

Pam - with the Mayoress, the Mayor's Attendant
and the Town Mayor!

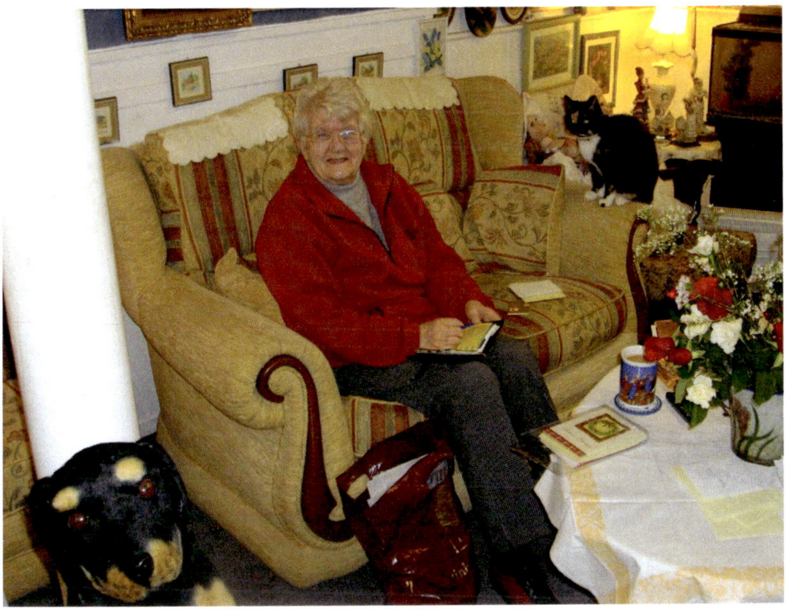

Frances - with Chloé, the cat

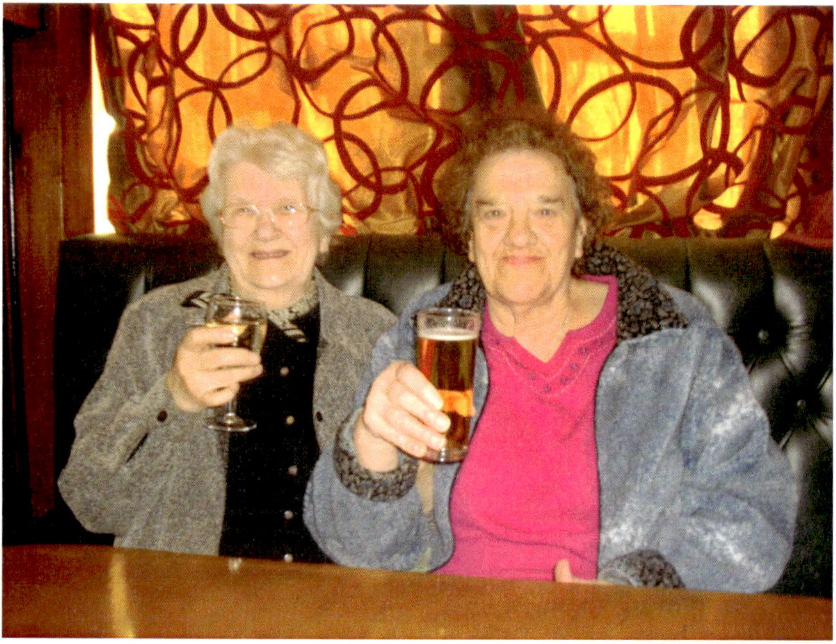

Befriender and Befriended! Frances and Joyce

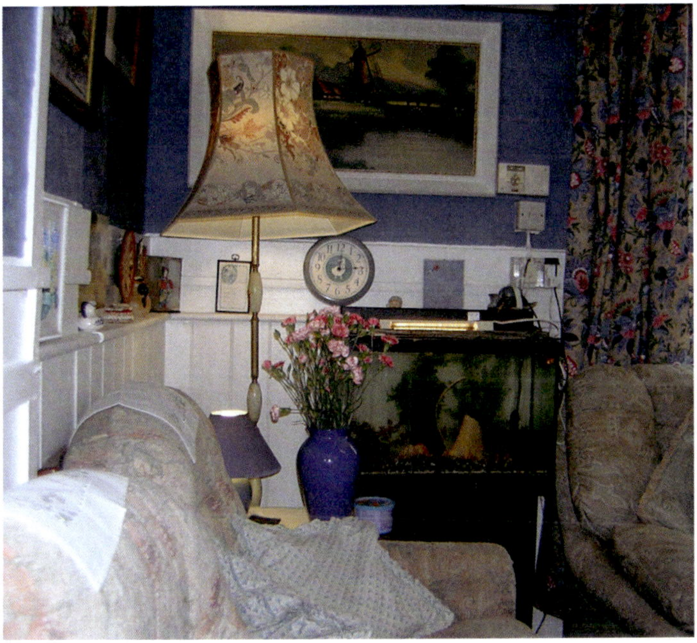

The Crisis House Lounge

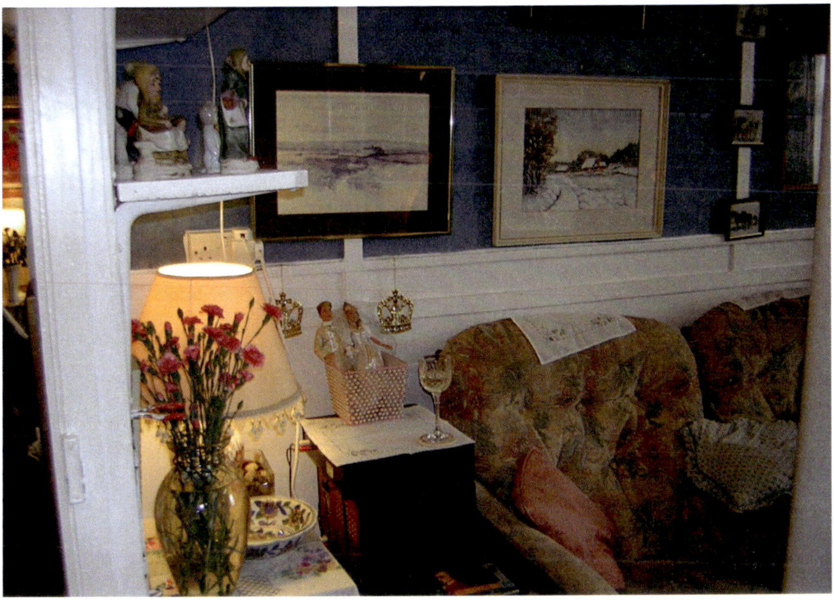

PART FOUR

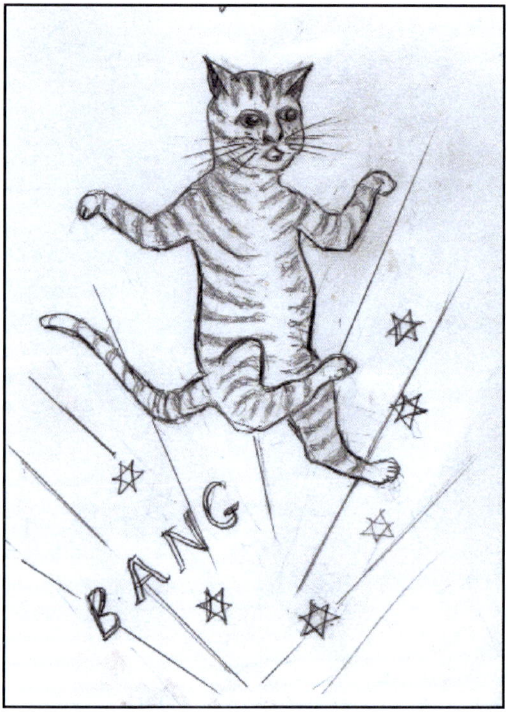

'Blew Him Up With Dynamite,
But Him They Could Not Kill'

The Battle For The Crisis House

Chapter 33

Fight The Good Fight

From the day that we walked through the door of the crisis house in March 1991, I knew that the mental health establishment would try to destroy us, but I was quite determined that they would not do so, and they haven't!

But we have had to fight! Once again, fighting for the crisis house, I shared some of the characteristics of Miss Bulstrode, Head Mistress of Meadow Bank School. When she was fighting for the survival of her school, 'She sat, cool and unmoved, with her life work falling in ruins about her.' At the time, I also shared Miss Bulstrode's belief, that my crisis house, like her school, was important in itself, and not just to me!

The most determined attempt at destruction, commenced on Valentine's Day – 14th February 2007. This was a Wednesday, when the drop-in centre does not open, so I received the telephone call at home. The Council Property Department needed an urgent meeting with us.

The meeting revealed that the Molly Millar pub – whose electricity supply we shared – wanted us to have a separate supply – because sharing overloaded their system. The Council was not willing to pay to lay a new cable, and so were closing down the crisis house in a week!

To say that we were dumb-founded, understates it. Even our Lease allowed us six months' notice. At the time, we had two mentally ill guests in residence, and a large number of vulnerable people who attended the drop-in centre regularly – to say nothing of our precious, and much loved, animals!

This particular lease, had only been issued the previous August, and our excellent solicitor, Ian Graham, from Clifton Ingrams, had actually suggested a six month, rather than the usual three month, break clause – precisely because vulnerable people need more time to prepare for change – than do people in full health. Bitter/sweet, irony, is it not – that the solicitor – who is not a mental health professional, has a better grasp of the needs of mentally ill people, than do the people who dare to call themselves mental health professionals?

We had an excellent friend, Ally Goodwin, who remonstrated with the property department, and who also found out that the brewery who owned the pub, had promised not to disconnect our electricity supply whilst vulnerable people were still using the premises – so there was no need for an immediate exit. We could have our six months.

We reached the inevitable conclusion that an attempt had been made to rush us out of the property, before we had a chance to consider all the ramifications.

I confess that there had, in the past, been times, when I wondered whether all the work that I put into the crisis house environment – the animals, the pictures, the embroidery, the comfortable furniture, were really appreciated. I need not have had such qualms!

The protest was seismic. 'We don't want to go to some miserable, cold, old hall, and sit on plastic chairs – staring at a bare wall! We want the animals! We want the fresh flowers! We want pictures! We want ornaments!' I reached the conclusion then - that there was not a stitch, nor a bloom, nor an artifact, nor a living thing, in the place - that had not been duly noted, and appreciated by our service users – a most affecting revelation for me!

I recall an amusing occasion, in our very early days, when the 'irate' social worker visited the crisis house, with someone, whom I presumed to be, a social work colleague. I showed them round – pointing out all the features that had been included, in order to promote mental health. This, you will recall, was the irate social worker, who claimed that 'crisis intervention is a very highly skilled branch of social work' – very highly skilled, my Aunt Fanny!

It transpired that the colleague was the then, County Solicitor, who was after me, for libelling the Social Services. I would have claimed 'fair comment', but the crisis house disarmed him, and he wrote, 'A very lovely place'. In the Visitors' Book.

Chapter 34

Outright Battle

At the time, we also had an excellent publicist, Ernest. He had experience of campaigning, and was able to get our cause highlighted by local radio, and television.

I have a vivid memory of the reaction of the television presenter. He walked into the crisis house, cast an eye over it, and then declared, 'I have seen lots of mental health facilities, and this place is immaculate!' He then stormed up to the Council offices to tell them so.

So the Council caved in – allowing us the six months' notice that we were entitled to, under the terms of our lease. Throughout this awful time, the excellent Ian Graham, gave us free legal advice and representation. The local Press was also excellent – with coverage every week, throughout the duration of the affair. Once we had six months, we got cracking on fund-raising – making enough money to supply our own cable and meter.

Our marvellous Patron, Lady Elizabeth Godsal, and her late husband, Alan Godsal, donated money from their Family Charitable Trust, to bring our fire safety system up to standard. So once the six months had elapsed, the building would be up to scratch, and there was no reason why we could not continue to occupy it. Or so one would think!

I would like to put in a word, here, in tribute to the late Alan Godsal. As we battled against the powers that be, I reached the conclusion that he was the ONLY person outside our own ranks, who could see what they were up to. He was the only one who saw things exactly as I saw them myself. How wonderful to have such a distinguished ally, a former High Sheriff of the County, on our side, and he, certainly, saved the crisis house from destruction.

We had not bargained for the local Social Services' employee. We had already experienced an attempt on her part to stop the local authority funding for the crisis house – in the summer of 2004.

She tried to pretend that our service had problems, but was defeated by facts. The facts, then, were that we, over the years, had won two top Mind Awards, a Department of Health Voluntary Sector Award, five local Civic Awards, and the Queen's Award for Voluntary Service. We pointed out to her, that these august people, do have other groups, hundreds of them, from which to choose! Why do they always choose us?

Now she was clutching at straws! She had convinced herself that the crisis house was closing down, and, discovering that we had the money, and were, consequently, able to get all the necessary work done, she simply flipped. She couldn't take it! She could not accept that we were to remain open.

I received her telephone call first thing in the morning of a July Friday, in 2007. She had been told that we had the money the previous evening, and had, evidently, hatched her plot the night before, and could not wait to put it into operation. She said that we were not to spend our money on the necessary improvements - because the council might be closing down the crisis house anyway – due to a number of complaints which they had received about us.

We knew about the one complaint. It had been submitted, the previous February, by the notorious Gabriela Rani. We had known Gabriela for fifteen years, and, in that time, she had caused serious trouble in every one of the twenty places where she had lived, and in every one of the places where she had worked!

One of our service-users reported to us at the time, that he had seen Gabriela Rani, sitting in a local pub, and trying to devise a plot to 'Get Pam out of Station House'. The welfare of users who needed our services, did not enter the equation – which was purely vindictive.

The Social Services' employee was unable to explain why she had waited six months to address this one complaint – since it raised concerns about the well-being of vulnerable people, and why one complainant had now increased into eight! Did they reproduce asexually by splitting?

The Social Services' employee had been hoping to present the thing anonymously on the grounds of protecting the complainants from our reprisals! But she could not do this, because we knew the people. Her real reason for the proposed secrecy, was that she knew that we knew, and that everybody else, knew, that Gabriela Rani was not a credible witness. In fact, she was a sad character, basking in her one moment of glory, and never for one moment suspecting, that she was being used!

This situation has echoes in the current 'abuse' bandwagon. Yes, it is about money, but it is also about being important, being in the limelight – for the first time in your life!

Gabriela had bullied some acquaintances, who suffered from learning disabilities, to add to her main complaint. We were able to give evidence that these people had never used our services, and did not, indeed, qualify for them.

As recently as September 2015, I have had to explain to a service user with learning disabilities, that, though he is welcome to drop-in for a cup of tea, he is not allowed to use our service all day long.

The reason is, that we do not cater for learning disabilities, we do not understand learning disabilities, and that such service users would take up a disproportionate amount of our attention - at the expense of service users with mental health problems.

We gave the council a detailed history of Gabriela's long record of physical violence, and the case against us collapsed.

Furthermore, the only reprisal that I could possibly make, was the one that I went on to make, that is, to prevent any malicious complainant, from further use of our services – thus meaning that they would have to rely on those provided by the main-stream. I consider that to be the greatest reprisal that I could inflict, but I could hardly expect the main-stream providers to agree!

At least, they could hardly come out and say so. Furthermore, professionals do not take on board that – with the adult freedoms – go the adult responsibilities. They intended to destroy the crisis house, but, if they failed, it did not occur to them to warn Gabriela Rani, that she would never be allowed to use our services again, and, sure enough, in due course, she turned up at the crisis house drop-in – only to have the door slammed in her face!

'Oh, she wailed, I was terribly ill then!' Her pleas fell on deaf ears.

Her cousin, Melville Rani, attends our drop-in, because he suffers from depression. He confirms that Gabriela is as mad as a hatter, and she, most certainly, does need a mental health service, but it's not going to be ours!

Although I considered Myles to have good potential as a counsellor, he, nevertheless, adopted similar thinking, and a similar stratagem - when trying to get Jeanette back into our ranks, after she tried to destroy us – when grief-stricken for the loss of her [imaginary] lover. This is the view that so many professionals, [Myles being a trainee professional], take.

The client is a child - not responsible for his actions. Not with us, he isn't. As Agatha Christie would have it, he has taken what he wanted, and is paying, says God!

It simply isn't on - to try to destroy a service, and then think that you can access it again, once you have recovered your temper. That is what small children do. The facts are, that if you burn a house down when you are mentally ill, then the house is burned down! Due to mental illness, your responsibility may be diminished, but the house is still burned down! It is no longer there for you to live in!

I recall that, in our early days, we had banned one particularly difficult service user – who had been in flagrant and persistent breach of our rules. A visiting Police Officer said, 'You would not be able to do that if you were Social Services'. All the more reason for not being, and what is the point of having rules, if one fails to enforce them?

Chapter 35

We'll Keep Self-Help Flags Flying Here

When the crisis house was under threat of closure, the then Leader of the Council visited, at our invitation. We wanted him to see what they were proposing to throw away.

He had read the Social Services employee's Report, and was, no doubt, expecting to find an appalling place: instead, he found an excellent one. 'But it looks good', he said. 'Of course it's good, I replied That's why she wants to close it down!'

I think that what so infuriates the mental health establishment, is the fact that our services are very valuable, and completely outside of their control. If our services were tenth rate, they would not mind so much – because such things tend to fizzle out anyway. Things that are excellent, and last, they perceive to be a threat.

In our battle, what the Social Services' employee, and the Council, did not bargain for - was the strength of the resistance. This came from all fronts - not just from our own service users, but from the wider community as well.

Faced with overwhelming resistance, the council had to give in. You have to laugh. This Social Services employee was in receipt of a salary of one hundred thousand pounds a year – out of the tax payers' money! 'She's not worth a hundred thousand pounds!' protested one of our trustees. To me, she wasn't worth tuppence! Don't pay them more, to try to improve things. Get rid of them.

This is the thing that these 'professionals' never acknowledge. When this Social Services' employee came to the crisis house in the summer of 2004, pretending that we had problems, and I told her that she was a load of rubbish to her face, her reply was, 'But you want our money!' 'It's not your money, I retorted, it's Council tax.' It is not THEIR money. It is OUR money!

Chapter 36

Victory - 'The Dog It Was That Died'

Magnanimous in victory, we agreed to attend a Council Training Course, as a face saver for them. It is good psychology, once you have won, not to leave your defeated enemy too angry. If they are 'training' you, then they can deceive themselves that they are superior to you, and thus have power over you!

One has to laugh. This course was suitable for basic grade care assistants, in care homes, and bore no relation to any of the work that the crisis house does. In fact, we remained as separatist as ever. Within a year of our victory, the Social Services' employee died very suddenly.

My sympathies have always been reserved for the many people who would have suffered, if our services had been destroyed by her. As I have mentioned elsewhere, the one thing that is never taken into consideration in these power struggles, is the welfare of the people for whom the services are set up! Society should restore social welfare to volunteers – with no other motivation than the desire to do good! Then the services would be sustainable.

Always analytical, I remain interested as to why the voluntary sector, when it is genuinely voluntary, is so much disliked by the so-called 'professional' services. I have reached the conclusion that it is because they are not 'professional' at all! With the exception of the medical people, they are claiming to have a specialist knowledge which they do not have. All their stuff is opinion, and, when it comes to opinion, yours, is as good as mine.

After two decades of constant harassment by the mental health establishment – either to join them, or to be destroyed by them – we have now experienced almost a whole third decade - with no harassment whatsoever. This might be because we are now totally self-funding, or it might be that people are superstitious! Perhaps they fear going the same way. 'The dog it was that died!'

Now, late in 2015, all Wokingham Council properties, including the crisis house, are coming up, once again, for a suitability assessment. It is highly unlikely that Crisis House will be found to be deficient, because we had a complete survey of the property done, as recently as 2007. We have already undertaken the minor improvements deemed necessary as a result of this survey. But the difference now, is that if major improvements need to be made, at least we have the money!

We have been told that all their properties are being thus reviewed, so I don't think that this is yet another, latter day, attempt to destroy us. If it is, we will win, as we did before, and they would do well to take note of the fact that, 'The dog it was that died!'

Chapter 37

Closing The Beds

Few decisions are made on the spur of the moment. Rather, they are made gradually – various strands coming together to make a whole – and then the decision can be made.

As soon as we were offered the Crisis House – which had been, in earlier times, a Victorian dwelling house, with bedrooms – I was quite adamant that, once we took possession, we were going to provide mental health beds there.

As I explained to an early visitor to the crisis house, a social worker from the mental health team, 'I have just been waiting to get my hands on a house'. 'Well, you certainly have your hands on this one', he replied, very impressed by our homely ambience, but not totally sympathetic, to my separatist stance!

Why was I so adamant? As I explained earlier, such passion can only be stimulated by personal experience. The following is my personal experience!

My younger brother and sister had both been diagnosed with schizophrenia in their mid-teens. My father's death coincided with the time of their breakdowns. In the natural order of things, one by one, we other siblings, left home for college, to marry, or to set up homes for ourselves.

As is commonly the case, my widowed mother was then left with the two mentally ill adult offspring, and, for some years, things jogged along not too badly. Not too badly, from my mother's point of view, that is. It was certainly not a life that I would accept, but she had always had a hard life, had always been too inadequate to cope, and so expected very little.

When undertaking some Post Graduate training at London University's Institute of Education, I encountered a very dedicated headmaster, who ran a school in a very deprived area. He maintained that the families whom he served were 'Blown about by life', and, unlike better off people, were not used to living in a routine way.

His mission was to enable them to acquire as many skills as possible. One of his families were Maltese, and were skilled in making lace. He got them to teach this to his pupils. I couldn't have agreed with him more. Once you have a skill, you cease to be an inadequate. Did he have more money and resources than other headmasters? No, more dedication.

Why was he so dedicated to deprived children and their families? Because he came from a deprived background himself, of course. I can assure my readers that one does not wake up one day, and say to oneself, 'For the rest of my life I am going to devote myself to the welfare of a remote tribe of native indians who live on a island in the southern seas!'

Dedication always springs from a personal motivation – even if some people, unlike me, prefer to take the professional route in order to deliver service to the cause to which they are dedicated!

'Blown about by life' would describe my mother perfectly. She never saw any way out of her adverse circumstances. No doubt that is why the four of her six children, who were well enough to do so, all did brilliantly.

My elder sister, Valerie, for instance, who started with no advantages whatsoever, achieved, through sheer graft, the position of Legal Secretary to the Queen's Solicitor, at Lincoln's Inn Fields.

Then there was little Jimmy, the youngest, the runt of the litter!

I can barely describe to you, you little runt, how much I admire the success that you have made of your life!

Brilliantly successful in business, he has, from early youth, made loads of money. He owns a big, six bedroom house, with its own swimming pool, and can afford to employ paid help in the house. Wow, what a success!

Another brother, Robert, also did very well in his career as an accountant. This book describes my own achievements!

We knew that we had to make our own way in life, and we did.

One day, when visiting my mother, I noticed that she was looking very old and tired. She was now approaching seventy, and I was thirty-two. So I decided that the time had come for me to assume responsibility for my brother and sister – in order to relieve my mother – since she was now getting old.

At seventeen, I did not want to take on the responsibility for my family. I wanted to be a teenager, and enjoy myself. Shakespeare, in his play, 'Twelfth Night'. describes perfectly, my feelings about my family situation, at the age of seventeen:

'O time, thou must untangle this, not I, it is too hard a knot, for me to untie.'

Time, certainly did, untangle it, and, at thirty-two, I was happy to accept responsibility. But even when such is the case, I come back to my eternal theme, about the Social Services, and their deficiencies. They always want to pile all the responsibilities for the mentally ill – onto their relatives. What do they think that THEY are there for, and why are we paying them?

You won't ever change my opinion. I sussed them out in the nineteen -sixties. They intrude into your home. They write a report on you and your family – all of which is their opinion, and not based upon objective facts, and is, in any case, of no use to anybody whatsoever. And then they leave you to it! Your situation remains exactly as it was before. They have done nothing to improve things. Wake up, society, and get rid of them!

My first step was to find my family better accommodation. They were, at that time, still living in the old, Victorian, house, in which we had grown up. It was in need of extensive modernization which they could not afford. So, very quickly, I got them all into a nice council house with all the modern conveniences. Oh, wonderful days of the past - when one could do just that!

You have been waiting for it, and yes, there is a funny story connected with this move. Firstly, I took my mother to see the house – just the two of us, together. I was perplexed to see that she was hedging. It was to be such a step up for them, that I was baffled.

Incredible, when you consider that the house was freshly decorated – it was still the days when councils provided a choice of wallpapers, and decorated as soon as the former tenants moved out – so that it was all clean, and fresh, for the incoming tenants!

It had a nice bathroom and a separate, indoor, toilet. The old house had neither of these. It had central heating. There was only one flight of stairs to negotiate. The old house had two. The rooms were good sized. There were communal gardens, and the council paid the gardener! The old house had big gardens – which my mother, brother, and sister, were incapable of keeping in trim.

Determined not to lose the opportunity, I roped in an old uncle, my mother's brother, to support me. My mother, like many in her generation, was named 'Florence' – after Florence Nightingale.

'Florrie, he remonstrated, this place is a palace compared with where you are living!' So we won. Why was my mother hedging? Because, for decades, she had treasured a fantasy that, one day, she would have a dream home. It wasn't going to happen, but the fantasy persisted. If she accepted this new house, better than before, but not fulfilling her dreams, then the fantasy would be destroyed!

I have experienced similar situations in the crisis house. There is an unwillingness to move on, into a better, but nevertheless, realistic, situation, because, then, you have to stop dreaming!

This move worked out fine for my mother and sister, but not for my brother. The old Victorian house had three storeys, and lots of space. He could walk around – muttering to himself – without bothering anybody. Not so, in the modern council house, with its paper-thin walls. So there was a lot of friction, and some violent incidents. Evidently, I needed to think things out again.

I approached the council – explaining the problem – and suggesting that we exchanged the three-bedroom house, for a two-bedroom flat, for my mother and sister, and a separate one-bedroom flat for my brother.

'Oh, no, was their reply. If you relinquish the house, you can only have one flat, in exchange.' What to do? My mother's health was now deteriorating fast, and I thought that the continued strain of coping with my brother, would probably kill her, so I decided to accept the two-bedroom flat for my mother and sister, and then to sort out my brother's accommodation separately.

So my mother and sister moved into a lovely flat, with total success, and my mother's health started to improve immediately. We even got her to take a holiday in a little cottage in Cornwall, and I encouraged both my mother, and my sister, to go on some 'Away Day' excursions, by rail, something that they had not done before.

My brother had used up a lot of their [very limited], finances – a very common situation when adult, mentally ill offspring, remain living with a widowed mother. I visibly wince at some of the situations that people live with. Freed from this, my mother said, 'Now we can afford to have fruit, and sweets'. I did wince at this revelation.

Fenella Bewley was the same. [Chapter 14: 'Everybody's problems but her own'.] Fenella never had any new clothes. Her limited income was all used up by her son.

Now, for my brother, Richard's situation. Local housing authorities move extremely slowly, so he was able to go on living in the house for a year, before they decided to change the locks – in preparation for moving another family in.

Nevertheless, the day for changing the locks, arrived eventually – as inevitably as tomorrow succeeds today! I told my brother that I would meet him at a little café, and then go with him to the Homelessness Section of the council – in order to secure him accommodation. So vividly is that day etched in my memory, that, although it was thirty-three years ago, I remember what I was wearing. It was a chalk-white Courreges coat – with a fine, grey stripe.

Busy doing nothing

'We're busy doin' nothin'
Workin' the whole day through
Tryin' to find lots of things not to do
We're busy goin' nowhere
Isn't it just a crime
We'd like to be unhappy, but
We never do have the time'

At nine a.m. we had coffee in the little café, and then set out. We went to the Homelessness Section of the Council, the Council Housing Department, the [then] DHSS, a hostel for the homeless, a charity for the homeless – you name it, we went there!

One and all – they provided us with nothing! At 5.30pm, we ended up back at the café – with nothing, zilch! I think that I was bewildered. I had never approached welfare services for anything, so I was bemused, that you could have all these people paid to do nothing! 'Busy Doin' Nothin' understates it! Decades on, and in a different county, nothing has changed!

Because of this experience, I always make a point, at the crisis house, of doing SOMETHING! It might only be giving somebody a small amount of money for electricity, or sending a befriender with them to the food bank, but I have determined, in our twenty-five years, that I wil never send anyone away with nothing!

'You are not going on the street, I said to my brother. We'll go back to the house, break the locks, and you will stay there until they house you.' Back we went.

I was just about to attack the lock with my steel umbrella tip, when a small boy appeared. 'You locked out, miss?' he said. Then his small hand shot through the letter-box, he turned the lock from inside, and in we went. 'Good boy', I said. My brother stayed in that house for a second year!

Finally, the great day came. It never rains but it pours. Evidently, my brother had reached the top of the local authority housing list.

Our twenty-first century equivalent, here in Wokingham, is the case of Glyn. In August 2015, after a wait of five and a half years, he has, finally, secured the tenancy, for a council flat!

My brother telephoned to say that he was being offered, either a one-bedroom flat, or a place in a shared house. What should he do? 'Take the flat with both hands, I advised. In a shared house, you have to liaise with other people, but a flat is your own, precious, place.' He took the flat – which was close to the rest of the family, but gave him the space, and the privacy, that he needed, and so this worked out fine as well.

I have reached the conclusion, after decades of experience, that schizophrenia is, very much, a condition of youth. When young, its sufferers seem to be so disadvantaged, compared with their healthy counterparts. Their relatives are desperate, seeing no hope for their future, while everybody else is doing so well!

Come middle age, settled in their flats, coping with daily life, and doing as well as they can, their life then, is not so different from everybody else's!

By then, the splendid marriages, with the full white works, have, frequently, ended in divorce. Einstein wasn't Einstein after all – only Fred Bloggs! The schizophrenic may not have had children, but he certainly does not envy Fred Bloggs his delinquent ones!

Then, come Autumn years, 'the creaking gate' scarcely describes the situation! As youngsters, we had a neighbour, Michael, who was always the life and soul of the party; he was in charge of the bar at my youngest brother's wedding.

Had you told me, in the nineteen-sixties, that our sister, Joan, would outlive our neighbour, Michael, I would have laughed in your face. Unfortunately, Michael died of a heart attack – aged only sixty-two. Joan is still plodding on – aged sixty-eight! Age – the great leveller!

Another of my brothers – I have three in all, and two sisters - agrees with me. This brother, Robert, who has always been very supportive of the crisis house, asserted that my sister, Joan, actually kept her flat in a better state than did a friend of his.

His friend was not mentally ill, but, after divorce, didn't bother with things, and let his house go to pot!

By contrast, although the schizophrenia sufferer needs the family to set them up, they can actually cope quite well, once this has been done.

My mother died, and, since I now had my brother, and my sister settled successfully, we were now free to move over to Berkshire, my husband's native county.

My experience taught me how vital it is for mentally ill people to have temporary accommodation available to them – while permanent accommodation is being arranged. This was why I was so determined to have the beds in the crisis house. In fact, we set up the first sanctuary bedroom on the very day that we took over the Crisis House, twenty-five years ago.

Three months had elapsed, and our beds were established, when an irate social worker from the local mental health team, turned up at the crisis house door. I did listen to his opinions – though – as a mental health 'professional' – he was banned from the Association – so these opinions were academic, and the conversation was conducted at the front door, because I did not invite him in.

I may complain about the inefficiencies of statutory services, but, at the same time, I am very much in the position of Agatha Christie's character, Vivian Dubois. I have profited from their incompetence!

Vivian Dubois was having an affair with Adèle Fortesque, and he was annoyed. 'He tore Adèle Fortesque's letter angrily across, and threw it into the waste-paper basket. 'Why have women got to be such damned fools? Surely common prudence...' But then Mr Dubois reflected gloomily, women never had any prudence. Though he had profited by this lack many a time, it annoyed him now.' Agatha Christie: 'A Pocket Full of Rye'. [Published: Collins: 1953.]

Had statutory services been thoroughly efficient, they would have established, before giving us the original lease and funding, for the crisis house, the basis on which we intended to operate. Once we were up and running, and successful, changing anything, became much more difficult, and they failed to do so.

The social worker said, 'You are stupid to think that you can run a crisis house with no professional support at all. Crisis intervention, he claimed, is a very highly skilled branch of social work!' Very highly skilled, my Aunt Fanny! Since social work isn't anything, other than opinion, you can't have a skilled branch of it!

'The hospital will dump people on you, and you will have suicides.' While he was ranting, I thought, wryly, of the 'very highly skilled crisis intervention', that my brother and I had received. Far from being highly skilled, it was non-existent!

I was intrigued to note that this social worker appeared to assume, that I would not be versed in the simple art of saying, 'No'. If I ever believe us incapable of providing a service, I always say so, and this refusal to take on things with which we cannot cope, has always stood us, in good stead, over our twenty-five years. It has also been a major source of annoyance, for Social Services!

At the same time, it is totally dependent upon our separatist stance. I consider it very dangerous, for one group of people, the referrers, to have any power over another group of people, the providers. While those who provide the service, decide who should use it, a service can be run appropriately, and safely, as ours always has been.

We are very safety-conscious. I recall an incident, when the Head of Social Services, had occasion to call in at the crisis house. This was the one who wrung his hands when we declined to have a partnership with him.

On this occasion, he told me that I had put community care back by twenty-five years. Why? Because I had complained to the local Press, that a known mentally ill arsonist was to be placed in some new supported flats, close to local schools, and to which one of our successful crisis house graduates, Jack Hayward, had just moved.

He maintained that this man was all right now that he had been back in hospital, and had been re-established on medication. Did the idiot think that, having failed to take his medication previously, he would not do so, once again, living unsupervised in the community? Known arsonists need to be placed in 24/7 supervised accommodation – indefinitely.

Had this man gone into those flats, and set fire to them, then HE would have put community care back by twenty-five years, and would thus have prejudiced the chance of Jack Hayward to make a success of the placement. Eighteen years on, Jack is still making a success of it!

I thought that I would treat this Head of Social Services to a bit of psychology, himself, so I said, 'The best predictor of future behaviour, is past behaviour'. That is just the point, is it not? If a referrer wants you to take someone, and fails to reveal the full history of past behaviour – fearing that you won't accept the person, if you know the truth, then that is very dangerous.

It is essential to know the person's history, but, even then, risk assessments only give a rough guide. Mental health never was, and never will be, totally predictable. The best that one can do, in a crisis house, is to eliminate obvious dangers, to be firm in refusal, and refuse to continue with an individual, if concerns as to their safety, arise.

We never took on dangerous people. They need nursing, or, at least, detention.

In ninety-nine cases out of a hundred, the people whom we did accept, didn't need 'very highly skilled intervention', even if such were possible, which it isn't. So often, they needed simple, practical, things – such as a roof over their head, some clean clothes, a hot bath, a hot meal. This is why organizations like the Salvation Army, are so marvellous, because they meet people's basic, and practical, needs.

I sent all the social workers about their business. I don't believe in social work, I believe in self-help. Their stuff is not a profession. It is opinion – in which case, my opinion is as good as theirs! I was adamant that we were to retain the beds, and, for twenty years, the service was very successful.

Certainly, the hospital and other referrers did try to dump people on us, but we did not accept unsuitable referrals, and if one proved unsuitable, we sent the person back to their referrer. Certainly, we had guests with suicidal ideation, and we prevented numerous suicides by intervening in their crisis, and giving them hope for the future.

The annual two thousand pounds, which we received from the local mental health budget, ceased in 2007. We continued to receive the tiny grant for our day service, but this was not adequate to fund the beds, so we had to close them down. All statutory funding, for all local small charities, ceased in 2010, so it was only the Gillian Homer Legacy that enabled us to continue at all.

The loss of funding was, however, only one strand, in the whole thread that leads one to make a major decision. There was also my advancing age, and the fact that move-on accommodation was becoming more difficult to obtain with every year that passed.

When we set up the crisis house in 1991, with their mental health priority, any guest who wanted a council flat - when their immediate crisis was resolved, could get one, within weeks. Then the weeks became months. Then the months became years. The current time, on the council housing waiting list for a single person, is seventeen years!

So the various strands came together, and led to our decision for closure. Instead, we now use money from our legacy pot, to fund temporary accommodation for people who – in the past- would have accessed a crisis house bed.

Awards: 1996 - 2016

Chapter 38

You Can Win 'em All

'The judges will decide, the likes of me abide.
A big thing, or a small. The winner takes it all.'

The years 1996 to 2016 were our Award winning years. They started with us winning the MIND Awards - instituted to celebrate their fiftieth anniversary. One was for running the best crisis service, and a second was for making community care work on a shoe-string.

The Mind awards

By 1996, the crisis house had already been in successful operation for five years, and had not, as I am sure that the local mental health establishment had predicted, suffered some terrible occurrence, and thus – either had to close down – or submit to professional interference.

So they started trumping up complaints. These provoked a visit from MIND's Regional Director. When he arrived, for the first time at the crisis house, of course he was impressed – everybody always is! The timing of his visit co-incided with the timing of MIND instituting Awards to mark their fiftieth anniversary.

Service users were on the committee which determined which local associations should receive these awards. I think that some MIND Officers might have doubted that we should receive two – the only local association to do so, but a majority of users on the committee insisted. As they have said consistently for twenty-five years, 'The Wokingham Crisis House is exactly what we need'. Our awards were, specifically, for providing the best crisis service, and for making community care work on a shoestring.

We travelled to Cambridge to receive our two Awards, and these were presented by the Mayor of Cambridge, and Marsha Hunt, one time girlfriend of Mick Jagger, who was over in England to promote a book which she had just had published – on her experiences of caring for a grandmother with dementia.

Further awards

In 1997, I received one of the first 'Civic Awards' - presented by Wokingham Town Council. Later in 1997, the crisis house received an Award from the Department of Health - from its 'Voluntary Sector Awards. This was signed by Paul Boateng, himself, the then Health Minister. This Award certainly did cause some fluttering in the dovecotes – do I mean 'fluttering', or do I mean 'fury'?

An amusing memory of this time is when the local director of Social Services visited, and saw the Award displayed on the wall. He literally beat his hands together. 'That's a national award, he pleaded. I want a partnership with you!' Ah, but we did not want a partnership with him! At a later time, I put it more bluntly to their Head of Adult Services. 'Working in partnership with you, would be like Eton College working with Borstal.' They were not amused.

Civic awards

The local Wokingham Town Council Civic Awards were instituted early in 1997, and they were to acknowledge voluntary service by the whole range of local charities. The Town Mayor of the time, Tina Marinos, explained at the Awards Ceremony – just how difficult it was to select organizations – because so many were doing good work.

However, they had tried to represent all areas of need. Thus, mine was for mental health, there was another for work with children, another for youth work, and so on. We had a splendid presentation ceremony in the lovely, Victorian, Wokingham Town Hall, where our photographs hang to this day. I joked with my colleagues that I can guarantee that I am the only radical separatist ever to have their picture hanging in Wokingham Town Hall!

It was our befriender, Sandra, who put Phil up for a Wokingham Town Council Civic Award in the year two thousand – for his successful holiday caravan project. By this time, the caravan at Selsey had been running holidays for three years, and was a very popular amenity. I attended the ceremony, and Phil was presented with the Award by Town Mayor, Fred Clarke.

In the year 2001, Dave received his Award. Dave had done a tremendous amount of work at the crisis house, and this included creating a new sanctuary bedroom. Such a service was vital because – once we started accepting guests who wished to resolve life crisis, and, therefore, needed to stay for months, rather than days or weeks, we were beginning to be short of emergency accommodation. He created a beautiful sanctuary, and its first use proved poignant.

Dave had literally just finished, and the room was ready for occupation. It was a quiet afternoon at the crisis house, so I just sat – relaxing and doing crosswords. Suddenly, there was a scuffling at the door. I went out and saw an old lady, in a very distressed state, sitting in the reception lounge. For details of her background, [Please see: Chapter 12: 'Playing Fair'].

The gist was that, the marital home having been sold over her head, she went to stay in London with her very severely ill, schizophrenic, son. He had become violent, so she had escaped through a window, and fled to us. Thank God that she had thought of the crisis house!

What was good about the situation, was, that because of Dave's hard work, we were able to provide her, immediately with crisis accommodation, while we sorted her problems out. Because she was so elderly, we took her to see a local doctor, before settling her in for the night, and both Frances and I stayed overnight because we considered her to be particularly vulnerable.

I pay few compliments to Wokingham Borough Council on their services, but, to be fair, their services for the elderly are excellent. Their Housing Department provided this lady with a local sheltered flat on the very DAY that we took her to see them.

Excellent service! We provided furniture, and household equipment – as we always did, when somebody moved into a flat. Nevertheless, I was still intrigued by the request of the local social worker who had been allocated to the lady. She telephoned me to say that the lady had no carpets! Really, why tell us? What was the social worker there for?

I attended the Awards Ceremony, when Dave received his Award from the Wokingham Town Mayor – an Award so richly deserved.

In 2002, it was Frances' turn to receive an award. By then, she had been giving the crisis house sterling service for six solid years – covering everything. She did befriending, crisis care, and, her favourite activity, as 'Mrs Steptoe', collecting furniture for people who were setting up in flats in the community.

I attended her Awards Ceremony – which was also attended by members of her Widows' Group – because the Award was also given for this service to the community.

Sadly, Frances, as I have already mentioned passed away at the age of eighty-three, in November 2012. We wanted a permanent memorial at the crisis house, so, in June 2015, we created a Memorial Garden in memory of Frances, and this was opened by our Patron, Lady Elizabeth Godsal. The plaque states: 'In loving memory of Frances Rowley, Founder, Wokingham Widows, volunteer, Wokingham Crisis House'.

This garden was part of the overall upgrading of the crisis house – which we undertook in 2014 and 2015 – and is a pleasant place where service users can sit and relax on warm, summer days.

Another Dave - Dave the Second, was the fifth in our ranks to receive a Wokingham Town Council Civic Award. He, again, did an enormous amount of work at the crisis house – creating a further sanctuary bedroom – as the demands upon our service increased all the time. I attended his Award Ceremony with colleagues, and his family came down from Glasgow to see him receive the Award in 2003.

Shirley was a stalwart befriender, and she received a Wokingham Town Council Civic Award in 2008. I attended the Ceremony, and, again, there were people from other charities – since Shirley also worked, among other things, for cancer research.

It is always good to be right up-to-date. In January 2016, we received the Wokingham Lions Club, Jenny Aggett Award - For our outstanding service to the local community. You can win 'em all!

These local awards are so precious - because they demonstrate the high regard in which we are held by the local community.

Our crowning glory, in 2003, was our Association's receipt of the Queen's Golden Jubilee Award for voluntary service.

This is the highest national award that voluntary sector organizations can receive, and is the equivalent of an MBE. Our members attended the Royal Garden Parties at Buckingham Palace - delighted that our voluntary service had received the royal seal of approval.

From applicants of thousands, only two hundred voluntary organizations were put up to the Queen for consideration; only five mental health groups were successful, and we were the only MIND Association in the United Kingdom to receive this Award.

Our visit to Buckingham Palace, can be included amongst our 'Happy Memories'. It was a lovely, sunny, day in July 2003.

We graced the occasion with beautiful dresses and hats. Everything was perfect, and yes, it had its funny moments – such as when we joined the queue to enter Buckingham Palace. Some American tourists passed by, and asked us why we were queuing. 'We are going to tea with the Queen!' we replied. 'Can we come?' they asked. We feared not. 'By invitation only!' The tea was lovely, and both the Palace, and its grounds, beautiful. A life-long happy memory.

When refurbishing the crisis house in 2015, we included the Queen's award logo in our external signage, so that now, visitors to Wokingham, coming out of the Station, see, as their first sight of the town, the proudly refurbished crisis house – displaying our Queen's Award.

PART FIVE

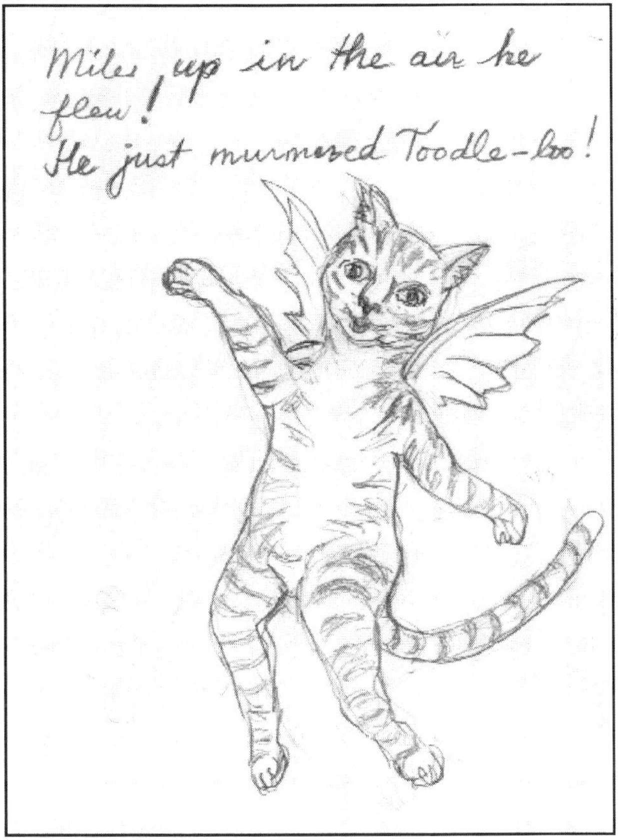

'Felix Keeps On Walking, Keeps On Walking Still. Miles Up In The Air He Flew. He Just Murmured 'Toodle-oo'. He Landed Down In Timbuctoo. And He Kept On Walking Still.'

Chapter 39

Travelling Around The United Kingdom

The crisis house opened at the end of March 1991. The nineties were a decade in which the deinstitutionalization policy – heralded by Enoch Powell's 'Water Tower' Speech in 1961, and making a beginning at implementation throughout the 1970's and the 1980's, accelerated dramatically.

At last, the old, Victorian asylums were closing down wholesale. There was, therefore, in this decade, quite naturally, a burgeoning interest in community alternatives.

From 1991 until January 2000, I travelled the length and breadth of the United Kingdom – giving talks about the Wokingham Crisis House, and, during that decade, we also welcomed visitors from the length and breadth of the United Kingdom and beyond.

I recall visiting Wales on four separate occasions – three times to North Wales, and once to South Wales. I made an important point on one of my visits to North Wales – which is a rural area with lots of small, isolated, hill farms, lots of depressive illness due to social isolation, and a high suicide rate.

I explained, that, in such circumstances, the concept of having one crisis house, based in Rhyl, may not be the best model of crisis service delivery. A mobile service with teams of crisis workers – visiting the farms – might meet the local need more appropriately.

On one of my visits to Wales, former crisis house guest, Adèle, accompanied me. She was able to tell the audience, how the crisis house worked to her advantage, 'from the horse's mouth!'

In April 1995, I spoke at the Scottish Mental Health Association's Annual Conference in Glasgow. I found their interest encouraging - because Scotland was slower to implement the deinstitutionalisation policy than was England.

Among other places visited, were the West Midlands, Northamptonshire, Kent, all parts of London, Shropshire, Middlesborough, Surrey, and Dorset. I managed to get to Cornwall and back in one day – taking the earliest train that left from Bracknell Station, giving the lunchtime talk at the hospital in Bodmin, and arriving back in Bracknell at 9pm.

All these places were looking for alternatives to the traditional mental hospital. In October 1991, I visited the Isle of Wight – to speak to their mental health service about the recently introduced Code of Practice, for the Mental Health Act.

So, is the crisis house a viable alternative to a hospital? The answer is that it is not! For one thing, we are selective. Our rules prohibit all anti-social behaviour, and we enforce them rigorously. Mental hospitals, by contrast, including our local one, have special wards for very disturbed, and violent, patients.

Secondly, we are totally voluntary, and embrace the philosophy of self-help. True, we occasionally accommodated Sectioned patients, but these were accepted when the Police sought us, as 'a place of safety', under Section 136 of the Mental Health Act – the less desirable alternative being a Police cell.

This Section is only of seventy-two hours' duration – giving time for the patient to be seen by a doctor, and by an appropriately qualified mental health professional. In our instances, the patients were then discharged from the Section, but had it been decided that they needed to be detained under Section 2 or 3, then they would have been admitted to a mental hospital. We could not accommodate people for the longer Sections.

So, if a crisis house is not an alternative to a hospital, what is its function? The answer is that it is a choice. It is an opportunity for a way out. It is the bottom rung of a long, long, ladder – leading up into the light of normality. Read my chapters on 'Success Stories'. It is a hard, hard, climb, but you can get to the top. They did!

Chapter 40

Visitors From All Around The UK And Beyond

At the time when alternatives to traditional mental asylums were being discussed, service users were of one voice. They wanted crisis houses in the community. The development of such crisis houses was MIND's official policy.

I recall a mental health meeting in London in 1994 – when leaders of a health authority pleaded with me to work with them – after I had described my work at the Wokingham Crisis House. 'Pam, they said, it's what they ALL say they want – and we have the money.' That is precisely the problem, is it not?

If one is dependent upon statutory money – and, particularly, large sums of it, the carpet can, so easily be pulled from under one's feet. One will never get user-friendly crisis houses with statutory authorities, but, in our early days, I had hopes of MIND – it being a charity. My hopes went unfulfilled! They tore my hopes apart, but, fortunately, they did not turn my dream to shame, nor did they kill the dream I dreamed. Felix kept on walking. Him they could not kill! Felix keeps on walking, keeps on walking still!

Nevertheless, throughout the entire decade of the 1990's, there was tremendous interest in crisis houses – at least in theory, and ours attracted visitors from all over the United Kingdom and beyond. As a break from my deathless prose, I have decided to make this chapter over to some of the visitors who have come to us over the past twenty-five years – with a selection of THEIR comments in the Visitors' Books.

1991 – 1992

Angela White, MIND in Camden, and Anna Neeter, Camden Mental Health Consortium, Crisis House Working Party Representative.

Derek and Margaret Williams, National Schizophrenia Fellowship, Enfield, Middlesex.
Comment: 'I thought the Sanctuary [local name for the crisis house] a good idea. The reality is even better'.

Justine Brener: Old Windsor, Berkshire.
Comment: 'A much needed amenity'.

Teresa Winship, Royal Berkshire Hospital, Reading, Berkshire.
Comment: 'Absolutely fantastic!'

Margaret Mitchell, Surrey Social Services.
Comment: 'Thank you for explaining your sanctuary to me. Great!'

Marie Laine, Bristol.
Comment: 'Excellent idea and work'.

1992 – 1993

Jenny Ticker: MIND in Harrow: Middlesex.
Comment: 'Great. Wonderful to see such a positive model of mental health care!'

Basil, Joyce, and Clare Bloodworth, Chateau D'oex, Switzerland.
Comment: 'Well done! May it be the first of many sanctuaries'.

Rick Allen, West Wickham, Kent.
Comment: 'Great vibrations here'.

Neil Ward, Chair, Safe House Committee, East Suffolk MIND, Ipswich, Suffolk.
Comment: 'Thank you for a warm, welcoming, and informative day'.

Susan Bell, Addlestone, Weybridge, Surrey.
Comment: 'Absolutely inspired. Excellent provision!'

Barbara Davy, Swindon.
Comment: 'Very interesting. Very friendly and helpful'.

Staff Nurse, Fiona Liddle, Horton Hospital, Epsom, Surrey.
Comment: 'Friendly, and very accommodating'.

Sean Gooding, Basingstoke Voices, Hampshire.
Comment: 'Very nice and interesting. Lovely people'.

Chris Borchard, Basingstoke Voices [a support group for schizophrenia sufferers], Basingstoke, Hampshire.
Comment: 'This place is fucking brilliant!'

Reg Gough, Abbots Langley, Herts.
Comment: 'Pam put a bar in the corner, and make the Wokingham hotel perfect!' [NOTE: We did!]

Jean Gough, Abbots Langley, Herts.
Comment: 'You are a perfect example of how community care could work'.

1993 – 1994

Caren Houghton and Kusher Score, Project 2000 Nurses.
Comment: 'Great use for our neighbourhood study. Thank you so much!'

WPC 3452 Payne, Wokingham Police Station.
Comment: 'Ref a place for a person who needs sanctuary'.

Sarah Banks, Shipley, Bradford, Yorkshire.
Comment: 'Very restful and calm place for a lot of support and thinking time'.

John Howard, Hounslow, Middlesex.
Comment: 'Very glad to meet friendly people, and find some time –

otherwise not available – but often desperately needed'.

Anthony Metcalf, Hermitage, West Berkshire.
Comment: 'Inspiration'.

Grier Thompson, Salford, Greater Manchester.
Comment: 'I hope to apply your experience back up north!'

Adrian Pullin, User Representative, Bristol.
Comment: 'A very vital service, much needed'.

Rosemary and Rory Meldrum, Harpenden, Hertfordshire.
Comment: 'Congratulations. You have done a wonderful job!'

Teresa Priest, MIND in Kingston, Surrey.
Comment: 'Lovely house and atmosphere. Very important'.

1995 – 1996

Dr Stephen Madgwich, Chalfont Surgery, Earley, Wokingham, Berkshire [local GP].
Comment: 'Good facilities. Need more of these in other areas'.

Carol Warner, Wokingham Social Services.
Comment: 'Excellent facilities, and what is needed throughout the country. Thank you for the opportunity'.

Graham Griffiths, Wokingham Adolescent Unit.
Comment: 'I was given a very warm welcome, and made to feel at ease. Thank you very much'.

John Redwood, MP, Wokingham, Berkshire.
Comment: 'Well done! Your hard work and enthusiasm do a lot of good'.

Geoff Glenister, PC 1773, Wokingham Police Station.
Comment: 'A wonderful facility in a wonderful town'.

Ros Williams, Kendal MIND, Cumbria.
Comment: 'Refreshing, mind-blowing, experience'.

Laura Pozzi, Ealing, Hammersmith, and Hounslow Health Authority.
Comment: 'An extremely interesting and useful afternoon'.

Nadia Hatul, Chiswick Oasis.
Comment: 'Thank you. A very homely place'.

Gabriel Mackintosh, Consumer Forum, Hammersmith, SW6.
Comment: 'What a lovely place. Hope we can tell you about a safe house in Hammersmith soon'.

1996 – 1997

Nick Spence, Crowthorne, Berkshire.
Comment: 'Very impressed with the services that are offered here, and hope that more centres are set up'.

Harry Dickinson, Fairmile Hospital, Oxfordshire [Consultant Psychiatrist].
Comment: 'Very pleased to visit'.

Dawn Wakeling, The Mental Health Foundation.
Comment: 'Thank you for talking to me, and being so welcoming. I shall keep you posted re our progress'.

Mary Eloise Noak, Finchampstead, Wokingham, Berkshire. [Psychologist].
Comment: 'Very interesting. Fills a crucial need in the community'.

Michelle Crouch, 'Concern for Mental Health', Ilford, Essex.
Comment: 'Very impressed. Homely. Obviously good work going on'.

David Samms, Swindon Mental Health Resource Centre, Wiltshire.
Comment: 'Challenging and very impressive'.

1997 – 1998

Tony Heyes, UK Federation of Smaller Mental Health Agencies.
Comment: 'Super. Thank you!'

Barry Miller, Kendal, Cumbria.
Comment: 'A wonderful set-up, very efficiently run, by charming and committed people. Keep up the good work!'

Peter Williams, Harrow, Middlesex.
Comment: 'Wonderfully relaxing. I could stay a month'.

Ronald Green, Bognor Regis, Sussex.
Comment: 'Thank you for an interesting, instructive, visit'.

Torsten Shaw, Nottingham.
Comment: 'Keep on with the anti-professional approach'.

Sharon Ryon, Arun East Community Mental Health Team.
Comment: 'Very inspiring. Thank you'.

Janet Jones, Placement Officer, Kingston Social Services, Surrey.
Comment: 'Thank you for your hospitality and openness. A project of great value. I'm impressed'.

Carol Mitchell, Herefordshire MIND.
Comment: 'Very impressed. Very real and open. Extremely friendly and welcoming. An invaluable service for people who need time out to access their lives'.

Margaret Yates, Radcliffe, Manchester.
Comment: 'Very friendly and homely. I feel as though I have known you for years'.

Chris Murphy, St Albans Hertfordshire.
Comment: 'All that I hoped it would be'.

Nasein Ulla, Black Women's Mental Health Project, Brent.
Comment: 'Very welcoming. Very good'.

Dave Middle, Mental Aftercare Association, Shropshire.
Comment: 'Very impressed. Some excellent ideas which we need to think about'.

1998 – 1999

Sian Morelli, Bridgend Link, South Wales.
Comment: 'Friendly'.

Alison Ashton, Psychiatric Student Nurse.
Comment: 'What a wonderful, informal, relaxing, beautiful home. The drop-in centre is a fantastic service for people to have a chat, and the Sanctuary is lovely and peaceful. Extremely well-run by knowledgeable, kind, caring, volunteers'.

Wendy Antrim, Vale of Clwyd MIND.
Comment: 'Excellent inspiration for a crisis house in our area'.

Brenda Singfield, Vale of Clwyd MIND.
Comment: 'The reality is even better than the literature. Excellent work'.

Craig Newnes, Shropshire Mental Health Trust.
Comment: 'Marvellous. The wine was particularly well-chilled'.

Paul Kelly, Shropshire Mental Health Trust.
Comment: 'This visit has been inspirational, and will live with me'.

Simon Heyes, 'Speak Up', Yeovil, Somerset.
Comment: 'It was very eye-opening, and the atmosphere and lunch were great'.

Val Radway and Frantz Fanon, Centre for Mental Health, Birmingham.
Comment: 'A great place. An oasis in time of trouble'.

Dr Anna Higgett, Mental Health Policy Branch, Department of Health, London, SE1.
Comment: 'A very enlightening and inspiring visit. Thanks for the welcome'.

David Crepaz-Keay, Chartridge, Buckinghamshire.
Comment: 'Merry Christmas, and keep the enemy at bay'.

Jonathan Passmore, 'Barnet Voices', North London.
Comment: 'A home from home. An inspiration for our crisis house in Barnet'.

1999 – 2000

Anna Patricia Hurley, Harrow Weald, Middlesex.
Comment: 'Tasteful, spiritual, artistic – Pam – an earth mother with intelligence, wit, and effective therapy'.

Alan Beadsmore, MIND [National Association for Mental Health].
Comment: 'Thank you for a great welcome. I found the service very welcoming, and providing a valuable community service'.

Simon Richards, Shropshire Health Authority.
Comment: 'Great to see and experience this super facility. Local people are lucky to have it'.

Janice Davis, 'Safe House', Corby, Northamptonshire.
Comment: 'Very impressive, lovely, friendly 'home'. Very positive service, valuable to users and people like myself'.

Les Clarke, Warwick.
Comment: 'Incredible. Absolutely unique!'

Rosalie Horner, Friern Barnet, London N11.
Comment: 'Long may you continue your wonderful work. It is so needed'.

Roger Dunn, London W14.
Comment: 'A wonderful, warm, experience. Stimulating conversation. Good luck!'

Ivan Moore, Kensington, London W11.
Comment: 'A very vibrant, stimulating, community refuge'.

Claire Hopkinson, Havering Social Services, Essex.
Comment: 'Very, very, impressed'.

2000 – 2001

Grace Agheghoubia, Regional Administrator, South East MIND, London SE1.
Comment: 'A warm, friendly, and lovely, atmosphere. Very well run and organized'.

Irene Burnett-Thomas, Broadstone, Dorset.
Comment: 'A pleasure to return to you where I enjoyed my voluntary work before I trained as a registered nurse [mental health] in Dorset'.

Janice Davis, USS Safe House, Corby, Northamptonshire.
Comment: 'What an achievement. You give hope and inspiration to projects like our own of what user-run projects can achieve. Many congratulations from all involved at Corby'.

John Mahoney, Department of Health.
Comment: 'Excellent – the type of facility I would want to use. Congratulations on your ten years'.

Thomas Lowden, Chairman, Paddington User Group, London W9.
Comment: 'Very impressed with its homely atmosphere. Very encouraging in our efforts to obtain a crisis house in Paddington'.

Mark Bunker, 'Second Step' Housing Association, Bristol.
Comment: 'Thank you for your hospitality. A very welcoming, relaxing, environment'.

Daniel Robinson, Chester-le-Street, County Durham.
Comment: 'I was very impressed. Did not know it would be like this. Very friendly'.

Sue Jackson, Patient Advocacy Liaison Service, Royal Berkshire and Battle Hospitals.
Comment: 'Incredible changes over the past ten years. Wonderful

progress. Congratulations, and keep up the good work'.

Roy Dickinson, Partners for Positive Change in Mental Health, Abraham Cowley Unit, Chertsey, Surrey.
Comment: 'Excellent, welcoming and warm environment. Thank you'.

Henry Daniels, Fontaines sur Saone, France.
Comment: 'Was welcomed with warmth and friendliness. Spent two happy hours in your company'.

Cathy Russell, Bonnet Bay, New South Wales, Australia.
Comment: 'Wonderful place to come and relax'.

Ann-Marie Stokes, Shropshire Community Mental Health Trust.
Comment: 'Very welcoming. Excellent service. Thank you'.

Gillian Bailey, South Wrekin Community Mental Health Team, Telford, Shropshire.
Comment: 'A grateful reminder of what it's all about. Thank you very much. A very enjoyable day with great hosts'.

2001 – 2002

Craig Newnes, Director of Psychological Therapies, Shropshire.
Comment: 'Fab. Keep up the good work'.

Kalli Mantala, Birmingham.
Comment: 'Great place, and very inspiring. Thank for letting us in!'

Elina Baker, Birmingham.
Comment: 'Thank you for your wonderful hospitality, and the insight into your innovative service'.

Lindsey Ridgeon, Crewe.
Comment: 'Thanks for the Chablis! Something I will take with me when I return to Liverpool!'

Ricky Handsworth, Berkshire User Group.
Comment: 'What an incredible amount of thought clear in every detail. I think this is a wonderful place'.

Peter Bestley, Bracknell, Berkshire.
Comment: 'Very interesting and inspiring. Very *sui generis*'.

Sandi Maddox, Shrewsbury, Shropshire.
Comment: 'Thank you all for your hospitality, and inspiration for

bending the rules, and other important things'.

2002 – 2003

Darren O'Brian, 'Network for Change', Leicester.
Comment: 'Great atmosphere. Keep up the good work. Lots of good ideas. You will get an invite to Leicester as soon as we open'.

Gabby Briner, Network for Change, Leicester.
Comment: 'A wonderful and welcoming environment. I only hope our crisis house gets this good. Thanks for lovely lunch and wine!'

Shaun Johnson, Network for Change, Leicester.
Comment: 'Really eye-opening. You've a wonderful place here! Thank you for the food and wine too!'

Bryony Rogers, Lancaster.
Comment: 'Well done! It's great to see and hear about the work you're doing'.

Joshua Howe, Bayhorse, Lancashire.
Comment: 'Fantastic. Really enjoyable to see people making their own waves'.

Martin and Mary Kibblewhite, Hereford.
Comment: 'Inspiring!'

Reg and Jean Gough, Abbotts Langley, Herfordshire.
Comment: 'Simply the best!'

Alex Welby, Classics Master, Wellington College.
Comment: 'Very impressed'.

Maureen Tyler, Phoenix Agency, Southend-on-Sea, Essex.
Comment: 'A very homely and safe environment. I have enjoyed my experiences here, and wish all well'.

Sarah Harrington, Student Nurse, Reading, Berkshire.
Comment: 'Lovely day spent here. What an amazing place. There should be so many more like this. Thank you!'

2003 – 2004

Danielle Ettia, Maidenhead Probation.
Comment: 'It was a pleasure to come here and see what excellent work has been put into making this a lovely home environment'.

Christina Young, Merseyside F.D.A. Self Help Group, Liverpool.
Comment: 'Fantastic. Lovely environment. Relaxing, inspiring, especially liked the cats!'

Janice Crane, Corby Safe House, Northamptonshire.
Comment: 'Great place. Always gives me inspiration'.

Julie Knighton, Service-User, Wellingborough.
Comment: 'Different'.

Joy Oliver, Northamptonshire.
Comment: 'A fine model and example to follow and be. All the best for the future. You will always be in my mind. Hope to see you again. Best wishes. Good for you!'

Zelyana Schonauer, Twyford, Berkshire.
Comment: 'Inspiring experience!'

Henrietta Catherine, Hove, Sussex.
Comment: 'Exciting to be in an environment which challenges the 'professionalisation' of mental health. Best wishes with everything'.

Milan Ghosh, Mad Pride.
Comment: 'All of you are 'bonkers'. That's good'.

Monique Klang-Joves, Chelsea Carers Group, London.
Comment: 'You are my kind of people. Excellent, good work.Safe environment for the right help for people in crisis. You've got the x factor'.

Matthew Gough, Voluntary Sector Mental Health Officer, Leicestershire.
Comment: 'Thank you for inspiring me and may you keep doing the right thing without distraction'.

Aron Oliver, Stow-on-Wold, Gloucestershire.
Comment: 'Very positive, friendly, and helpful to many'.

2004 – 2005

Tim Stratford, Woking, Surrey.
Comment: 'Just like coming home again'.

Mike Sarson, East-West Detox, Reading, Berkshire.
Comment: 'Very impressed with this wonderful, spiritual, supportive, warm community'.

Joan Penrose, Stanmore, Middlesex.
Comment: 'Your house gets better and better. If only its goodness spread one way or another to as many needy souls as possible, as soon as possible!'

Hilda Wright and Noreen Rice, Hillingdon Primary Care Trust.
Comment: 'We are so impressed with the service provided here. The atmosphere is so warm and welcoming, and one can only imagine how it feels to arrive here when you are in emotional/physical distress. Clearly, it is highly successful at empowering people in making their own choices. The unconditional regard demonstrated by all the 'staff' towards the guests is so evident that it is humbling to witness. Thank you so much for allowing us this experience'.

Lady Elizabeth Godsal, Vice Lord Lieutenant, and High Steward of Wokingham.
Comment: 'A marvellous organization and I am most impressed with everything at Crisis House'.

Gordon Foxley, Henley-on-Thames, Oxfordshire.
Comment: 'Great work by a dedicated team of helpers. Keep it up!'

Pandy [Karen], Crowthorne, Berkshire.
Comment: 'A wonderful, warm, home. Very impressed with all the hard work done'.

Rob Warriner, Walsh Trust, Henderson, New Zealand.
Comment: 'A wonderful afternoon with some very special human beings: inspiring and uplifting!'

2005 – 2006

Edward Matt, Director of Operations, CNWL.
Comment: 'Thanks for an inspirational time. The visit has helped to give me back some of the enthusiasm I had when joining the mental health services. I am really grateful'.

Daphne Carbery, 'Tandem', Oxford.
Comment: 'Lovely atmosphere. I shall take away lots of ideas and tips. Thank you for the opportunity'.

Kris Scott, 'Tandem', Oxford.
Comment: 'Lovely place and fantastic hospitality. Really informative. Thank you so much'.

Peter Davies, Yapp Charitable Trust [a funding organization].
Comment: 'How wonderful to find a winner'.

Francine Shaw, Windfall Films, London.
Comment: 'A very enjoyable lunch and afternoon. I feel charmed. More of these, please!'

Sally Parnell, Burnley, Lancashire.
Comment: 'Congratulations on continuing to provide a super crisis house which is really warm and peaceful , and thank you for your hospitality'.

Carl Jacques, Carshalton, Surrey.
Comment: 'Thank you. Lots of food for thought'.

Barbara Charvet, Hereford.
Comment: 'Most inspiring and interesting to hear your views. Thank you for giving us so much time'.

Sarah Davey, Herefordshire.
Comment: 'Wall to wall wisdom. Absolutely amazing.. What commitment and inspiration'.

2006 – 2007

John Findlay, University of Durham.
Comment: 'Good luck'.

David Grey, Psychotherapist, Dulwich, London, SE21.
Comment: 'Congratulations on the wonderfully calm and welcoming atmosphere that you have created here'.

Mike Paxton, Slough Mental Health User Group, Berkshire.
Comment: 'Lovely ambience you've created here. Stress free. Just what we need. [They better not try to close you down.]'

2007 – 2008

Annabel Lee, Committee member of crisis house project, Slough, Berkshire.
Comment: 'What a wonderful place for respite and therapy. Thank you for your time and generosity'.

Ruth Morris, Mentoring and Befriending Foundation.
Comment: 'I had a really interesting couple of hours talking to the befrienders about the services provided – really welcoming with lunch

and conversation. An amazing project'.

Sandra Burrows, Winchester area Community Action.
Comment: 'It is such a warm, friendly, place, and I had a lovely visit. Thank you all very much'.

Paul Fine, St Lewes, East Sussex.
Comment: 'What a lovely place, and a warm welcome. It's worth having another episode of mental illness just to stay here. I'll return –ill, or not!'

Ken Fish, KTMC, Ltd.
Comment: 'Really impressed with the house, and the great way there is support and atmosphere that helps everyone. Superb! Superb!'

2009 - 2010

Tony Barber, Ex Wokingham Town Mayor.
Comment: 'Wonderful to see the Drop-In, and clients in such good form'.

Tania Appleton, Student Mental Health Nurse.
Comment: 'Very interesting and homely place. Very welcoming, and well thought out'.

Mel Cox, Voluntary Action, Wokingham Borough.
Comment: 'A truly excellent facility. Truly hope we can assist you in finding new funding streams'.

2010 - 2011

P. Shand, Neuro-partnerships.
Comment: 'Feel very inspired. Thank you very much for a wonderful visit'.

Niamh Donnelly, KCA, Station Road, Wokingham [Community Drugs and Alcohol Service].
Comment: 'Looking forward to a neighbourly relationship'.
NOTE: They have one. Many of our service users use both services.

Carol-Anne Bidwell, Wokingham Borough Council, DAAT.
Comment: 'A most fabulous service – truly inspiring'.

Ruth Underwood, London N19.
Comment: 'What an inspiration to meet you. Thank you for providing sanctuary for people in need'.

Peter Lucey, Wokingham Town Mayor.
Comment: 'Uplifting and sympathetic. Thank you'.

Elaine, Wokingham Town Mayoress.
Comment: 'Wonderful'.

2011 – 2012

Jason Wear, Community Mental Health Team, Old Forge, Wokingham, Berkshire.
Comment: 'Very pleasant and welcoming'.

2012 - 2013

Martin and Yvonne Bishop, Wokingham Town Mayor and Mayoress.
Comment: 'A very interesting visit. You are doing a wonderful job in our community'.

2013 – 2014

Christina Ioannou, Wokingham Volunteer Centre.
Comment: 'Exciting visit. Very helpful. Warm and calm place. Lovely people'.

Nicole Strudley, Healthwatch Wokingham.
Comment: 'Lovely to see a service daring to be different. We are happy to publicise your work'.

Nick Durman, Health Watch, Wokingham, Berkshire.
Comment: 'Great to meet you. Fantastic community service'.

Matt Smith and Michael Maclennon, Bracknell, Community Mental Health Team, Berkshire.
Comment: 'Very friendly and helpful'.

2014 – 2015

Alan Bunce, *Wokingham Paper*.
Comment: 'Amazing Place'.

Canon David Hodgson, Minister, All Saints Church, Wokingham.
Comment: 'Delightful new garden and welcome here'.

Charlie Doolan, School of Psychology, University of Reading.
Comment: 'Lovely to meet you all and see where our students volunteer. Thank you for your hospitality!'

So there you have it – 'S'wonderful! S'marvellous!' – from Avon, Berkshire, Buckinghamshire, County Durham, Cumbria, Devon, Dorset, Essex, Gloucestershire, Greater London, Greater Manchester, Hampshire, Herefordshire, Hertfordshire, Kent. Lancashire, Leicestershire, Merseyside, Middlesex, Mid Wales, Northamptonshire, North Wales, Nottinghamshire, Oxfordshire, Shropshire, Somerset, South Wales, Suffolk, Surrey, Sussex, Warwickshire, West Midlands, Wiltshire, Yorkshire, France, Switzerland, Australia, and New Zealand.

Twenty-five years' adulation. Am I happy and gratified? Well, in one sense I am. At least I have not wasted my middle age. What we do, is exactly what the mentally ill need. But there is bitter/sweetness as well.

After twenty-five years, if MIND had put its policy into practice, such crisis houses could now be established the length and the breadth of the UK. And, it is particularly galling for me to reflect, that, though hard work, crisis houses are not difficult to establish and continue – if people are committed.

Is it really so difficult to go around the charity shops – selecting beautiful pictures and ornaments? It isn't even costly! Is it really so difficult to make sure that the house has fresh flowers? Pets obtained from Animal Rescue Centres cost nothing! Comfortable furniture will be donated, if one can be bothered to collect it.

There are times when I truly believe that our statutory services are beleaguered with bone idleness – a culture in which people won't even water plants, if there is no additional funding. I have said it before. I do not wish to see Social Services improve. I wish to see them abolished!

Chapter 41

The Involvement Of The Local Community

When we received the Queen's Award for Voluntary Service – which was in the first year that it was instituted, in 2003 – part of the selection process involved a local, regional, committee, as well as the, central, Queen's Golden Jubilee Committee. They considered local opinion of a service to be very important, and I agree with them.

From the day in 1991, that the Wokingham Town Mayor, Jeanne Burnett-Wilson, opened the crisis house, we have always involved local Town Mayors, Borough Councillors, representatives of other community groups, and, of course local services users, relatives, and any local residents who are interested in our work. The following are their comments in the Visitors' Books – over the past twenty-five years:

1991 – 1992

These visitors just signed:

Chris Davies, Senior Care Manger, Wokingham Locality Team. Sue Jackson, Citizen's Advice Bureau, Wokingham. John Binmore, Police Sergeant, Wokingham Police. Neil Davies, Trinity Church, Lower Earley. Charles Kenderdine, Joint Service Manager, Social Services, Wokingham Mental Health Service. Albert Dunham, Mayor's Attendant, Town Hall, Wokingham. Robert McBain, Wokingham Methodist Church. Joyce Baldry, British Red Cross Centre, Wokingham. Mavis Harding, British Red Cross Centre, Wokingham. Beryl Bray, Wokingham Mental Health Team. Peter Falham, Community Psychiatric Nurse, Wokingham Mental Health Team. Jackie Palmer, Job Centre, Wokingham. Ann Fugeman, Woodley Social Services, Wokingham. Pat Gillespie and Erin Day, Samaritans. Jackie Maslin, Community Support Worker, Wokingham. John Starkey, Wokingham Social Services. Geraldine Ryder, Wokingham Social Services. Andrew Batt, *Wokingham News*. Natalie Firman, Reading MIND. Bob Wyatt, Town Mayor of Wokingham. Diana Bone, Job Centre, Wokingham. Sharon Allesbrook, Reading MIND.

1993 – 1994

Most of these added comments:
David Hamilton, Winnersh, Wokingham.
Comment: 'Thanks for sharing your views'.

J.H. Brown, Bracknell.
Comment: 'Helpful'.

John Hangley-Hobson, Berkshire College of Nursing.
Comment: 'Very good atmosphere'.

David Spender, Wokingham.
Comment: 'Very interesting'.

Brian Connington, Wokingham Mental Health Team.
Comment: 'Your service is excellent'.

Jenny Ames, Reading.
Comment: 'Thanks for all your help and time. Most appreciated'.

Johanna Brown, Bracknell.
Comment: 'Thank you for your help'.

John Hoggett, Reading.
Comment: 'Very Nice'.

Mary Kadisz, Wokingham.
Comment: 'Very restful'.

Joyce Baldry, British Red Cross, Wokingham.
Comment: 'Very bright and happy. Well done, new rooms'.

Laurie Tytel, Wokingham Social Service.
Comment: 'What a difference from what it was [when he ran it!] Many thanks'.

Val Canty, Community Psychiatric Nurse, Wokingham Mental Health Unit.
Comment: 'A bright, cheerful, place, a good welcome, tour, and cup of tea. Excellent!'

Vicky Williams, Student Nurse, Fairmile Hospital.
Comment: 'Friendly and warm atmosphere. Warm reception'.

Elsie Hudson, Wokingham Town Mayoress.
Comment: 'Very interesting and instructive'.

Philip Hudson, Wokingham Town Mayor.
Comment: 'I know where to come now!'

Ray Stagles, Caritas [local charity for young homeless].
Comment: 'A superb facility!'

Shirley Manson, Crowthorne.
Comment: 'Best wishes to all concerned'.

June Russell, Crowthorne.
Comment: 'Thanks for sharing your lovely home with me for this little time. Will be back'.

Douglas Thomas, Bracknell.
Comment: 'How nice to know there is a warm welcome for those in need'.

Lynn Vass, Social Worker, Wokingham Mental Health Team.
Comment: 'A very welcoming atmosphere'.

Gareth and Liz, volunteers, Bracknell Samaritans.
Comment: 'Thank you from the whole branch'.

Jenny Barrie, Bracknell.
Comment: 'Very peaceful and restful'.

Margaret Jackson, Reading.
Comment: 'A really restful and peaceful house. Very pleasant people and very friendly'.

Dave Cheeseman, Wokingham.
Comment: 'Lovely people and beautiful place'.

Geoff Pugh, *Wokingham Times*.

Ann-Marie Thompson and Andrea Fairclough, Wexham Park Hospital.

Jane Wood, Wokingham.
Comment: 'A wonderful place'.

Sue Duffy, Wokingham.
Comment: 'Friendly and cosy'.

Teresa O'Leary, Wokingham.
Comment: 'Very nice house'.

Eileen Higgins, Wokingham.
Comment: 'God bless the work'.

1995 – 1996

Mary Reinach, Wokingham.
Comment: 'Superb effort. Nothing but praise for everything'.

E. Jenkinson, Windsor.
Comment: 'Just like home from home. Very good'.

V.W. Jenkinson, Windsor.
Comment: 'It is very clean and comfortable, and the pictures look very nice – gives a friendly touch'.

D. Jenkinson, Bracknell.
Comment: 'Very impressed'.

Roy and Chris Howell, Maidenhead.
Comment: 'An inspiration!'

Justine Brener, Old Windsor.
Comment: 'Very inspiring'.

Tony Churchill, Wokingham Social Services.
Comment: 'An excellent and unique model of crisis provision'.

Janet Phillips, Student Nurse, Berkshire College of Nursing and Midwifery.
Comment: 'Nice to know places like this exist for people in need'.

Melanie Fairs, Berkshire College of Nursing.
Comment: 'Nice to see people care, and there's somewhere to go in need'.

Joyce Ward, RELATE, Wokingham.
Comment: 'Very welcoming atmosphere'.

Anne Davies, Wokingham Town Mayor.

Lieutenant Ruth Hardy, Salvation Army, Wokingham.

Jean Bell, Deaf and Hard of Hearing Team, Wokingham.

Averil Burton, Wokingham.
Comment: 'I'm really looking forward to coming here again'.

Reginald Burton, Wokingham.
Comment: 'A well run establishment!'

Trevor Allwright, P.C. 2442, Wokingham Police.
Comment: 'Keep up the excellent work'.

John Murphy, Student Nurse.
Comment: 'A very useful asset for the community'.

Andrea Phillips, Wokingham.
Comment: 'Very comfortable, safe, peaceful, environment'.

Gabriel Mackintosh, Hammersmith Consumer Forum.
Comment: 'Thank you very much. What a lovely place. Hope we can tell you about a safe house in Hammersmith soon'.

1997 1998

Claire Nelson, Student Nurse, Wokingham.
Comment: 'Lovely house. Very useful'.

Marina Cahill, Reading.
Comment: 'Very nice, friendly, atmosphere. Very helpful house'.

Kieran Piggott, Reading.
Comment: 'It was extremely nice to see people in such pleasant, friendly, surroundings. I hope to see many more of these houses opening up in the future'.

Nick Spence, Crowthorne, Berkshire.
Comment: 'Very impressed with the services offered here, and hope that more centres are set up'.

Sue South, Job Centre, Wokingham.
Comment: 'Peaceful, friendly, atmosphere'.

Barbara and Ray Stagles, Wokingham.
Comment: 'A lovely, welcoming, shelter. Thanks for the invitation'.

Tina Marinos, Wokingham Town Mayor.
Comment: 'You are doing a great job. Well done!'

Stella Nichols, Wokingham Mental Health Team.
Comment: 'Welcoming and cosy atmosphere'.

Ken Adams, Brookside Group Practice, Wokingham.
Comment: 'Very impressed'.

Gill Oates, Student Nurse with Wokingham Community Mental Health Team.
Comment: 'Fantastic work being done. Long may it continue'.

Mohammed Bockare, Student Nurse, Wokingham.
Comment: 'Very impressed with services offered. God bless you!'

Mary Organ, Paramount Housing Association, Reading.
Comment: 'Interesting to find out about you'.

Jack Earnshaw, Wokingham Town Mayor.
Comment: 'A lovely, friendly, home for all'.

1999 – 2000

Daisy Coates, Student for Learning Disabilities, Wokingham.
Comment: 'Extremely helpful, and provides a comfortable atmosphere for all'.

Keith Padarath, Student Nurse, King Edward Seventh Hospital, Windsor.
Comment: 'Very enjoyable and rewarding experience. Loved it'.

Steve Glenister , Slough, Berkshire.
Comment: 'Good, independent, crisis intervention'.

Mike Paxton, Slough User Group.
Comment: 'Very impressed. Also, very homely'.

David Hodgson, Rector, All Saints Church, Wokingham.
Comment: 'Very hospitable'.

Jan Derkatsch, Homelessness Officer, Wokingham Borough Council.
Comment: 'A peaceful sanctuary in the midst of a busy town'.

Ruth Wilson, Duchess of Kent House, Reading.
Comment: 'Homely, welcoming, place of sanctuary'.

Jane Masson, Tilehurst, Reading.
Comment: 'Such changes from my visit in 1991. Many congratulations'.

Sandra Noake, Julie Render, Simon Lock, Sanctuary Housing [Seaford Court], Wokingham.
Comment: 'Very impressed'.

Sue Dart, MIND in Bracknell.
Comment: 'Thank you for your hospitality. I hope we meet again'.

Val Keen, Centrepoint, Berkshire.
Comment: 'An inspiring project'.

Sarah Robins, Reading.
Comment: 'A place of peace and sanctuary. Welcome for everyone'.

Lindsay Adams, Mental Health Project Worker, Wokingham.
Comment: 'Thanks for being inviting and showing me around. Hopefully, we'll have much more contact'.

Susan Wattam, Caversham, Reading.
Comment: 'Brilliant place'.

Fred Clarke, Wokingham Town Mayor, Elsie Clarke, Town Mayoress, and G.F. Runce, Mayor's Attendant.

Tim Jones, Wokingham Borough Council.
Comment: 'Keep up the good work'.

Simon Williams, Wokingham Borough Council.
Comment: 'Great atmosphere. Thank you'.

V.A. Carter, Wokingham.
Comment: 'Very homely and friendly. Places like these are very good for disturbed people'.

Cheryl Page, Woodley, Wokingham.
Comment: 'A true sanctuary'.

Liz Tait, Wokingham Community Mental Health Team.
Comment: 'A very impressive, homely, service'.

Helen Glover, Wokingham and District Counselling Service.
Comment: 'Very interesting and informative'.

John Fisher, Caversham, Reading.
Comment: 'I fully endorse every person concerned'.

Lee Whitehead, Berkshire Health Authority.
Comment: 'Very homely and welcoming. Helped clear up what you do. I leave feeling positive about the service'.

Annie K. Bluebell Ward, Fairmile Hospital.
Comment: 'Lovely place. Impressive'.

Louise Cassidy, Student Nurse, Reading.
Comment: 'Lovely, homely, place. Run very well. Perfect for anyone to drop in'.

Hilary Withers, Wokingham.
Comment: 'Very cosy atmosphere'.

Jo Harrison, Wokingham.
Comment: 'Very homely and friendly. Keep up the good work'.

Victor Rosewell, Wokingham.
Comment: 'A genuine home-from-home feeling, with truly dedicated staff'.

Stella Cairnes, Wokingham.
Comment: 'Thank you for your wonderful company'.

Tom Hall, Wokingham Community Mental Health Team.
Comment: 'A warm welcome, and lovely atmosphere. Thank you'.

Sue Hetherington, Chief Executive, Wokingham Primary Care Group.

2001 – 2002

Charles Kenderdine, Wokingham.
Comment: 'Congratulations on all you've achieved. We look forward to further advances during this new century'.

Janet Lucas, Community Priest, All Saints Church, Wokingham.
Comment: 'A marvellous achievement. Many congratulations, and God's blessing on you all for the next ten years'.

Joan Grayell, Sunninghill, Berkshire.
Comment: 'Such a warm, welcoming, place, which must be a real haven'.

Tony and Doreen Barber, Town Mayor, and Town Mayoress of Wokingham.
Comment: 'Many congratulations. Wonderful work. Best wishes for the future'.

Dee Tomlin, Chairman, Wokingham Borough Council.
Comment: 'Thank you for inviting me. I am delighted that you are doing so well. Nice to see you all today'.

Johnnie Hoggett, Reading.
Comment: 'Long may you thrive'.

Tony Heyes, Crowthorne, Berkshire.
Comment: 'Glad to be invited. Always the most welcoming place I go to'.

Bob Wyatt, Wokingham Borough Councillor.
Comment: 'Well done for all your excellent work'.

Pauline and Jim Murphy, Wokingham.
Comment: 'Many thanks. What a wonderful place full of wonderful people'.

Paul Whitelam, Reporter, *Wokingham Times*.
Comment: 'Keep up the good work. Thank you for showing me round – it was very informative'.

Linda Barnes, Wokingham Town Councillor and Deputy Mayor.
Comment: 'Very enjoyable visit. I had no idea that such a cosy and welcoming house existed behind the exterior. Wish you all every success'.

Sarah Dalymore and Lindy James, Supporting People Team, Wokingham Borough Council.
Comment: 'Very informative and welcoming'.

Jill Vance, Wokingham[North] Student Social Worker.
Comment: 'Wonderful environment. Great support. Fantastic philosophy. Thank you for allowing me to visit'.

Karen Paige, Student Social Worker, Wokingham.
Comment: 'Really refreshing and stimulating. I love all the pictures'.

Peter Morton, Community Mental Health Team, Wokingham.
Comment: *'Vive la différence!'*

Linda Barnes, Wokingham Town Mayor.
Comment: 'A very entertaining evening. Thank you'.

Andrew Wareham, Reading College for Social Action Video.
Comment: 'A wonderful environment full of interesting objects and people'.

Diane King, Deputy Town Mayor, Wokingham.
Comment: 'A calming and friendly environment. Best wishes to everyone'.

Linda Barnes, Town Mayor, Wokingham.
Comment: 'Another very enjoyable visit'.

Pauline Tin, Berkshire Healthcare Trust.
Comment: 'Very interesting, and lovely sandwiches'.

Paul McRobert, Wokingham Community Mental Health Team.
Comment: 'A most interesting and inspiring home'.

Joseph Shenni, Reading School of Art and Design.
Comment: 'It's a very nice place – welcoming. People are very relaxed, and seem to enjoy living here'.

Jean Blomfield, Wokingham Community Mental Health Team.
Comment: 'Offering a different perspective towards support required. Welcoming and enlightening'.

Naomi Jefferies, Nursing Student, Reading.
Comment: 'I was given a great deal of information to help me with my work which was very helpful. It was very welcoming and interesting'.

Christine Chessell, Deputy Town Mayor, Wokingham.
Comment: 'Keep up the good work, and may you go from strength to strength'.

Richard Bull, Berkshire Probation Service.
Comment: 'Keep up the good work'.

Claire Pritchett, Student Nurse, Thames Valley University, Slough.
Comment: 'Very impressive and friendly service'.

Danny Miller, Wokingham Town Mayor.
Comment: 'Delighted. Great people. Great job being done. An honour to know you'.

Iain Brown, Chairman, Wokingham Borough Council.
Comment: 'So good to see such a caring environment which gets people back on their feet. Well done everyone'.

Pat Jones, Head of Community Care Development, Wokingham Borough Council.
Comment: 'Thank you for showing us round, and making us welcome'.

Francis Dumbuya, Social Worker, Wokingham.
Comment: 'A very impressive setting with a friendly atmosphere'.

Sarah Bishton, *Wokingham Times*.
Comment: 'A homely, warm, friendly, place. An asset to Wokingham'.

Brother Colin Payne, Pillars of Friendship Lodge [Masons].
Comment: 'Pleasure to have visited. Carry on with the good work'.

Brother Zarak Goodwin, Pillars of Friendship Lodge.
Comment: 'We need places and people like you'.

Councillor and Mrs Angus Ross, Chairman, Wokingham Borough Council.
Comment: 'Thank you for your hospitality and interest. All best wishes for 2007'.

2007 – 2008

Karl Relton, Wokingham Baptist Church.
Comment: 'Marvellous visit'.

Rebecca Reid, Student Nurse, Wokingham.
Comment: 'Fantastic, lovely feel. Many thanks'.

Brian Willis, Wokingham Town Mayor.
Comment: 'A very enjoyable visit. Inviting and homely. Good luck'.

Barbara Bench, Wokingham Town Deputy Mayor.
Comment: 'Very entertaining and enjoyable visit. Best wishes for a successful future'.

Jo Hadfield, Clinical Psychologist, Wokingham.
Comment: 'Thank you for being so warm and welcoming. Wishing you all the best'.

Margaret Stronach, Wokingham.
Comment: 'Thank you for your support and advice, and a good cup of tea!'

Mike Paxton, Slough Mental Health User Group.
Comment: 'Lovely ambience you've created here. Stress free. Just what we need. They had better not try to close you down!'

Susanne McGregor, LSHTM.
Comment: 'Lovely people. Lovely place. A privilege to spend time here. There should be places like this'.

Susan Stanley, REAP Resettlement, Reading.
Comment: 'Love it!'

Brian Willis, Wokingham Town Mayor.
Comment: 'Have a wonderful and enthusiastic 2008. You do a great deal of good work for the community'.

Julie Quarrell, Wokingham Borough Council.
Comment: 'Had a really good morning. Shown around and given a lot of information on the service provided by the dedicated team. Many thanks'.

Julian McGhee-Sumner, Wokingham Deputy Town Mayor.
Comment: 'Very interesting visit. Very enjoyable. Well done'.

Peter Lucey, Wokingham Town Mayor.
Comment: 'Uplifting and sympathetic. Thank you'.

Elaine White, Deputy Mayor.
Comment: 'Wonderful Thank you for inviting Peter and I'.

Jason Wear, Wokingham Community Mental Health Team.
Comment: 'Very pleasant and welcoming'.

Sarah Till, Wokingham Mental Health Team.
Comment: 'Wonderful place run by caring people'.

Martin and Yvonne Bishop, Wokingham Town Mayor and Mayoress.
Comment: 'A very interesting visit. You are doing a wonderful job in our community'.

Chapter 42

Feedback From The Guests Themselves And Comments On Anniversaries

Spreading the word was important, and the comments of visitors from all over the United Kingdom and beyond, and comments from the local community, are all vital. Even more important, are the comments of those on the receiving end of the service – the crisis house guests. Here is a selection from the years when the beds were in operation

1991 – 1992

Benita.
Comment: 'Thank you for your kindness, Wokingham. God Bless'.

Ivan Granville Culquehan.
Comment: 'Thank you'.

1993 - 1994

Stan Wheeler.
Comment: 'Thanks for all your support'.

Magnus Runce.
Comment: 'AOK'.

Lauren Wilkinson.
Comment. 'You are all looking good. See you soon'. [Visit after leaving.]

Jack Hayward.
Comment: 'Very glad to meet friendly people and find some time otherwise not available, but often desperately needed'.

1995 – 1996

Agnes, Aurelia and Heather Runcie.
Comment: 'Lovely and cheerful, friendly, place'.

Magnus Runce.
Comment: 'Thank you for letting me stay, and thank you for your kind hospitality'.

Edwina Schaley.
Comment: 'Thanks for a wonderful opportunity to recover in the sanctuary. It's a marvellous place'.

Rob Jenkins.
Comment: 'Thanks for all your hospitality'.

1997 - 1998

Geoffrey Coley.
Comment: 'Super, smashing, Great. Just what I needed. Thank you for your help. Best wishes'.

Gavin Morris.
Comment: 'On the wings of love. Spiffing'.

Joan Morris.
Comment: 'Super. Thank you'.

1999 - 2000

Kath Alexandra.
Comment: 'Excellent help'.

2002 - 2005

Marcus Chain.
Comment: 'Lovely to see Crisis House again. Very nostalgic as ever'. [Former guest: 2001 – 2002.]

Leona Bridport.
Comment: 'Thank you to Pam and Frances for letting me stay in the crisis house, helping me to improve my life'.

Ambrose Meyer.
Comment: 'A blessing and gift from above from God to be helped by an angel. Eternally grateful. All my love and best wishes'.

2006 – 2007

Sylvia Kane.
Comment: 'What would I have done without this house, and all the support I have been given! Thanks, Pam, for all you have done, and to

everyone else'.

Chapter 43

Comments From Visitors On Crisis House Anniversaries

Ten Year Anniversary

Justine Brener, Old Windsor.
Comment: 'A dream come true! I came to the opening ten years ago together with Kath Lewis and Anne Davies, and am delighted to visit with them today'.

Kath Lewis, Wraysbury.
Comment: 'There have been many improvements over the last ten years. Congratulations'.

Anne Davies, Weybridge.
Comment: 'I agree with the other girls. It's wonderful. Congratulations'.

Mary Reinach, Wokingham.
Comment: 'Superb effort – an achievement out of this world!! All the best to all'.

Joan Grayell, Sunninghill.
Comment: 'Congratulations and best wishes. Such a warm and welcoming place which must be a real haven'.

Shirley Foley, Wokingham.
Comment: 'Congratulations. I'm glad to have been a small part of it. Here's to the next 10'.

David Crepaz-Keay, Buckinghamshire.
Comment: 'A ten year tribute to one woman's vision and single minded determination. It shows what can be done. Congratulations and best wishes'.

Gloria Wright, Harrow:
Comments: 'Inspiring. Congratulations. Long may you continue this excellent system of encouraging us'.

Joan Penrose, Harrow:
Comment: 'Your vision in practice continues to be a great inspiration to us all. Your provision of a real home to everybody here is a tribute to

your determination and courage. As you go from strength to strength, you will either demolish or outlive all your critics!'

Pauline and Jim Murphy, Wokingham.
Comment: 'Many thanks. What a wonderful place full of wonderful people'.

Rosemary Moore, Addlestone.
Comment: 'Love it all. The cats, the tea, the people, the computers'.

Fifteen Year Anniversary Open Day

John Redwood, MP, Wokingham.
Comment: 'Happy Anniversary, and many thanks to all the volunteers'.

Gordon Storey, Deputy Lord Lieutenant, Berkshire.
Comment: 'Well done on fifteen very successful years'.

Iain and Carole Brown, Chairman and Lady, Wokingham Borough Council.
Comment: 'Congratulations on fifteen years' splendid support in the community. Here's to the next fifteen years!'

Rex and Joyce Baldry, British Red Cross, Wokingham.
Comment: 'Wonderful to see these people again'.

Tony Barber, Ex Town Mayor, Wokingham.
Comment: 'You deserve all the plaudits and thanks of the community'.

As I mentioned earlier, of course I am pleased with the adulation that the crisis house has attracted over decades, but I do wish to emphasise one point.

I am not a team player. No way! I am a Prima Donna. No doubt about it! – To quote Miss Jean Brodie – 'It's the corps de ballet that has the team spirit!'

Yes, but one can't stage 'Swan Lake' WITHOUT the corps de ballet, and one individual cannot run a crisis house. Team work is absolutely essential – even if it is NOT consistent with one's temperament, and so I am pleased that so many visitors acknowledge and thank our team.

PART SIX

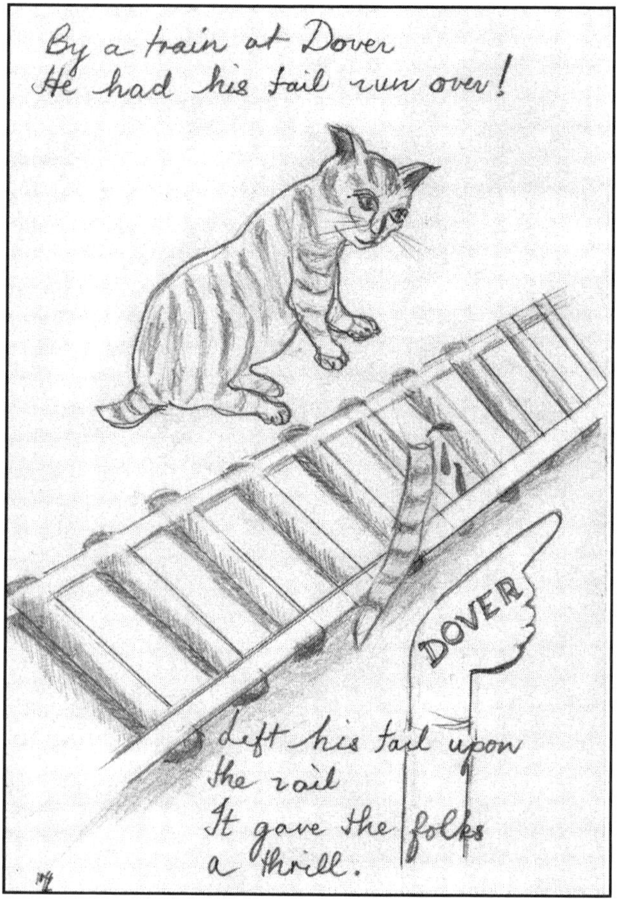

'Felix Kept On Walking, Kept On Walking Still. By A Train At Dover, He Had His Tail Run Over. He Left His Tail On The Rail. It Gave The Folks A Thrill

Chapter 44

Early Experiences In The Crisis House

The traditional mental hospitals offered a twenty-four/seven service. Modern 'Care in the Community' does not. We demonstrated this truth cogently when battling for the crisis house. On Good Friday 2007, I took a Press photographer around all the mental health services in Wokingham, such as they were, and, with the exception of the crisis house, they were all closed!

So the first thing to note about a crisis house, is that it is a twenty-four/seven commitment. From first days, I worked closely with the local branch of the Samaritans. Frequently, a mentally distressed person would turn up at their base in Bracknell – late in the evening. The Samaritan volunteer would be able to offer support and counselling, but the provision of beds was not within their charitable objects. This is where we came in. If the person had nowhere to sleep, the Samaritan would telephone me, and, together, we would go over to the crisis house. By now, it was, frequently, midnight!

This is where good organization kicked in. Each sanctuary bedroom was equipped with pyjamas, shaving gear, toiletries, slippers, dressing gowns – in fact anything that the person, who usually had only what he stood up in – needed to stay the night. I would make a cup of tea – or a meal if it were earlier in the evening – and then I would suggest that the person had a good night's rest, and we could get down to sorting out all the problems in the morning.

Most such guests did not need overnight cover. They were just emotionally exhausted, and needed to sleep. On the few occasions that overnight cover was required, we had a team who would provide this – always on a same/sex basis, but, in practice, such occasions were few.

Thus we accommodated – with referrals usually from either the Samaritans or the Police – and usually on a short-term basis – a great number of individuals in crisis.

These included - a man whose irate girlfriend had, first, torn up his redundancy cheque, and then, thrown him out on the street, an eighteen-year-old schoolgirl, who had had a row with her mother, and didn't want to go home, a nineteen-year-old who was suicidal, because he had lost both his lodgings, and his job within a space of two days, and a pregnant eighteen-year-old who had been sleeping in a field – having come down from the North to seek out the father of her unborn child.

They included a man who suffered from schizophrenia – who had come down from Manchester to stay with his father, but found that his father had gone away on holiday. There was another girl, who had been thrown out by her mother, and a young man who had absconded from a home for people with learning disabilities. Another young man was suicidal because he had been dismissed from his employment – having committed credit card fraud.

There was another young man, who had been involved in a family row, but whose father actually came to collect him after a few days. We accommodated two brothers with mild learning difficulties, for a night – until the Housing Authority assumed responsibility. Yet another young man with schizophrenia ran away from the crisis house, and had to be rescued by the Police, and admitted to hospital under a Section of the Mental Health Act.

It was also through the Police – under a 136 Section – that a young mother, her toddler, and her baby were admitted. The mother was mentally ill, and they were escaping from domestic violence. The plan was that they should stay for two nights – giving the social services and housing authority time to find them accommodation. At least – a quarter of a century ago – the authorities would find them something – even if it was less than ideal. Nowadays, you get nothing, and that was one of the reasons that we closed our beds!

I remember vividly that it was May Bank Holiday weekend. The Council had arranged bed-and-breakfast accommodation for this family, and I was just locking up the crisis house for the long weekend, when the telephone rang. It was the lady. 'Could they come back and stay in the crisis house, because the bed-and-breakfast accommodation had no pictures on the walls!'

I had to smile. Admittedly, the crisis house probably has a thousand pictures in total, and, yes, they are an important part of our therapeutic ambience, but hardly an essential, in emergency accommodation. I have included this anecdote in 'Funny Stories'.

Yet another lady – with a son who suffered from epilepsy – arrived via the local Samaritans – both having been the victims of domestic violence. Yet again, they were housed by the local housing authority within days. Another young man was accommodated for just one night. In a quarrel he had threatened to kill his mother. He just needed a bed for the night, prior to an interview for accommodation at the local Y.M.C.A.

A lady [we'll give her the benefit of the doubt], was referred by the Samaritans. She was homeless and roofless. I settled her in for the night, but when I arrived at the crisis house next morning, she had disappeared.

Then, two days later, she reappeared. [Guests were always given a set of keys]. 'Two nights ago, I met a gentleman, she said, but last night I didn't, so I came back.' We liked to think that we were accommodating, and accepted all sorts, but I don't think that temporary accommodation, for unemployed prostitutes, was ever envisaged in our remit!

Another young man was brought in by the Police, because he was refusing to leave his mother, who could no longer cope with him. Another lady presented a crucial situation, because her social worker was taking the view that, since we had accepted her in crisis, she had then, become our long-term responsibility. We improved his education, to a satisfactory conclusion.

This social worker caused us some mirth, because he appeared to be in a state of high anxiety. 'I shall have to have someone with me when I see her, he bleated, because she is coming on to me, sexually!' I don't know whether anyone provided him with a nursemaid. We didn't!

I have vivid memories of yet another social worker, who arrived to interview one of our early crisis house guests. Aged about twenty-two, she looked like a bit of chewed up string! 'Will they get a breakfast?' she inquired, wearily. Fancy looking like that, at that age! At twenty-two, I was raring to go – bursting with enthusiasm!

All such experiences ratify our position, that it is so important to ban professionals from the service at the very beginning. Given the chance, they would dump anyone and everyone onto the volunteers – who would be helpless, if the professionals had any position of power within the organization.

In those days, people who were vulnerable, were invariably given accommodation by the housing authority. We accommodated one man who suffered from a brain tumour, and, sure enough, bed-and-breakfast accommodation was provided after a night's respite with us.

Yet another man, was admitted for sanctuary, and, on this occasion, we felt that – due to severe mental illness – he needed overnight cover. This we provided. Our volunteer became concerned that this man was very paranoid, and suicidal, so he contacted a local doctor.

The belief, held by some local mental health professionals, was utter nonsense, that we would not contact doctors if we felt that their services were needed by guests, and several have been called to the crisis house over the years. It is professional interference in the working of our services that we will not tolerate, and not legitimate professional intervention – when this is necessary.

Thus, having won the battle for the crisis house, we were quite happy to amend our Rule Number 10 from 'No professional intervention' to 'No inappropriate professional intervention' – one of the measures that the Council required, if they were to continue with our Lease and our funding. No one determined who should decide whether a particular professional intervention was appropriate or inappropriate, and, in practice, we carried on exactly as before!

One man was yet another example of somebody disliking the accommodation that the authority provided. They all liked the crisis house, but, alas, we could not accommodate them all, nor forever. Surely, the answer is to set up more crisis house – and long-term ones, as well as short-term!

The Police frequently have to use the 136 Section, because it is the only way in which they can access a service for the person. One mentally ill lady was admitted to the crisis house on this basis. She was terrified of her family, and did not want to return home.

The drill, in such circumstances, was that the person stayed with us for the seventy-two hours duration of the Section, giving time for them to be seen by a doctor, and a suitably qualified mental health professional. Then, if they were homeless, or, as in this case, had no safe place to live, the local authority would provide them with temporary accommodation, under the Housing Act.

After three days, we had completed all the legal formalities, so I wished this lady well, and sent her up the road to the council housing department. A sigh of relief, another good job done! Not a bit of it. Ten minutes later, her retreating back became her advancing front. The council had asked, 'Could she stay longer, in the crisis house?' Answer, 'No.' We are crisis accommodation, only.

Fortunately, she was able to arrange accommodation with a friend, and so did not have to return to an abusive situation.

On other occasions, social workers had asked guests, 'Is Pam turning you out?' and since I was not, thought that they would not have to bother to find accommodation for people. They always struck me as being so stupid. Is not the whole point of a crisis house, the fact that it is to resolve crisis? It is a temporary measure, while more permanent solutions are achieved. But I had forgotten, of course. The client is a nuisance. If he can be dumped somewhere indefinitely, then nobody has to make any effort on his behalf!

Another occasion when I called out a doctor, was when a lady was referred by a local emergency housing project. I was told that she was fit to stay in the crisis house, but doubted this, once she had arrived. We insisted that the authorities took responsibility for her!

During these early years at the crisis house, today's heavy legislation regarding children was not in force, and we were able, quite frequently, to accommodate a mother with young children.

One lady arrived with an eight-year-old, and an eighteen-month-old. Our lady befriender, stayed the night with them, to give support and help. Alas, we can no longer allow children on the crisis house premises at all, because so much extra legislation is now involved.

The next example, is the one where we nipped inappropriate referrals in the bud. A lady had been referred by the mental hospital, and our volunteers went to collect her in our minibus. As soon as they met her, they had reservations about the suitability of the situation. She stayed for one night, but, next day, I told the mental health team that they must find her alternative accommodation.

A social worker. from the mental health team, came to the crisis house, and cast doubts upon our judgement, but to no avail. We insisted that alternative accommodation was found, and it was! I have stated elsewhere in this narrative, that, despite a twenty-year battle – lost, at last, to the power of money, I would swear that the local mental health establishment are miffed that we have closed our beds. It was not the beds that they objected to. It was their inability to CONTROL them!

This social worker's visit created a hilarious situation – because she was a particularly inept specimen of the breed. There is no private office in the crisis house, so her telephone call – presumably to some higher authority – could be overheard by all and sundry. She was saying, 'I don't know whether this person needs to be under supervision'.

One of our volunteers at the time, had both a very low opinion of Social Services, and a very loud voice. Oblivious to the feelings of the social worker, she yelled, at the top of her voice, 'That stupid cow doesn't know whether the lady needs to be under supervision! You can see that she needs supervision. I can see that she needs supervision!' No wonder that they never felt very comfortable – on the rare occasions that they got through our door!

Sometimes, the Samaritans would refer a couple [or a trio, if you include the unborn baby]. One such couple, neither of whose parents would accommodate them, stayed for just five nights while a flat was organized. They were very grateful for this crisis service.

I would swear that one young man was referred to us purely because the crisis house is clean!! It was the first thing that we did, when we moved into the building, in March 1991. Scrub the place from top to bottom. Get rid of all the grime of years – left by the previous tenants – the Social Services mental health team!

This man was obsessional about cleanliness, and would be very distressed, if he had to stay in a place that was dirty. He stayed in our clean sanctuary for a month – perfectly happily – and then moved into a bedsitter provided by the Council.

One guest was a lady who illustrated my belief that social work is not a profession. It is composed of sitting in meetings, and of making reports that are of no use to anybody!

This lady had been employed as a hospital social worker, but, due to a schizophrenic breakdown, was dismissed from this employment. She came to us for a few nights – just to get some respite from the pressures that she was suffering at home. When sufficiently recovered from acute illness, her husband insisted that she return to work. That was just the problem. She had no skills - because social work isn't work!!

First, I suggested office work. No good. She couldn't type. She couldn't use a computer. She had no idea of office organization. Filing was a mystery to her, and she didn't have the most basic information technology skills, that even children acquire in these days.

What about shop work? No good! She would never cope with the busy check-out! She ended up with dementia care, and she failed to cope with that as well, but she lasted for a time – simply because they are so desperate to get people to do this work, that practically anybody will be accepted.

Once this lady reached the age of fifty, her husband relented – to my relief. She was a nice lady, and it seemed a shame, that she was thrown, for the first time in her life, into the real world of work, when in her late forties!!

These stories cover some of the earlier, and shorter, stays at the crisis house. As the years went on, we accepted more and more people who needed to resolve life crises, on a longer-term basis. This was largely the reason for our opening two additional sanctuaries in the 2000's.

The value of the crisis house, as a community mental health facility, was recognised in certain quarters, from our earliest days. We had only been open a few months, when a mental health service user, whom we knew, escaped from the Secure Unit at Epsom Hospital, and turned up at the crisis house, complete with his suitcase, ready to stay in one of our sanctuaries!

'Shouldn't you be at Epsom?' I inquired. 'I escaped over the wire!' he explained. After making a cup of tea, I telephoned his Consultant. I did not think it necessary to involve the Police, but, with the Consultant's consent, simply telephoned Epsom Hospital, and three of their staff came over to collect their patient.

They joined us for a cup of tea, as well, and commented, as we have been saying ever since, that such little community mental health facilities, are needed everywhere.

Throughout my decades in mental health, I have found that there is much less hostility towards me, from the medical mental health professionals – as compared with the social workers. This is because we present less of a threat to them. The administration of medication is an absolute essential in mental health care: we can't do it, because we are not medically trained. Therefore, we do not, as our member, bluntly, put it, 'threaten their pay packets!'

In our early days, we ran an evening support group, at the crisis house. Here, we learned that some people accept such bizarre situations, that one would think that any escape route, even living in a hostel, and going out, scrubbing, for a living, would be preferable!

One evening, a timid little blonde woman came to the group – accompanied by her friend, who was quite normal, but who was living with an alcoholic husband.

The blonde lady explained that her husband was so paranoid, and feared so greatly, that she would go off with other men, while he was out at work, that, each morning, he would tie her up, and then lock her in a room, only untying her when he came home in the evening.

She could not escape, and he had only let her out, on the occasion that she came to us, because she had a female friend with her. 'Readers, what do you advise? Would you not run away that very night, and make a living anyhow, anywhere?'

I come back to Agatha Christie. In 'Why Didn't they Ask Evans?' [Published: Collins: 1934.], Roger Bassington-ffrench, asks a similar question of Lady Frances Derwent – when they are discussing the dilemma that Moira, Dr Nicholson's wife, is in. Moira claims that her husband is trying to kill her, so that he can marry Roger's sister-in-law, Sylvia Bassington-ffrench.

'What are we going to do about Mrs Nicholson?' [Lady Frances] asked abruptly. 'What do you mean, do about her?' [asks Roger.] 'Well, the poor thing is terrified to death. I do think you're callous about her, Roger.' 'I'm not really, but people who can't help themselves always irritate me.' 'Oh, but do be fair, [says Lady Frances]. What can she do? She's no money, and nowhere to go.'

Roger said unexpectedly, 'If you were in her place, Frankie, you'd find something to do. Yes, you would. If you really thought somebody was trying to murder you, you wouldn't just stay there tamely waiting to be murdered. You'd run away and make a living somehow . . . You'd do something.'

Frankie tried to think what she would do. 'I'd certainly do something,' she said thoughtfully. 'The truth of the matter is that you've got guts and she hasn't', said Roger with decision.

It was only a story, but so telling. Such situations do exist in real life. One can scarcely believe that anyone would tolerate such a situation, but they do!

Another lady, from those times, had a happy resolution to her problems.

This lady was very attractive, cultured, and smartly dressed. She said that she had only realised just how bad her living situation was, when her husband died. Her husband, who suffered from paranoid schizophrenia, had a very good, highly paid, job, as a merchant banker, in London. They had lived in a big house in Maidenhead – by the river.

His was a 'compartmentalising' illness. He was only disturbed in one compartment of his life – his marriage. At work, he behaved completely normally. At home, his jealousy of his wife, and his terror that she would go off with other men, while he was at work, led him to isolate her completely. She wasn't even allowed to talk to other women.

This lady said, that it was only after her husband had committed suicide, in the exhaust fumes of a car, shut up in a garage, that she realised that he had isolated her, completely, from everybody. She was left without contact with any other soul in the world.

This story has a happy ending. Six months after she first contacted me, she rang to say that she was doing very well, had joined two choirs, and was rebuilding her life.

Chapter 45

Lucy's Story (Written in Her Own Words)

My BiPolar Experience - A True Life Experience of a Mother and Grandmother in her late fifties.

"As a school girl of 16, back in the 1960's, facing my GCSE's, I was under such extreme pressure, that I flipped, as I was expected to get 9 GCSE's. One night I could not face going to school the next day so I took my first overdose of Aspirins. I actually woke up my parents and told them what I had done. Although I wanted to die at that time, I must have had a pang of conscience, to tell them. They took me to A&E at out local Hospital in the West Midlands. When I was discharged I went to a Psychiatric Hospital. I'm not too sure how long I was there, but it was weeks rather than months, and I continued to see my Psychiatrist as an out patient on Saturdays, when I had a job, so I didn't have to have time off work.

Not everyone with BPAD (Bipolar Affective Disorder) suffers the exact same symptoms, but the outcome is usually the same. The very nature of the condition means, that although it is usually manageable with proper medication, it will never go away, and therefore, it is for life, so you have to learn to live with it, the best way you can.

I usually suffer from very extreme Lows, and can also feel suicidal. I have only suffered one Manic High, in 2001, and I was hospitalised in Fair Mile Psychiatric Hospital to adjust the dosage of Lithium, which I am still taking today, in conjunction with other medication.

In 1982, when my oldest son was born, I suffered with Post Natal Depression. In 1984, when he was 2 years old, I attended Eldon Road Day Hospital, Reading, Berkshire, where I was diagnosed with BPAD, and he was looked after by a wonderful childminder. I was extremely lucky because my husband's firm paid for the childminder, so he could go to work, and not stay home to look after both of us.

Not everyone with BPAD has to be hospitalised, but the law of averages says that during their lifetime, it's possible that they may have to be in hospital to stabilise their medication.

In June 2007, I was admitted to the Royal Berkshire Hospital, after taking a near fatal overdose, then onto Prospect Park Psychiatric Hospital. This was not a cry for help; I genuinely wanted to take my own life at that time. Having gone through a Divorce, bought my own house, and just getting my life back on track, my boss made me redundant, and at the time, I didn't know anything about Benefits. I was worried how I would manage with no income coming in, and this is what drove me to take the steps that I did.

Part of getting to grips with BPAD is accepting that your Extreme Mood Swings can be so extreme that you are not aware that anything is wrong, if you are Manic. Other people are telling you that you are as high as a kite. But you can't see it, because you feel so elated and euphoric.

Over the last seven years, as a family, we have suffered various personal crises. I suffered a near fatal car crash (2004) with a double tyre blow-out on the fast lane of the M4 near Swindon. I was also diagnosed with a near fatal Pulmonary Embolism (2002) and admitted to the Royal Berkshire Hospital as an emergency admission.

I think that I have always suffered from Depression, but until my first breakdown and overdose when I was 16 years old, no one realised it.

Depression and all forms of Mental Illness are one of the worst conditions that anyone can suffer. They look "Normal", whatever that is, and no-one knows what they are suffering inside their mind and heart.

Mental torment is far, far, worse than any physical condition. I can say that, because I suffer from a chronic back condition, and my knee joints, fingers, and toes, have Arthritis. I have also undergone a full knee replacement operation, which was a total success. People are more sympathetic if they can see what is wrong with you, i.e.: you use a walking stick or have a bandage or sling on, etc.

When HIV/Aids first came to light, people were ignorant about it. Mental Illness has been around since Victorian times, but it is still so misunderstood by most people.

It is part of 'getting better' process to keep busy, by setting yourself simple, but achievable, tasks to do each day. There's nothing wrong with watching T.V., as I find when I am on a BPAD Low. It helps to distract me from my problems. It's really a question of finding out what's right for you and acting on it. We are all different, and what suits one person will not suit another. Don't be afraid to ask for help from the professionals.

I have been lucky that I have had so much help and support from my Social Worker, Psychiatrist, GP and family and friends.

I also attended two different 'Drop-Ins' up to four times a week, I only go to one now. I did go to ten pin bowling, as a group, and then we went out for lunch.

The 'Drop-Ins' also arranged day trips, cinema trips, a walking group and free college courses. I have been on a Digital Camera course, and I really learnt a lot from doing a Tai Chi course, which I find a great source of distraction.

When we are talking, it's amazing how many of us have lost some of our friends. I think it could be because they don't fully understand mental illness, and therefore, they back off.

When I got divorced, I moved away from my marital home to live on my own, it was really very strange, and also very frightening, as I had to learn how to deal with running my home single-handed. I managed all through the Divorce to stay well.

When both my Social Worker and Psychiatrist, feel that I am ready for work, they have suggested that I try some voluntary work first, even if it's only half a day. It should help to build up my confidence and self esteem - which goes down the pan, when I am on a BPAD Low?

During 2008, it was obvious to me, that Mum might not survive Christmas; I think she knew it herself, and so put all her affairs in order. Mum and Dad lived in Somerset for the last 20 years. Unfortunately, for me it's 125 miles each way, and on a good day, I can get there in 2-3 hours.

Mum, who was a retired General Nursing Sister, was never the same again, after she fell and broke her hip in 2004, and whilst in hospital, she caught Clostridium Difficile. It was not as widespread then, as it is now. She finally lost her battle with life, and passed away in September 2008. Not only did she have C.Diff, she also caught M.R.S.A. whilst in hospital. Mum was always very slight, in build, and when I first visited her in Hospital, she didn't even recognise me at all. It was very hard for me to keep visiting, as she kept asking for me, and when I tried to explain that this was me, she didn't, or couldn't, know me.

Dad stayed in his bungalow alone for about 6 months. He had been going to this Care Home for a number of years, for a week's respite, every 6 weeks, so it was all familiar to him, when he moved in as a permanent resident.

I tried to visit him as often as possible, but that's dependent on my mood, as I have to drive there. I need to be well enough to undertake the journey. Dad had always understood my illness, much more than Mum.

Looking back, it was a shame that, although Mum was a General Nursing Sister, she never understood my illness, Dad, however, did. He actually had Vascular Dementia, but was still able to recall his War Stories. My Partner, at the time, took a video of Dad relating various

War experiences. We contacted the Imperial War Museum in London, and together with a photo of him in uniform, and some relevant background information, this appears on their Internet Web Site, which is available to view for the I.W.M. We will go to visit the Museum one day.

You may be asking yourself, if this is relevant. Well yes, I think it is, because actually, it will show you how I coped with organising events like Mum and Dad's Funerals, which for anyone was a very stressful situation, but made far worse because of my condition, contacting friends and family, and booking the Undertakers etc.

I hope that my story has helped you to understand that there is life after BPAD, although you never fully recover, from BPAD; it is for life, and you have to find a way to cope with it, within your own limits. It's a simple case of managing it the best way that you can.

The relationship that I mentioned earlier, took its toll on me, and I had to finish it. (We never actually lived together.) He didn't take it well, and was sending me abusive and threatening texts. I did not reply.

In October 2010, I lost my Dad, we were very close, although he lived 125 miles away. We went to visit him as often as we could, usually once a month. I feel very empty, but he had a long life, living till he was 92 years young. I will miss him so much, but he will soon be with Mum. Arranging his Funeral was easier this time, as he lived in a great Care Home, so there was no house to sell.

I would like to thank Wokingham Mental Health Team, (CMHT), my Social Worker, and my CBT Therapist, my Psychiatrist, and GP. I have now been discharged from them, as I have been stable for 3 years, and got a part-time job. Also the CRS Group, and of course my family and friends, and The Wokingham Crisis House, and anyone else involved in my welfare.

Many famous people suffer from this condition, below is listed just some of them;-

Robbie Williams
Frank Bruno
Carrie Fisher
Rick Stein
Vivienne Leigh
Madonna
Kenny Everett
Stephen Fry
Angus Deayton
Spike Milligan
Caroline Aherne
Kerry Katona
Norman Wisdom
Tommy Cooper

I am dedicating this to my late Mum, who lost her fight with life in September 2008, and also my Dad, who, 2 years later, lost his final battle with life.

I hope this story is of some comfort to those of you who suffer, or care for someone, with this condition, or any other Mental Disorder. If it helps just one person to come to terms with their illness, it's been worth writing this.

Since completing this, I have got myself a Part-Time Admin Assistant position, and look forward to a bright future. I had been job hunting for over 2 years, before getting this position, and was in fact wondering if I would ever work again. My Line Manager understands my condition and she is very supportive.

Unfortunately, I was made redundant in August 2013, and am still looking for another job. I now volunteer at The Wokingham Crisis House 2/3 days a week, to try to help people with all kinds of mental illness plus Drugs and Alcohol abuse.

Here are some interesting Web sites to visit for more information:-

www.mdf.org.uk	The Bipolar Organization
www.depressionalliance.org	Support & understanding to anyone affected by Depression
www.mind.org.uk	National Association for Mental Health
www.rethink.org	National Association for Mental Health
www.samaritans.org	Samaritans

I actually started writing this back in 2007, when over a period of time, I couldn't sleep, when suffering from several very bad BPAD episodes. Over the next 5 years, this is the finished result. You may think I have taken a long time to complete this, but I sometimes only scribbled notes down on scraps of paper, in the middle of the night. When I felt able to make sense of it all, I started to write this in booklet form.

Thank you for finding the time to read this, and I hope it has shown you, THAT YOU ARE NOT ALONE and, maybe, some of my coping strategies will help you, Good Luck for your future."

What I like about 'Lucy's Story', is the way in which she sets out, with supreme common sense, to cope with all the problems of daily life – despite her illness. To me, she is the personification of my statement in the 'Conclusion' of this book, that you have precisely two choices. You can either sit down and moan for the rest of your life, or get up and make the best of it. Lucy chose the latter!

Chapter 46

The Crisis House Today

Crisis work never abates, never lets up! When we had the beds at the crisis house, we would get just enough time as a guest left – to clean the room, and make up a fresh bed – before a new guest in crisis arrived. So we certainly are helping to resolve life crises throughout 2015 and 2016. Will we have further success stories? I certainly hope so!

Neville Sandford

Neville Sandford came to us in the Autumn of 2014. He was homeless and roofless, and had been sleeping in a tent in the woods. Fortunately, through the kind offices of the Salvation Army, he obtained a place in a local youth hostel, so at least he had a roof over his head, for the forthcoming winter.

Neville is intelligent, personable, well-mannered, articulate – and is quite severely mentally ill, with depression – though this is not immediately obvious. He attends the drop-in centre regularly, and greatly appreciates the asylum ambience that the crisis house provides. No pressure!

By contrast, at the youth hostel where he lives, Neville is put under constant pressure to sort himself out – probably because they do not understand the full extent of his mental ill health. Neville, should be in mental health supported housing, but our Wokingham hostels have closed.

I use this analogy repeatedly. One cannot walk with a broken leg. One needs complete rest so that it can heal, and then supported exercise once healing has taken place. By the same token, one cannot function with a broken mind. One needs complete rest while the mind heals, and then supported rehabilitation, once healing has taken place. Far from rejecting the medical model of mental illness, I find it both a useful, and an accurate, model to adopt!

Neville has a background of severe family problems. His father abandoned him and his mother, when he was an infant. Neville's father died recently, but Neville, now aged twenty-five, had had no contact in the intervening years. Neville's mother used to take in paying guests in order to make ends meet – so Neville – during his growing up years, felt that they got his mother's attention at his expense. Nevertheless, Neville did well with his education, both in school and in college, obtaining a large number of GCSE and NVQ passes.

When Neville's mother met a new partner, he was no longer able to live at home with them. I have encountered this situation before. Sometimes, the adult son reminds his mother, of the man who abandoned her – hence the rejection. Sometimes, having slaved to rear the child alone, she feels that he is now an adult in his twenties, should be self-sufficient, and that she, herself, is now entitled to some life.

Repeatedly, in mental health work, one encounters the fact that people who have not been given the nurture, support, and encouragement, which they need to achieve maturity, fail to do so, and go on, needing and craving, the care which they did not receive in childhood and adolescence. This is why I recommend adult fostering as a good service in mental health.

If you read [Chapter22: 'Have you seen my childhood?'], you will conclude that adult fostering would probably have been the only service adequate to deal with such a severe case. Unfortunately, it was not, then, available.

In recent correspondence with our MP, John Redwood, I put forward the idea of adult fostering, as a suggestion for local community care. He liked the idea, and said that he would suggest it to the local authority.

Adult fostering is not the same as supported lodgings. Supported lodgings are often found for youngsters leaving 'care'. Such youngsters are usually all right, mentally, or may have only emotional problems. They need lodgings, because they have no family to return to, but can fit in quite well with ordinary families.

For adult fostering, you need couples in early middle age, with plenty of time, money, and the wife not having to go out to work. These are people with a nice, big, house, who wanted children, but never had any.

Now in their forties, they are experiencing a gap in their lives. They see a future stretching ahead – well off financially, but not emotionally. At the dinner parties, they gaze wistfully into space, while everyone else relates, with enjoyment, the latest news about their children, or grandchildren.

Such couples may now feel that they are too old to take on a child, but might feel able to take on a profoundly physically, or mentally, disabled adult. A very severely disabled, mentally ill, adult, could tear an ordinary family to pieces, or, a frequent occurrence, absorb so much of the parents' time and attention, that other family members feel neglected.

Adult foster parents take on only one individual. They have a strong, formerly, frustrated, need to be parents, and so, nurturing one high-needs individual, can prove most satisfying to all parties involved.

In early adult life, Neville drifted into homelessness, and also became drug, and alcohol, dependent. Despite this, he has not given up on life. He is intending to study Media, at college, in the near future, and I am hopeful that he will be a success story!

On 25th September 2015, Lucy Farmer and Neville Sandford made the new DVD of the crisis house which, on publication, is to accompany this book. As well as being useful for us, this was a good introductory stab at media work, for Neville.

Norah Chessling

Norah [then named Hank] first came to us in 2008. She was both depressed and drug-dependent. We helped her to obtain a flat, and she got into voluntary work – progressing on to paid work which he sustained successfully for a number of years.

Norah came back to us in 2015 – having suffered a further breakdown, due to work stress, and the fact that she had been repressing transgender issues. Hank [now Norah] explained that, despite all the stigma, it is actually LESS stressful when one 'comes out' as transgender.

Norah has been accepted by Charing Cross Hospital for their Gender Reassignment Programme. The patient has to live as a woman for two years, before surgery can be considered. Hormone treatment is also included in the Programme. Norah needs a lot of emotional support throughout this process – which is being provided, both by her parents, and by us. We are optimistic that Norah will be a success story. She has already made the first steps towards recovery, by going back to work, part-time.

Currently, Norah is explaining to us, that the transgender issues are not the ones causing her the most distress. More distressing, is her inability to get any effective help and treatment from the local mental health service. She has continuous suicidal ideation, and is in despair – that her needs are so complex that nobody wants to take her on.

So we have referred her to a local private psychiatric hospital. We have done this a number of times, now that services are so diminished, and we consider it to be a good use of our charitable funds. As Agatha Christie would have it [of Meadow Bank School], 'You pay through the nose, but you get what you pay for!'

One useful thing that one gets from the top consultants at the private psychiatric hospital, is a report – detailing the patient's needs. This can be used by us when advocating for services for the individual.

Marian Brewer

I have described Marian's problems with the Bedroom Tax in the chapter on Advocacy.

I hope, through obtaining for her the Personal Independence Payment [PIP], to enable Marian to find a place to live in quieter and more congenial surroundings.

Marian will take her, severe, neurotic illness with her, wherever she goes. There is no miracle cure, so, if she becomes a success story, it will be in terms of RELATIVE success. This is so often the case, with mental health.

Our aim is that her life – while not idyllic – will be better than it was before. She will still have problems with relationships, [having, when she came to us, ended up with no relationships at all!], but she will have us, and, as Phil Green said all those years ago [Chapter 6: 'A Therapeutic Environment', and Chapter12: 'Embroidered on silk'.], we are like an extended family – the family that all these mentally distressed people never had!

Jimmy Jenkins

Round and round in circles

'In and out the windows, in and out the windows,
in and out the windows, as we have done before.
'Round and round in circles, round and round in circles,
round and round in circles, as we have done before!'

It is frightening to face the fact, that, in September 2015, it is now getting on for a year, since Jimmy's sister approached me for help.

He suffered from a severe paranoid personality disorder, and had returned to Wokingham from Somerset – in order to escape a knife threat there. His sister, Holly, had found Jimmy sleeping in a field. The Council were refusing to house him, but the local mental health team had agreed to assess his mental health.

I reassured Holly, that our charity would pay to accommodate Jimmy in bed-and-breakfast accommodation – while this assessment was being carried out.

The assessment was undertaken by social workers – who have no training in mental illness. They concluded that Jimmy, who is profoundly mentally ill, did not qualify for supported, mental health housing. This reflects the Minister of Health's comments to me, all those years ago, about doctors being used to making objective judgements, while social workers are not.

Doctors, if they had diagnosed you with cancer, for instance, would never say that you did not have the disease – though they might say that you had to wait for some of the less urgent treatments.

By contrast, social workers' 'assessments', co-incide with the services that they have. If they want to meet adoption targets, you are a deficient parent! If they have no supported housing available to you, then you are not mentally ill!

Interestingly, Jimmy's case is one of the many, where the man in the street can see what he needs, while the 'professionals' can't or won't! On 23rd September 2015, Lucy, Neville, and I, attended the launch of the new charity, 'Wokingham in Need', at the local Salvation Army Hall. One of their helpers, without any prompting from us, said that she knew Jimmy, and that he needed to be in mental health supported housing. You don't need qualifications to see it. All that you need is common sense.

We took the matter up with our MP – who suggested that we obtained a specialist's report on Jimmy's mental health. We did this, going to the top, and the distinguished, Consultant Psychiatrist, whom we paid to examine him, confirmed that Jimmy was, indeed, seriously mentally ill, and in need of priority housing.

This was still refused by Wokingham Borough Council, and he was offered only an amount of money, for the deposit on accommodation, which he would have to find for himself.

Jimmy was incapable of doing this, so he went back on the streets, and has been on the streets ever since. The Council's Homelessness Officer sent him a letter – reams and reams of rubbish – citing every reason under the sun for NOT accommodating him.

What we need to do, is to get rid of these bureaucrats, restore welfare services to dedicated volunteers, and put the money into practical facilities – such as supported housing.

Carrie Jean Layley

Right back where I started from

'California, here I come – right back where I started from!'

In the good old days – before welfare was handed over to the state – there existed charities, run by dedicated volunteers, known as Prisoners' Help Societies.

On discharge from prison, such a society would help the individual, by finding them somewhere to live, new clothes, a job, and, in fact, everything necessary - to prevent a relapse into crime.

Agatha Christie, is very good, at giving us insights, into such little snippets of social history.

For instance, in 'The Big Four', [Published: Collins: 1927.], Hercule Poirot interviews the recently released prisoner, Robert Grant.

'When did you come out of prison?' asks Poirot. 'Two months ago.' 'How did you obtain this job?' 'Through one of them Prisoners' Help Societies. Bloke met me when I came out.' 'What was he like?' 'Not exactly a parson, but looked like one. ....Said he hoped I was repentant, and that he'd find me a good post.I went to old Whalley on his recommendation.'

Then Poirot said, 'Saunders gave you a pair of boots, didn't he?' Grant looked very much astonished. 'Why, yes he did.'

This little exchange, I find most revealing. Before we had the Probation Service, it is evident that charities looked after people who were discharged from prison. They were found jobs, accommodation, clothes, shoes, and in fact, everything, that they needed. It was all practical, and it was all delivered on an entirely voluntary basis. Extraordinary, is it not, that we tax-payers, get the services that are necessary when we DON'T pay for them, but we don't get any services when we DO pay for them!

Frequently, nowadays, former prisoners leave prison, with no welfare arrangements being made for them at all. Such was the case with Carrie-Jean Layley.

Carrie - Jean suggested that her parents contact me, to see whether I could help, and I agreed to do so. I had known Carrie-Jean for many years. She was a heroin addict, in prison for the shop-lifting, which financed her drug habit. On discharge, her flat was to be repossessed. Some elderly friends had agreed to accommodate her temporarily, and our charity agreed to pay removal costs, and storage for her furniture.

Both parties were aiming to help out temporarily – thus giving the

Probation Service, time to find Carrie-Jean accommodation. 'Hope springs eternal in the human breast!' Months passed. We had agreed to store her furniture for six months. Still nothing was arranged for her, so we extended this to nine months! Then the elderly friends, who suffered ill-health, themselves, had to ask Carrie-Jean to move out. Ill health or not, this is invariably the scenario.

Friends are willing to rally round TEMPORARILY. They do not want house-guests for months on end, and who can blame them? The inevitable happened. The authorities had done nothing. Carrie-Jean would have been on the street once again, so she had no alternative but to go and stay with the inveterate heroin-addict, Ewan. Back on the drugs she went, back to shop-lifting she went, back to prison she went. 'California, here I come. Right back where I started from!'

I read the court report on Carrie-Jean's case in the local newspaper, and I was frustrated by the arresting Police Officer's comment – that stealing will always be dealt with robustly, and heavy prison sentences, imposed.

If Carrie-Jean's addiction were dealt with, she would not be stealing, but one can't conquer addiction, if one has nowhere suitable, and stable, to live.

In the days of the Prisoners' Help Society, their volunteer would have ensured that Carrie-Jean had suitable accommodation – away from the drugs sub-culture, and that she was given all the support needed to complete the detoxification programme, successfully. Carrie-Jean was back in prison because of negligence, because statutory welfare does not exist. The bureaucracy is there, but the practical facilities are not!

Carrie-Jean came to see us, at the crisis house, in early September 2015. She had been discharged from prison, but under strict conditions. Carrie-Jean confirmed the truth of all my earlier comments.

IF they had housed her on her former discharge from prison. IF they had provided the support needed, she would not have fallen back on accommodation with an inveterate heroin addict, would not have returned to using the drug, would not have shop-lifted to fund her drug habit, would not have gone back to prison. Round and round in circles, as we have done before! California, here I come, right back where I started from!

Fortunately, Carrie-Jean's parents have agreed to accommodate her while she undertakes yet another period of detoxification, and there is even the possibility of residential rehab - which finally commenced in December 2015. 'But why not before?' one asks. The bureaucracy is in place, but the service is not!

Bank Holiday Monday at the Crisis House: 31st August 2015

It is Monday 31st August 2015, and the crisis house drop-in centre is open. I always open on Bank holidays, because there is nothing else available, for the mentally ill, on these days.

Such occasions always remind me of the time when we were fighting for the crisis house. On Good Friday, and on Easter Monday, 2007, I took a Press photographer around the mental health services, such as they were, in Wokingham. They were all closed. Now, whether something is any good or not, may be, to some extent, a matter of opinion. Whether a place is open or not, that's a matter of fact!

Of course, Bank Holidays, are quieter than regular days, but one can still get some useful work done. I used this one, to fill in Neville Sandford's PIP [Personal Independence payment], application form. The PIP form is not quite so daunting as its predecessor, the Disability Living Allowance Application Form, but one still wades through forty pages. No severely mentally ill person [and you have to be severely ill, in order to qualify for this benefit], could cope alone, with filling it in. Our advocacy service is essential.

Relative peace and quiet, also enabled me to get talking with Wes. Wes has been coming to us for about eighteen months. He suffers from some degree of learning disabilities, as well as anxiety, and social phobias. He is homeless, and was one whom we paid to accommodate in bed-and-breakfast accommodation, during the most freezing weeks of last winter.

We got talking, and it transpired that Wes, aged twenty-eight, does not like twenty-first century pop music. He is an Elvis Presley, Rock 'n Roll fan – as are all his family – including his parents, and his grandparents. They all belong to Rock 'n Roll clubs.

'There is nothing that I don't know about Elvis', Wes continued. He went on to prove his point, and it was no idle boast. Going back to the early 1950's, Wes knew all the songs, and later, all the films, right through the whole history of Elvis.

On Bank Holiday Monday, Wes proved my point. Take an interest in a mentally ill person, and the trouble to talk, and listen, and you will get a remarkable response. Wes also confided, that Social Services had always been in his life, and had always been completely useless. One almost gets to the point of saying, 'Well, they would be, wouldn't they!'

Daniel Rendell also came in on the Bank Holiday. He is so over-medicated, that he can scarcely articulate his words, and, indeed, spends most of his time, asleep, but, at least, he attended. Getting out of your four walls, and getting to a place where there are other people, is always the first step towards recovery, when one is battling severe mental illness.

In September 2015, we were saddened, when a friend of the crisis house, dropped in, with the news that his former partner had died, of alcoholism. She was a lovely lady!

I remember the first occasion, in 2011, when this couple first visited the crisis house. They said that it reminded them of America, where crisis centres abound. Access to these is available, twenty-four/seven, and they are run by volunteers. Why does America have such desperately needed services, while we do not? I suspect that the answer is, that they are a self-help culture, and not bounden, as we are, to things run by the state.

Then, she went on to make, her most telling, point. 'This is a marvellous place, she said, and, what I can hardly believe, right on our doorstep!' That, twenty-five years on, is the sad truth about the Wokingham Crisis House. By now, all mental health sufferers, should have access to such a service, right on their doorstep. It could have been done. It wasn't!

At the end of September 2015, Ellie came to us, once again, in crisis. Ellie's problems stem from a situation which is very common in these days of easy divorce. Once again, I bring Agatha Christie into the picture.

In 'The Moving Finger', [Published: Collins: 1942.] Megan says to Jerry Burton, that she is not wanted by her family. Furthermore, as an intelligent, and perceptive, girl, she knew why. They were a complete family without her.

Megan's father went to prison for blackmail. Her mother re-married. She married the solicitor, Richard Symmington, and they had two boys. Neither mother, nor stepfather, wanted Megan. She reminded her mother of the man who had disgraced her, and her stepfather had no biological bond with her.

In Agatha's inimitable prose, when Jerry asked Richard Symmington for his stepdaughter's hand in marriage, 'the frozen halibut thawed'.

What a relief! He could get rid of Megan, and respectably, too!

We have experienced this situation many times in the crisis house, and Ellie is not the only one, experiencing this, amongst our current ranks. Her parents divorced when she was ten. The stepfather never wanted her, and she has experienced emotional problems ever since.

Going back to the nineteen thirties, not only was divorce very difficult, and very expensive, to achieve, but were one's spouse committed to a mental institution, and thus considered, legally, unable to give consent, divorce was unobtainable. The strictures imposed by this situation are dealt with in Agatha Christie's novel, 'Three Act Tragedy'. [Published: Collins: 1935.]

Easier divorce has, no doubt, freed many people from a life of misery. The 1968 'Marriages Act', which was on the Statute Book by 1970, relaxed things considerably, bringing in, for instance, the concept of 'irretrievable breakdown of the marriage' – thus leading to the 'quickie' divorce.

On the other hand, in the days when divorce was a social disgrace, and very difficult to obtain, most children were raised to adulthood by both their biological parents, and a biological mother or father, has a natural bond, even with a difficult child. Frequently, a non biological parent simply doesn't want the hassle.

We are, of course, being sympathetic, and supportive, but Ellie is now in her forties, so I fear that it is very much a case of the hard, but the only realistic, choice that faces her. 'You can either sit down and moan for the rest of your life, or get up and make the best of it!'

Chapter 47

Problems Encountered

At the time that the local mental health establishment was trying to destroy the crisis house – throughout 2007 – there were a lot of jokes in the local Press that 'the crisis house was in crisis!' The Press were highly supportive of us, so we took it all with good humour and equanimity. In fact, the crisis house was NOT in crisis. As a service, we were easy to solve – because we did not have a problem. Before one can justify closing something down, one has to pretend that there is something wrong with it, and that is what happened to us!

The attempt to demonstrate that there was something wrong with our service, and thus to create a problem, was, as the late Alan Godsal explained, 'a put-up job'. It was an attempt to justify closure. The motive was three-fold – and it is interesting that in all these political manoeuvres – the welfare of the people involved – never enters the equation.

The late Social Services' employee did not care a scrap about the mentally ill people, who were suffering because their sanctuary had become insecure. All she cared about, was her own career, and the fact that our services were preferred to hers! This is why I believe in the abolition of Social Services. Restore services to a simple level – where ordinary people, deliver welfare out of the goodness of their hearts – and you will get the services that the mentally ill actually need. The people who deliver them, have no other motivation than a desire to do good, and to serve their fellow men and women.

Three motives for the desired closure! First, they cannot control us. We are independent and separatist. Secondly, we are a centre of excellence – showing up mediocrity, or worse, wherever it is encountered locally. Thirdly, and the strongest motive of all, if one demonstrates, as we do, that welfare can be delivered by volunteers, where does that leave them – their careers, their fat salaries, their pensions, their cars?

In times of austerity, it could give local councils, ideas, too terrifying to be contemplated! As one of our service users put it very recently, cogently, if somewhat crudely, 'You threaten their pay-packets!'

It is never a good idea to offer just one service – provided by the State. Do so, and that service can be tenth rate in peace! Choice, and healthy competition, is always essential – in order to ensure that standards are maintained.

So we did not have the problems that they alleged, but, over twenty-five years, we have encountered plenty of problems – because problems, and their solution, are what a crisis house is about.

When the new road was being built, and we were sitting in a state of dereliction – at one point, literally surrounded by water – like the house on stilts in a child's history book – local people felt sorry for us, but we did not feel sorry for ourselves.

We have a lovely, big, Victorian house, and – although parts are a bit rickety – it is fundamentally sound. In a context, where many charities have to cope in a bit of, cramped, office space, I consider us to be fortunately placed.

Nevertheless, in ideal circumstances, it would have been better to have two adjoining houses – one for the residential part of the service, and one for the day drop-in. Guests, after a while, began to regard the crisis house as their home, and drop-in service users were regarded as an intrusion!

On the other side of the coin, people wishing to access the upstairs library, and internet, could find encountering guests in their dressing gowns – an embarrassment.

There is no doubt – that now that we have discontinued the beds – the facilities are much improved for drop-in service users. They now have a games room [a former bedroom], ready and private access to the library and internet, and a completely private counselling room, [a second former bedroom] – where they can sit with just one confidante, or, in peaceful solitude – if they so wish. All this is not to say that crisis beds are not still desperately needed. They are!

On the whole, throughout the years, crisis house guests got on well together, but there were, inevitably, some personality clashes. Again, it tended to be this thing: 'If only I could have this house to myself. It is so perfect for my needs – in the heart of Wokingham, and close to everything. If only I didn't have to put up with the other guests!'

One notorious former guest, Gabriela Rani, actually got her GP to write to me – more or less suggesting, that I should get rid of Gabriela's fellow-guest, because he disturbed her sleep!

This guest had reversed the biological clock, and so was up and about at night, and although the bedrooms had heavy fire doors that shut out sound effectively, Gabriela still wanted sole use of the house, uninterrupted sleep, and perfect conditions. I had to point out that it was a four bed crisis house, and not a private residence!

By contrast, there was Leona – of whom I have such fond memories. Leona was a guest from 2003 to 2005. She suffered from depression, body-dysmorphic syndrome, and alcoholism.

Leona accepted the crisis house with all its limitations, never criticized anything, and never gave us a moment's trouble. She was a realist. You can't have everything on your terms. So many, over the years, have wanted the service on THEIR terms – with all the freedom and advantages, inherent in a voluntary service, but with none of its disadvantages!

I shall always retain a soft spot for Leona. At the time that I was striving to accommodate the heroin addicts, some of my colleagues thought that I had gone mad, but when I restored Ambrose and Sylvia to worthwhile, addiction-free lives, Leona commented, 'To be proved right, is not usually regarded as a sign of mental instability'. Heart-warming, and memorable words!

Our association has always operated strictly within the framework of its ten rules. These are:

1) No abuse of alcohol
2) No abuse of drugs
3) No violence
4) No stealing
5) No racial harassment
6) No sexual harassment
7) No abuse of the premises
8) No smoking
9) No disturbing the peaceful enjoyment of others
10) No intervention by professionals.

As a sweetener to the local mental health establishment, when we won the battle for the crisis house, we amended Rule 10 to 'No inappropriate intervention by professionals' – a happy concession for us to make, because we, not, they, decide what is appropriate. We can, and have, called doctors out to see guests in the crisis house, if we deem it necessary, but the amendment does not prevent us from enforcing our separatist stance.

When I set up the crisis house, I considered the rules very carefully. I could not research successful models, because there were none! However, I included rule 9, because this was referred to, as being very useful, by Judi Chamberlin in her book 'On Our Own', [Publisher: MIND, London: 1988.] It enables one to deal with situations, where a person is causing severe distress to other service-users, but is not in actual breach of any of the other nine rules!

In twenty-five years, some of the rules have been broken, and some guests have been asked to leave because of this, but it has only been a handful. There has been some abuse of the telephone, very little abuse of alcohol, very little abuse of the premises. One instance of abuse of the telephone, resulted in a hilarious situation. [Chapter18: 'One person, one vote'.]

Plenty of fish in the sea

Naturally, with mentally ill people in crisis, being particularly vulnerable, problems often arise, in finding partners, and forming relationships.

I always advise our service-users, not to look for romance, or for partners, at the crisis house. Do they take my advice? I fear not! There are times when I think that our advice and information service, should simply be renamed – our 'information' service. People only take advice, if what you are suggesting is what they want to do anyway!

Nevertheless, I stick to my point. If one meets a prospective partner at a dinner party, or at a golf club, in fact – in any normal social settings – one COULD meet someone with severe problems. The difference is – that – at the crisis house – severe problems, are GUARANTEED!

I see the temptation clearly. It is so much easier, just to grab the person sitting next to you in the drop-in centre. This requires no effort, and one has a fellow-feeling, because he has mental health problems – just like you. For an example of this, that was foiled by the service-user about to be grabbed, [Chapter 19: 'I can if I try'.]

It is easy, and fatal – because those mental health problems are then compounded. By contrast, if one makes the effort to smarten oneself up, [not always easy - bearing in mind the depleted energies, that go with depression], and, taking courage in both hands, go out into the normal world, one may then meet a partner, completely outside of the mental health milieu. For a recent example of this being done successfully, [Chapter 11: 'Back to normality'.]

The only circumstances in which I would not advise against mentally ill people getting together in relationships, is where the couple are so disadvantaged by severe, and chronic, mental illness, that they stand no chance whatsoever, of finding a normal partner.

Then, they may as well settle for each other – rather than be alone. We have experience of this scenario working quite well – albeit in a limited way. We celebrated Henry and Amelia's wedding, on this basis, in April 1995. More than twenty years later, they are still married – albeit with all the problems that both having a diagnosis of schizophrenia, imply!

For most of those twenty years, they have not lived together, but, emotionally, they ARE together. Both have suffered bouts of mental illness during this time, but they are not WORSE off than they would have been – had each stayed alone, so, as far as is possible in the circumstances, their marriage can be accorded a success.

So, if the crisis house is not a place to find romance, where is? Unlike many of my generation – for whom the conventional way to find a partner, was at a party. or a dance – I am not entirely prejudiced against the modern idea of internet dating – which is – after all - only a technological version of the old-fashioned marriage bureau, or 'Lonely Hearts' column. Of course, such dating can be dangerous, but so can meeting anybody – anywhere! One has to exercise discrimination and judgement – whoever, and wherever, one meets.

Perhaps I have become unromantic in my old age, but I consider the process of finding a partner, not essentially different from that of buying a house! The estate agent sends you dozens of specifications. One has a list of 'Essentials' and 'Desirables'. One quickly eliminates those with obvious dry rot, or rising damp, and then one sifts through the 'Possibles'.

This, as I see it, is the great ADVANTAGE of internet dating. As one popular site has it – there are 'Plenty of fish'. One does not have to grab the nearest person – warts and all. We have experience at the crisis house, of people finding suitable partners in this way, but, to do so, they did put lots of effort into it.

Here, in 2016 - 2017, I am still advising young service users, against the trap of romance with the unstable.

Young Jason, aged just twenty-one, is a notable example. He got involved with an extremely unstable girl, Sunny. She was clinging onto him like a limpet, and he saw no way of escape. 'At your age, I advised him, you don't need to get tied down with anybody, least of all with Sunny. Go out and enjoy your youth. Thirty is the age to think of settling down.'

Then there was Neville Sandford – hoping to go to college. A girl he knew slightly, invited him for a weekend, and at a loose end, he accepted. As soon as he was through the door, she was talking of marriage. Good old Neville didn't need my advice. He ran for his life!

In seeking partners, one might be choosy, but one must also be realistic. Gabriela Rani, constantly asserted that she wished to marry into the aristocracy. Our advice, that she could not do so, because they marry each other, fell upon deaf ears. Now, at fifty, she is unmarried!

An incident in the drop-in centre brought this truth home to people, in a poignant way. Nicolette walked into the crisis house one day. She suffered from mental health problems, thought to be brought on by cannabis abuse, but was extremely attractive, with long, blonde hair, emerald green eyes, and a slim figure. Before becoming ill, she had represented Southern England in gymnastics. All the pairs of male eyes, young and old, followed her around the room.

'Wait', I laughed. Not five minutes later, an extremely good looking young man, with blond hair, and blue eyes, and a great physique, walked into the room, and claimed his fiancée. Like goes with like. He was the son of a doctor from Henley, and ran an antique furniture business. Nicolette had trained in interior design. They went together like peaches and cream, got married, had two children, and are happy to this very day.

'*Implacable Venus toute entière à sa proie attachée*': Racine

My book celebrates twenty-five years in the crisis house with lots of eulogies, but balance can be given to the text, if I describe just one, total failure! The lady concerned, came to us in order to escape from a failed marriage – to a husband, who, amongst other problems – was a transvestite. She told us her history. Her first marriage – to the father of her daughter – was to a lodger in her mother's house. He was serving in the British Army, but turned out to be an I.R.A. terrorist, and was arrested shortly after his daughter was born. They never saw him again.

Husband number two, was an alcoholic – whom she also found at the Army camp. He was the father of her son, and while she was pregnant, slept with numerous women at the camp, and so infected her with venereal disease.

Husband number three, was the worst. He was an extremely violent schizophrenic, as was his son, from a former marriage, and beat the lady so severely that she ended up in a battered wives' refuge.

It was on coming out of the refuge, that the lady met husband number four. This was the transvestite. He seemed safe and gentle – compared with her previous husband, and she actually stayed with him for some fifteen years. But the marriage, though not violent, presented numerous other problems. She came to us, to escape them!

Against my advice, while staying in the crisis house, this lady got involved with a psychopath, who did not want her as a partner, but who was content to exploit her. He died in violent circumstances.

At the time of his death, the lady had already moved into a flat. Her next relationship was with a murderer. This man had pushed a man under a London Tube train, and his victim died. He served his sentence for murder, but, on release, had difficulty finding work and accommodation.

My lady came to the rescue. He moved in with her, and lived in her flat for free. He did find some work in a pub, and, because he was earning, the lady was no longer entitled to Housing Benefit.

When, after a year, she was presented with a huge bill for rent arrears, he walked out, and left her to be thrown out on the street.

I remember relating her story – with wry humour – at a talk that I gave, at a mental health meeting in Shrewsbury. 'When you consider ordinary social life, I said, it must be quite difficult to find a murderer. She found one – and just up the road!'

I did manage to get this lady Disability Living Allowance, and accommodation in a sheltered complex for the elderly – which she resented – considering herself, still too young for such accommodation, but I thought it would afford her some degree of protection. Needless to say, she got herself involved with one of the male residents!

Particularly amusing, were two, conflicting, conversations, that I had with this lady. One was about work. 'I don't know why, she protested, that they are trying to get me back to work, at the age of fifty-three, when youngsters are out of work, and have no intention of getting a job.'

The second was about relationships. 'Sex, she averred, is going to be part of any relationship that I have. I am only fifty-three!' So she was too old for work, but still young enough for sex!

I know when I'm licked! I was not going to have any success with this lady – who is now, sadly, prematurely deceased. Features of the case that interest me, go right back to her meeting her first husband. What was missing? EFFORT! She simply grabbed the nearest man – her mother's lodger – who was living in the same house.

Psychoanalysts, would no doubt explain, that this lady's low self-esteem, could be traced, right back, to rejection in childhood, so unconsciously, in adult life, she actually sought out partners who would abuse her.

I remember an interesting discussion which I had with Myles. [Chapter 32: 'Investing In The Young - Students At The Crisis House'.] He was a trainee counsellor, and I explained that it was not unusual, for us to have a guest who had been PHYSICALLY abused, and who, on leaving the crisis house, was determined that this would not happen in future relationships. A year on, we agreed, one would find them back in a relationship, which WAS abusive, but not in the same way. This would explain the lady's marriage to her fourth husband!

I agree with the psychoanalysts, but my approach is pragmatic. If one is to become an abuser, because your parents abused you, because their parents abused them, because their parents abused them – one could, eventually, trace it all back to Adam and Eve! Do what Maurice Santereau did. [Chapter 10: 'What starts as disaster can end in triumph'.] Break the cycle!

Yet another way to handle the problem, is to avoid sexual relationships completely – contenting oneself with children, and grandchildren. This was the option taken by Petula. [Chapter 11: 'Free of abusive relationships'.]

In my twenty-five years' of running the crisis house, I have experienced no physical aggression from anybody, and very little verbal aggression. There was verbal aggression from the lady who refused to believe that her would-be partner had been a promiscuous homosexual.

One young man was quite verbally aggressive, when I suggested that the answer to his homelessness, would be solved if he got a job!

I have so little to do with the statutory services, that they have had little chance to be verbally aggressive. One social worker retorted that a client's sexual relationship was not my business - when I had told her it was not hers!

One social worker, a particularly, notoriously useless, one, did yell 'For you! For you!', repeatedly over the telephone – when I was explaining to her the inappropriateness, of her proposed referral. No doubt about it, they could not disguise their anger, that they could not control those beds!!

Among service users – or rather – a relative of one – there was a notable exception. Sonia came to the crisis house – referred by Leona. She had been sacked from her job - due to alcohol abuse, and was homeless. She stayed in the crisis house, for nine months, got romantically involved with another service user, and made no progress. This being the case, I suggested that she move on.

As with all other homeless new guests, I had filled in for her a Housing Application form, for Wokingham Borough Council, but it transpired that she had thrown this away – evidently intending to live, for free, in the crisis house for the rest of her life!!

When I suggested that Sonia, having made no progress, should move on, she suddenly developed a broken leg! She was wearing a plaster cast – which, apparently, was miraculously removed when she was walking about town!

It was a Bank Holiday weekend, [it always is!], so I told Sonia that she could not stay in the crisis house – with leg broken – or even just, ankle sprained – because her fellow guests might wish to go away for the weekend, and I could not impose upon them, to stay and look after her, nor leave her alone – in case she fell in the shower, and could not get help.

Sonia had a sister, Joan, who visited her regularly, during her stay at the crisis house. This sister had three young children, and lived in a three-bedroom Council house in Finchampstead.

'Telephone her, I said to Sonia, on the Friday afternoon, and tell her that I am sending you to her in a taxi – to stay the long weekend. I shall then meet you at the Council Offices on Tuesday.' At this juncture, I assumed that Sonia had submitted her Housing Application form!

She telephoned Joan. 'Out of the question! Sonia said. Joan says that it is out of the question!' I had no other choice. The Council's Homelessness Officer, I knew from bitter experience, would do nothing. I could not leave Sonia alone in the crisis house, nor could I turn her out in the street. The user with whom she had become romantically involved, suggested that I fix up a rota of people to look after her over the weekend.

This may have been a valid suggestion - were the broken leg genuine, but since I believed it to be a ploy, to stay in the crisis house, I thought it better to confront the problem head-on, so I placed Sonia in a taxi, and locked up the crisis house for the weekend. The telephone rang continuously, but I did not answer it.

As arranged, on Tuesday morning, I met up with Sonia and sister, Joan, at the Council Offices. Then it started. Joan was literally screaming her head off – that I was unprofessional – though what is unprofessional, about requiring a healthy relative, to take responsibility for her sister, I failed to see. I had to take responsibility for mine, and it never occurred to me, to place the onus upon anyone else!

She continued to scream, and one of her taunts was to ask why MIND had nothing to do with us. I did not reply with the truth – which was that they had become a bureaucracy – tied up with statutory services, and that it was we, and not they, who had severed the connection.

Nor did I respond by asking why, if we were as black as painted, she was so anxious for our organization to continue to assume responsibility for her sister?

While this rumpus was going on, the Council's Housing Officer became involved, and it then transpired that Sonia was not even registered for housing. I then left them to it.

The Housing Officer telephoned me at the crisis house – begging me to take Sonia back. I refused, but – since the dilemma was not caused by him – I offered to pay for one week's bed-and-breakfast accommodation for her – while he sorted things out. Very important, this, in a crisis house. If you have a problem, deal with it head-on. If you give in, you will only be faced with the same problem, again, in three months' time.

Needless to say, Joan, full of righteous indignation, complained to the Council. A colleague and I saw their Complaints Officer, and a social worker. I explained, firmly, that Sonia was her family's responsibility, and not ours! 'Oh, bleated the social worker, we may agree, but what do you do if they won't take responsibility?' Not take them back into the crisis house, that's for sure!

At that time, the local mental health service, did have some kind of support team, which, full of their own self-righteousness, supported Sonia in her bed-and–breakfast accommodation. Payment for this was continued until she was found more permanent accommodation in Reading. So my actions achieved quite a lot for Sonia. What would they have offered, if I had approached their Homelessness Officer, that Friday afternoon? I can guarantee you – it would have been nothing!

Some weeks later, Sonia came to collect her belongings from the crisis house. I recall that the Police came with her, but there was no need for this, our relations were perfectly cordial, and I always liked her. Liking somebody, however, is not justification for allowing them to take up a room in a crisis house, for the rest of their life – when there are other needy people who could make better use of it.

Although Joan's tantrum was unpleasant, though, of course, water off a duck's back to me, I found her stance, nevertheless, interesting. It is this belief in entitlement. I don't think that she had ever worked. She was involved with drugs as a teenager. She, and her three children, all by different fathers, lived on benefits, in a Council house, all provided by we, tax-payers.

The concept of personal responsibility never entered her head. The concept that 'Somebody is always paying', was an alien idea to her. Yet such a mindset must be learned. She wasn't born thinking it!

So I concur heartily with Iain Duncan-Smith's Benefits Reforms. They may come too late for Joan's generation, but personal responsibility will, at least, be instilled in the forthcoming generation!

Chapter 48

Addiction

'Two, Four, Six, Eight. Who Do We Appreciate?'

I had no experience of heroin addiction, until Ewan arrived at the crisis house in February 1999. He explained that he had recently returned from a heroin detox in Eastbourne - where he had also spent some time in a mental hospital.

It was four years, and a failed marriage, later, that Ewan actually came to stay, as a guest, in the crisis house. Then I found out all about heroin addiction. When he came to stay with us, Ewan found some work, so I offered to sort out all his clothes, and hang them in the wardrobe – in case he felt too tired to do so, at the end of the working day.

At the bottom of the pile of clothes, I found a plastic bag containing white powder, a syringe, and a burnt spoon. I did not know what they were, and the burnt spoon, in particular, intrigued me. The Classics master from Wellington College, who was visiting that day, enlightened me. It was drugs!

From that day on, my education improved at a rapid rate of knots!! First, I discovered that heroin addicts reproduce asexually – by splitting! First, you have one, then you have two, then you have four, then you have eight! In the end, I had to remonstrate. 'Ewan, I said. We have a four bedroom crisis house. We can't accommodate every heroin addict in Berkshire!'

Nevertheless, it was through Ewan, that the twins came to us – with a tragic outcome. [Chapter 23: 'A waste of a young life'.] With people under the age of forty, dual diagnosis, is now very common. They will suffer from mental health problems, compounded by drug or alcohol problems, or both.

At the crisis house, we either get a wave of heroin addicts – or none. They are in a sub-culture, and flock together. Seventeen years after first walking through our door, Ewan is still injecting heroin. He appeared in a 'Court Report' in the local paper, quite recently, pleading 'guilty' to shop-lifting to fund his habit.

Throughout the years, and with what is now a lot of experience of heroin addiction, I have known of only two addicts to free themselves of heroin addiction, they were Ambrose and Sylvia! [Chapter 9: 'I want my life back'.]. I have also known only two recover completely from alcohol addiction. As a result of my experience, the following letter appeared in the *Wokingham Times* [Thursday May 1st 2014], and this remains my position.

Letter to *Wokingham Times*

"Do readers have any views in the drugs debate? My experience at the Wokingham Crisis House inclines me towards legalisation.

True, the crisis house has been successful in getting addicts off heroin, and back to useful lives, but only with a lot of hard work, and when the people concerned wanted to change. We have had no success at all when they didn't.

People at all times throughout history, and of all cultures, have used mind-altering substances – either to stimulate them – or to relax them – the latter being of particular relevance in mental health.

Our current laws, where some of these substances – nicotine and alcohol – are legal, and others – heroin, cocaine, amphetamine, and cannabis, et alia, are illegal – defy logic. Logic demands all or nothing.

It is, in any case, a losing battle. As the speakeasy illegal drinking bars of Prohibition America illustrate, people always do, and get, what they want – despite prevailing laws.

Trying to change unwilling addicts, takes up a lot of our precious public money – not to mention the precious time of doctors and the Police – both of whom are already overworked.

Legalisation, and take the personal consequences – as people already do with nicotine and alcohol – would seem to be the answer."

Mental health and addiction go together, and, this being very much the case with Ewan, the drugs and alcohol, are used as an anodyne to dull the pain inflicted by life.

Ewan's father left him, his baby brother, and his mentally ill mother, when Ewan was just four years old. His mother could not cope – leaving her vallium tablets within his reach, and he fed them to his baby brother – believing them to be sweets.

Fortunately, the child survived, but, in due course, Ewan was placed in a special boarding school for emotionally disturbed children – and this was miles away from home. When he left school, and returned home, he therefore had no local mates. He soon got embroiled in the local drugs sub-culture – trying various jobs, but never sticking with anything.

Ewan's marriage, at the age of twenty-eight, was to a Turkish immigrant, who wanted to obtain British citizenship. She paid Ewan, six thousand pounds, to marry her, and he spent it all on drugs! After the regulation two years of marriage - required to qualify for citizenship, she divorced him – and that was when he came to stay with us.

Elsewhere in this text, I have asserted that mental health is never 'plain and simple'. I don't believe that Ewan, was entirely free from feelings of attachment to his wife – nor she to him - though there is no doubt that the 'marriage' was a commercial arrangement. Where you have human beings, you will always have complexity!

Our accommodating of people who used hard drugs, was one reason why Wokingham Borough Council's Social Services' employee, was threatening to withdraw our funding in the summer of 2004.

I pointed out to her, that all I had to do, was to throw the heroin addicts out on the street [although I had no intention of doing so]. It wouldn't solve the addicts' problem, nor the Council's problem, nor society's problem, but it sure would solve MY problem!

National MIND, at the time, adopted a stance, similar to that held by the Council, so we sent them about their business. A mental health charity is there to help the mentally ill, and not to reject them.

The only circumstances in which an addict will be motivated to detoxify from either drugs or alcohol, are those where a better life is awaiting them if they do so.

Larrie illustrates my point. He is a heroin addict who visited the crisis house when we were supporting Kurt Haddow. [Chapter 10: 'Good with computers'.]

Larrie explained, that, as a child in junior school, he was too frightened to enter his house, after school. He would wait for his sister to return from senior school, and then they could go in together.

His father was an alcoholic. Because her husband did not work, Larrie's mother had to work full time. In the early evening, Larrie was too frightened to enter the house – in case his father was – either violent – or out cold on the floor. What a life for a child! Is it any wonder that he turned to the oblivion provided by heroin?

Thus, it is only if you had a good life before taking heroin, as Sylvia did [Chapter 9: 'I want my life back'.], that the motivation is there to get that life back – as she did.

We are all agreed that Ewan will never come off heroin, because his life, from infancy, was awful, and he sees no prospect of things being any better in a drug-free future!

Chapter 49

Advocacy

If you asked me what is the most valuable service provided by the crisis house, then there is no contest, the answer is 'asylum'. It is wonderful to see severely distressed and disturbed individuals, come into our drop-in centre and relax. A cat will climb onto their lap, and they will stroke it. One can observe the stress fading away. Pets as therapy – you can't beat it.

Pets are, however, a lot of hard work. I am constantly cleaning out cat-litter trays, bird cages, and fish tanks – to say nothing of staggering over from Bracknell to Wokingham – with heavy cat litter, and cartons of pet food.

As I sit, sipping my sherry, I am amused. People want to take over my role? I don't think so!

The drop-in centre is also very useful as a safe bolt hole. People, so ill, that they can barely get out of bed and dressed, can then, at least, get out of their four walls, and meet other people in a place which is undemanding, and accepts them exactly as they are. Here, they can heal in their own good time, until they are ready to face the world once again.

Jerry Burton, in Agatha Christie's novel: 'The Moving Finger', makes this point cogently. 'The Moving Finger': [Published: Collins: 1942.]

'Dogs, he explains, are wise'. 'If sick, they crawl away into a quiet corner and lick their wounds, and do not rejoin the world until they are whole once more.' Jerry was recovering from a flying accident, but the advice applies to mental ill health, just as it does to physical illness.

In addition to providing asylum, the crisis house does also have a more active function – advocacy. Over the years, I have completed more Disability Living Allowance Application Forms, than I have had hot dinners! These were sixty-four pages long, and far too daunting for any applicant to complete.

When once watching 'Prime Minister's Question Time', I observed David Cameron himself, acknowledge to Parliament, that he had filled the forms in, on behalf of his disabled son, and that he had found them daunting.

The new PIP [Personal Independence Payment] Forms are a bit shorter, but one is still ploughing through forty pages – still asking the same questions over and over again. Mentally ill people need an advocate, to undertake such tasks on their behalf. They are not well enough, to pursue their legal rights and benefits, for themselves.

It is always rewarding when a simple piece of advocacy, such as applying, successfully, for Disability Living Allowance, on a service-user's behalf, makes a seismic shift in their circumstances – for the better.

One such, was Jeremy March. Jeremy had been diagnosed with schizophrenia, and was prescribed medication. He explained that he had attempted to cope on three different university campuses, but had failed on all three. However, he had managed to complete a chemistry degree course with the Open University.

Due to mental illness, he was unable to work, so he was renting his own house out, to get an income, and was living, not altogether harmoniously, with his parents.

By obtaining High Rate Disability Living Allowance for Jeremy, he accessed sufficient extra income to resume living in his own house. This made an enormous difference to his quality of life.

I am so glad that Jeremy saw the alternative of the Open University. I do wish that Celia had done the same. [Chapter 23: '*Mens Sana in corpore sano*'.]. There is always an alternative route to the same goal!

I recall watching a 'Songs of Praise' Programme, in which a man explained, that he had wished to be a minister in the Church. Not academic, he had been unable to pass examinations in Latin, Greek, and Hebrew, so the path to that ministry, was closed to him. However, he was artistically talented, so he pursued a career in creating stained glass windows for the Church. He said that he was thus serving God, using his talents, and was satisfied that he was in a ministry of a different kind!

On occasions, advocacy involves attending a Tribunal with the mentally ill person. The following letter, and also an excellent article, appeared in the local Press – describing one such Tribunal.

Letter to the press - 'I query the stance on Bedroom tax'

"Recently, I attended a tribunal to support a mentally ill lady who was appealing against being charged 'bedroom tax' – her inability to pay resulting in her accruing hundreds of pounds in rent arrears, and the consequent threat of eviction from her two-bedroom flat.

The local authority officers present at the tribunal, took the view that since the lady qualified only for the middle rate care component of Disability Living Allowance, a high level of day care, but only occasional night care, then she did not need a second bedroom, and thus did not qualify for exemption from this tax.

They stated that the council usually only exempts from bedroom tax people who qualify for the high rate of the care component of Disability Living Allowance. I query the council's stance. A person qualifying for the high care component of Disability Living Allowance does not in fact require a second bedroom where their carer can sleep overnight, because a person needing a lot of care during the night has to have a waking carer in the same room with them in order to receive the frequent care necessary in the circumstances.

Such people may well require extra space in which to store oxygen cylinders, wheelchairs, dialysis equipment, etc, but it is actually people like the lady appealing to the tribunal who need a second bedroom so that they can get day care from time to time as needed – with their career sleeping in.

Other of our members who are falling foul of the new legislation, and being evicted from their homes, are those under the age of 35 who were previously entitled to Housing Benefit to rent a flat, but who are now allowed to rent only a room. The problem here is that mentally ill people often lack the social and organisational skills necessary to cope in shared accommodation, and thus such situations quickly break down.

I agree with the reform of the benefits system, and the Crisis House has never done other than encourage people back into work. Nothing is better than work for relieving depression, and nothing is worse for it than having too much time to sit around thinking about one's self.

However, getting back to full-time work, and achieving total independence from welfare benefits, is an ambition which applies more to people with less severe mental disorders. Frequently, severely mentally ill people who, in the past, would have spent their lives in protective institutions, are now only able to survive in the community at all, because they have flats to themselves, where they can experience some degree of asylum, not having to cope with other, possibly unsympathetic people, and where, like my lady, they can accommodate a carer, day and night, if necessary."

Advocacy can include all sorts of things – not just benefits entitlement, but Housing, and custody of children. It was when representing a service-user, with regard to the latter, that I was almost rendered speechless – a rare phenomenon indeed!

Violet was not a fit mother. I never maintained that she was! She had been sexually abused as a child, and had been placed in care. As soon as she came out of care at sixteen, Violet started having children. When she came to us, aged twenty, Violet already had a three-year-old son who had been removed for adoption. She had miscarried a second child, and was now expecting a third, another boy.

Violet had a nice solicitor, a mother of three herself, to represent her. This solicitor agreed with us, that Violet should be admitted to a 'Mother and Baby' unit, where she could be taught parenting skills. We agreed, because – when people are young – learning, growth, and development, are still possible. But it didn't happen. The child was adopted.

Then Violet became pregnant again – with a girl. I agreed to support her once again, in an endeavour to obtain a place for her in a 'Mother and Baby' unit. I prepared a detailed report, and submitted this to Violet's new solicitor – her previous one being on sick leave. I telephoned this solicitor, to find out what she thought of my report, and I could hardly believe my ears. It was like telephoning the counsel for the defence, and finding oneself in contact with the prosecution!

This solicitor informed me that I should not have had access to the papers for the Family Court, whose proceedings were held in secret. [Shades of the late Social Services' employee – who wanted to keep complainants' names a secret, so that she could pretend that the complaints were credible!]

I told her that, in a democracy, they should not be held in secret. She replied – 'That is the law!' Fortunately, due to campaigning by the *Daily Mail* Newspaper, changes to the law in this area are now taking place!

I went on to say that Violet should have the opportunity, of learning parenting skills, in a 'Mother and Baby' unit, and it was her reply to this suggestion, that rendered me speechless. 'That would cost Wokingham Borough Council a lot of money' she said!

This woman was Violet's ADVOCATE! Do you think that the expense to Wokingham Borough Council – or rather – to the tax-payers – is VIOLET'S point of view? That view, the view of the Council, and local tax-payers – is the view to be expressed by the COUNCIL'S solicitor.

In fact, other than me, Violet had no advocate, while Wokingham Borough Council, had two! The system required that she be given legal representation, so they appointed the required solicitor, and ticked the box. Who pays this solicitor? We, the tax-payers!

They had no other intention, than to take the child from Violet, and her views did not enter the equation. After this baby was adopted, Violet miscarried another pair of twins.

Violet realised that she was never going to keep the child that she yearned for, if she stayed in Berkshire, so she decided to move up North – where she had relatives. For once, it appears that geography has solved the problem.

Violet, pregnant once again, successfully completed the parents' training programmes, and has been allowed to keep this baby – no doubt under supervision. She has also, now, married, so some, much needed, stability has come into her life. I am very glad, because I am convinced that, when people are young, there is nearly always scope for growth and development.

The essence of advocacy is that one represents the person's point of view – whether one actually agrees with it, or not. The advocate is there, because the service-user is vulnerable, possibly inarticulate, possibly, due to illness, unable to grasp, and marshal all the facts, but, nevertheless, has a point of view, which needs to be presented to the Tribunal.

Over the twenty-five years, I have thus attended Court, and represented people at Child Custody Hearings, Criminal Proceedings, Housing Benefit Appeals, and, as the Press statements show, representations regarding the infamous Bedroom Tax.

We have a current situation illustrating the damage that this tax can cause an individual. Marion first came to the crisis house in 2015. She suffers from a very severe neurosis, hyperacuity, and physical problems as well – a very ill lady!

Marion coped reasonably well in her three-bedroom Council house – where she had brought up her daughter, and continued living alone – once the daughter had left home.The house was quiet, and she had a garden – a great asset, when one is mentally ill.

When the bedroom tax was introduced, Marion could not afford to pay for two spare bedrooms – being too ill to work, and living on benefits – so she exchanged the house for a one-bedroom flat. Her new situation was dire – noisy, and with uncongenial neighbours. In desperation, she exchanged again – and went out of the frying pan into the fire!

Marion now lives in a one-bedroom downstairs flat. The people above her, clomp across the ceiling like an army marching! The people in the flats on either side, shout through the walls. She feels unable to use the shared gardens, and even placing the dustbins out, causes problems!

Marion is living in a personal hell, and why? It is because modern society, unlike the society of Victorian times, does not acknowledge that the first and foremost need of the mentally ill, is the need for asylum! Why were all those Victorian, mental asylums, built in the heart of the country? Yes, it got the mentally ill away from normal society, but it also provided asylum for them.

This is why I fought for the crisis house. The Crisis House is a mid-Victorian build – with good, thick, walls – remember my brother? It is never noisy. Even when the new road was being built directly outside the building, with cranes, at times, right up to our windows, we scarcely heard a thing. Here is peace and quiet, sanctuary, asylum.

Marion has a physical problem with her ears, so that all noise is magnified. In modern buildings, one can hear the next door neighbour flick the light switch! Other, former, guests of the crisis house have made the same complaint, when they have moved from us into modern flats – though I don't remember any other situation being quite so dire as Marion's.

I have encouraged Marion to get away for a break, when she can, and this has been visibly beneficial. I have also offered to help her to apply for Personal Independence Payment [PIP]. With this extra money, she would be in a position to move into a house or bungalow, with her own garden, and some degree of isolation, thus relieving the worst of her symptoms.

With the bedroom tax, there is always a queue of people wishing to exchange larger properties for one bedroom flats, so Marion would not find it difficult to get an exchange – once she has the extra money needed to pay this tax.

We have actually observed the improvement to an individual's quality of life, that better housing can achieve.

Marcus Foreman hated his noisy flat in Bracknell. His description of the place, was very similar to Marion's description of hers. Eventually, he achieved a transfer to a bungalow – with a garden. When well enough to work, Marcus was a chef, so he is very into cooking. In his garden, he can grow his own herbs.

Marcus suffers from rapid cycling bi-polar affective disorder, so peace and quiet, in his living environment, are very important for his mental health.

Not to be fobbed off

The case of the Jamie Jervis suicide, illustrates how important it is for advocates not to be fobbed off by the mental health system. Persist, as I did, and you will get satisfaction at last!

Sean came to see me at the crisis house. He wanted to know if there was anything that I could do. His friend, Jamie Jervis, who had been a Sectioned patient in the mental hospital, had been allowed out on weekend leave – with no arrangements being made for his care, had turned up at Sean's house – where he had proceeded to take an overdose, and had died!

I explained – that since Jamie had been a Sectioned patient – then there was a lot that I could do. I started, by trying to get the facts from the health authority – only to be fobbed off, with the reply that they were confidential. Then I went to the Mental Health Act Commission, then to the Health Secretary, then to the Health Ombudsman – who referred me back to the Mental Health Act Commission.

I was put in touch with their Complaints Officer, and I told him that, having been pursuing this case for a year, the buck was going to stop with him! Sure enough, it did. He ordered a complete investigation.

Jamie's Inquest revealed that the Section 17 papers, which have to be signed – in order to allow a Sectioned patient leave in the community – had not been signed. No arrangements, whatsoever, had been made for his care, so both Consultant Psychiatrist, and Hospital manager, were dismissed. The social worker was disciplined, but, being of lower status, kept her job.

In my representations, to all the authorities involved, I demanded written care plans for patients – which had to be signed – thus ensuring that the person had a place to go to, a carer, medication organized, GP informed, etc. These were introduced, and exist to this day.

I could not criticise the Mental Health Act Commission Complaints Officer. Some months later, he telephoned me, to explain that the hospital staff had received extra training. Had I seen any improvements? The written care plans were certainly an improvement, but so much of this negligence is not cured by training. It is a change of heart that is required in our mental health services. In a service, properly run, by dedicated volunteers, it would be seen that the patient got proper care, because people WANTED him to have proper care, not because they had been trained, like performing monkeys!

I have noticed that the 'professional' services place all their faith in training. Does it never occur to them, that, often, employees fail to carry out their responsibilities, not because they don't know how to, but because they are too lazy to do so, too feckless to do so, too uninterested to do so. Give the services back to dedicated volunteers. Lazy, feckless, uninterested, people, are not going to volunteer, so, with a totally voluntary service, quality is guaranteed!

Here, in September 2015, we are dealing with two local cases of negligence on the part of the mental health services. The Inquest on Theresa's husband, has already taken place, and five points of negligence – including neglect by both the hospital, and the mental health crisis team, have already been established. [Chapter 28: 'Lucy and Theresa'.]

The second case, involves the suicide of a man, who was under the local mental health team, but whom their staff refused to deal with, because of his use of alcohol. How can such a refusal be justified? A very high proportion of twenty-first century mental health cases, involve dual diagnosis.

This man was found, dead, in a scruffy bedsitter, with which he had been provided. He hadn't even been supplied with a bed! Oh, sweet, nostalgic days, when we had the crisis beds at the Crisis House, and specialised in setting people up, to succeed, in the community.

Wonderful Frances, wonderful Dave, driving around in that minibus, and collecting furniture. We always fitted their flats with a nice, new carpet – nothing else gives a room such an uplift! Then we used to find curtains to match the service user's choice of colour, and we would polish up the furniture, so that it gleamed!

The idea was, that when people left the crisis house, and moved into flats, they would see their new premises, as a step up, and so would be setting out on a positive note – to make a success of their new life in the community.

On 7th September, this man's mother came to see me at the crisis house. She knew that nothing could bring her son back, but she expressed, an understandable desire, to prevent such a tragedy happening to other families. What could we do? His Inquest was to be held in January 2016.

I told her that we have to get rid of them! I think that she was surprised. No doubt, the Inquest will conclude, that lessons will be learnt, and that extra training is necessary. Alas, lessons will not be learnt, and training is not the answer. The answer, is the abolition of statutory Social Services, and restore society's welfare to the voluntary, and I mean, voluntary, [unpaid], sector.

This lady complained that the officials with whom she had spoken, were dismissive, had no interest in her son, and were only interested in their pay cheques. The answer? Don't have pay cheques. Have volunteers!

Her comments echoed those of Holly, with regard to Social Services attitude towards her brother. She said, 'They have no interest whatsoever in Jimmy as a person'. Of course they have no such interest. All they want is the pay cheque. The mentally ill person is a, scarcely tolerable, nuisance!

Chapter 50

Children And Mental Health The Strain And Stress

If you come into Wokingham, by train, the first building that you see, as you walk out of the station, is the crisis house – fortunately, now, smartened up, and looking as proud as the whole redeveloped area.

But, if you come into Wokingham, by car, St Paul's splendid church tower, is the sight on the horizon, to greet you. St Paul. Who could be more inspiring?

St Paul, not fashionable, nowadays, but, in my opinion, the greatest of all the saints, pronounced that he wished that everybody could be, like him, celibate. But he went on to say, 'But if he cannot contain, let him marry. He has not sinned. Better to marry, than to burn.'

St Paul knew that, for the human race to continue, there had to be, in nature, a force that was irresistible to the majority of people. That force is the motivation to reproduce. But that is just the point. It has to be a majority, and not a totality, of people who do so.

As I have explained, if there is one thing that I cannot stand, in life, it is a busybody. Such was the case of Aubrey Bennett and Archie Smuts. Aubrey had always been highly promiscuous, whereas Archie was just about to become a forty-year-old virgin!

So Aubrey interfered. 'I am going to make sure that you experience sex before you are forty', he asserted, 'so I shall pay for a prostitute from the firm that I use regularly, to have sex with you as a fortieth birthday present!'

All went as arranged, and Archie later confided to me that he would infinitely have preferred a Mars Bar!

The lesson. Listen to St Paul! Anybody who wanted and needed sex, would not wait until the age of forty to get what they wanted, and there are plenty of people, including Archie Smuts, who are happy to remain celibate for their entire lives!

I frequently reassure people who come to the crisis house, that it is not necessary, for everybody, to follow the conventional path – of marriage, and children. As my following narrative illustrates, there are people, who would have done better – not to have pursued this path.

Strangely enough, I regard the debate about the desirability of celibacy for the priesthood, as one of the very few issues, where each point of view, is equally valid.

The Roman Catholic view, is that – because their priests are unmarried, then they can devote the whole of their lives, to the service of God, and of their parishioners. A very valid argument! It is a fact, that the demands of a family, limits how much time one can give to serving the wider community. Single priests, can be available to those needing them, at any time of day or night.

This ready availability is described cogently by Agatha Christie in her novel, 'The Pale Horse'. [Published: Collins: 1961]. She writes:

'Mrs Gerahty opened the door of the presbytery.' ...There was a small boy on the doorstep. 'Is this the priest's place?' 'Is it Father Gorman you're wanting?' 'He's wanted. Woman says she's dying. This is the Catholic place all right, isn't it? Woman says the vicar won't do.'

Mrs Gerahty reassured him on this essential point, told him to stop where he was, and retired into the presbytery. Some THREE MINUTES' LATER a tall, elderly priest came out, carrying a small leather case in his hand.

Give welfare back to charities and churches. What happens if you ring the statutory service crisis line? Often, you get an answerphone message. Frequently, no one bothers to get back to you. They are not a crisis service; they are a bureaucracy.

In contrast to the Roman Catholic position, the Church of England, and the Free Churches, argue that it is desirable for their ministers to be married – with children – thus giving them insight into the concerns, worries, and pressures, experienced by ordinary families, and thus, placing them in a better position to give the families the help, and support, that they need. An equally valid argument.

I honestly have difficulty in deciding which argument is the more telling. If I had to choose, I would probably plump for the view of the Roman Catholics – which is ironic – because I am a confirmed member of the Church of England.

People who, like me, have never had children, cannot pronounce on the strains and stresses inherent in parenthood. We haven't done it, and we, simply, don't know.

What I can state, with authority, is that parenthood often brings people into mental health, who would probably not have come into it, had they not had children. This is especially the case, if a child is born, handicapped, or if an infant dies.

Take the case of Rosa, who was one of our early drop-in users. She had, as a young woman, been a dancer, and used to speak, with fond nostalgia, of her dancing years.

After marriage, and children, with no support – her husband being thousands of miles away – serving in the armed forces, Rosa had a breakdown, came into the mental health system, and stayed in it.

Then, there is Rosamund. She was attending the Crisis House, when it was a statutory mental health facility. We are going back as far as the early 1980's.

Rosamund's story, is that her mother suffered from schizophrenia. She went into a mental hospital, when Rosamund and her sister were teenagers, and never came out. Their father could not cope, alone with the girls. Rosamund's sister, Sarah, was mentally handicapped, and so went into supported accommodation.

Rosamund, who was running wild, went into an approved school for girls, run by the Salvation Army. This was in kent. At eighteen, she left school, and returned to Berkshire. The Salvation Army Officer got her a job, as a ward maid, at the Royal Berkshire Hospital. This was in September 1968.

By December 1968, Rosamund was married, and pregnant! Her husband was a thirty-five year old businessman. They had three children – two girls and a boy. The boy was born with defective kidneys – necessitating a lot of extra care. The marriage broke down, as did Rosamund, and she came into the mental health system – following in her mother's footsteps.

Had Rosamund not experienced the strain of bringing up three children – one of whom was chronically sick, and then the breakdown of marriage, and lone parenthood, she might have avoided mental ill health, herself.

Another such guest in the crisis house, was Dionne Black. Her mother suffered from schizophrenia, went into a mental hospital, and died there – eleven years later. Dionne herself, was a bright young girl – gay – in the traditional meaning of the word!

She married, and had two boys – suffering from post partum psychosis, after each of the births. Dionne never recovered fully. She stayed in the crisis house for some months in 1994, awaiting supported housing, because her husband did not want her back. Crying, she said that he had described her as, 'A waste of space in the world'. Naturally, a divorce ensued. Twenty-one years later, Dionne is still under mental health care.

Shirley's was a somewhat different situation. The strains and stresses in her marriage, were caused by her spending money, which she did not have, on private education for her son and daughter. She got the family into crippling debt, and, as a result, suffered domestic violence from her husband – hence, her fleeing to the crisis house, for safety!

Edwina Schaley, had never been mentally ill, until she gave birth to her two sons. Evidently, in her case, the strains and stresses of working as a nursing sister, were nothing, compared with the strains and stresses of giving birth to, and coping with, two boys!

With both Gavin Morton, and with Cynthia Topping, it was the death of a child, which triggered their mental illness. Gavin described it, poignantly, as, 'Not so much illness, as grief'. This was also the case, though in far more horrific circumstances, with the Tildesley family. [Chapter 26: 'The loss of a child'.]

The best people to help the parents of a handicapped child, are, not statutory Social Services, as Cynthia Topping's encounter with a social worker, so cogently, illustrates, but self-help organizations, set up, and run, by the parents themselves.

In Wokingham, we have the excellent Peapods, which supports families with a handicapped child, on exactly, this basis. We are also lucky to have a local branch of MENCAP.

Another, excellent, voluntary organization, is Homestart. Homestart, provides experienced parents, to help struggling parents – who have at least one child under the age of five. This is the way forward, and get rid of statutory Social Services. Some of their social workers have never had a child, and have no clue as to the strains, and stresses that child care involves.

I saw an excellent television programme, revealing what daily life was like, for parents with a handicapped child. One such mother, had had a relationship with a man, who went off, as soon as his, severely handicapped, daughter was born.

I have rarely seen anyone with a life as soul destroying as this lady's. The child, aged twelve, was profoundly physically, and mentally, handicapped. She was unable to speak. She could only utter grunts. She was doubly incontinent – requiring the constant changing of nappies. She was like a baby to handle, but, being twelve years old, was big, and heavy.

Her mother got, not one moment's respite. It was all go, all the time! All that the Social Services were offering her – was one evening off, per month!

Because I have never been a mother, I fail utterly to understand why anyone would put up with such a life. Were I in the situation, I am convinced that I would place the child in an institution. This woman was a mother. Life was hell, but she accepted it!

Then, the programme showed a couple from Oxfordshire. Again, they had a profoundly physically, and mentally, handicapped, child, who had to be lifted with a hoist.

The sad thing, in this instance, was that the couple had found a private special school – able to cater for the child's multiple, and complex, needs. The school had an excellent headmaster, who was willing to give their child a place.

Oxfordshire County Council would not pay the fees. This couple were frustrated beyond measure. They knew that it was the right place for their child, and that it would relieve them, but they could not access this service!

What infuriates me, is that so many Social Services' employees spend their lives sitting around in meetings. We taxpayers, pay them to do nothing, when that money could, more appropriately, be applied to families such as this one.

Gavin Morton's first marriage broke down, because his twins were born, handicapped. One died, and one had multiple needs. His first wife did find a suitable special school for the surviving child, but she had to move to Derbyshire to do so.

Where there is a family predisposition to severe mental illness, as in the case of Rosamund, and in the case of Dionne Black, it appears that childbirth, and the strain of bringing up the children, is the trigger that brings out inherent mental illness in the next generation.

Thus, I stand by my advice to Sadie Minton. Sadie first came to our services in July 1987 – having just come back to Wokingham. She had been at Art College in Brighton, had got pregnant, and had had an abortion. From time to time, after that, Sadie would raise the subject of having babies.

One day, Sadie came into the drop-in centre, and said, 'Pam, everybody has babies, don't they?' I was unable to agree. Our current guests, Gavin and Jean, had a baby, Christian, but that did not mean that Sadie had to have one.

It transpired that Sadie was pregnant – from a casual encounter with an Asian man. 'Pam, said Sadie. I don't think that I could cope with a baby!' 'It's funny that you should say that, Sadie, I replied. Because I don't think that you could, either.'

I then put her in touch with the British Pregnancy Advisory Service – and, very excellent, their service is. The person gets counselling before the proposed termination, the termination itself, and then, counselling afterwards.

Sadie's only reaction to the whole process – was relief. She had not really wanted a baby. The pregnancy was simply the biological result of a loveless encounter. Sadie would not have been capable of raising the child, who would, inevitably, have gone into care – probably to be 'messed up', as one of their social workers, so damningly put it, by the likes of him!

Thus, the termination was a satisfactory solution, for everybody involved.

True love

'I'll give to you, if you'll give to me, true love, true love.
For you and I, it will always be, true love, true, love.
For you and I have a guardian angel on high, with nothing to do,
But to give to you, and to give to me – love forever, true.'

Gabriela Rani was very angry, when I advised her that, at the age of forty-two, she was too old to have a baby. She had been lamenting the fact that, in early middle age, she was still unmarried, and without children.

Gabriela was unmarried, because, due to mental illness, her concept of the state of marriage was delusional. Her two younger sisters were both married, with families. They had married ordinary people. One was a kitchen fitter, and one had a small business.

Such, was not good enough for Gabriela. She wanted to marry into the aristocracy. In her delusional state, she was incapable of considering what daily life would be like – with somebody from a completely different background, nor could she see that the thing was impossible, anyway. It wasn't going to happen.

King Cophetua and the Beggar Maid are the stuff of fairy stories. On the rare occasions that such a thing happens, and they are rare indeed, there is always a special reason. The ordinary woman, who has attracted the aristocrat, is, invariably, exceptionally beautiful, and exceptionally talented.

Thus, the American actress, Grace Kelly, married Prince Rainier, of Monaco. Grace was extraordinarily beautiful, and, not short of a bob or two, herself! Did she have IT? She most certainly did! Strictly speaking, she was not Royalty, but, she, nevertheless, came from the glamorous Royalty of Hollywood!

Fifty-five years later, Prince William married the beautiful Kate Middleton. Why did he marry somebody from a successful business background? The answer is, that the twenty-first century Monarchy is, to a large extent, a successful heritage business. It costs the country a lot of money, but it brings in even more!

My husband is Windsor, born and bred, so we are frequent visitors there. If you doubt the veracity of my words, you only have to visit Windsor in the summer. You can hardly move on the pavement, for all the American and Japanese tourists – all fascinated by our Monarchy, and all bringing in lots of money!

Back to mundane reality, Gabriela was colossally overweight, severely mentally ill, and, in fact, could never have coped with raising a child – at any age. Children are very demanding, and, since Gabriela was unable to cope with the ordinary demands that daily life placed upon herself, a child would have been the straw that broke the camel's back. Thank God that it never happened.

I have had the point of view put to me, that the great majority of the world's marriages are arranged marriages, and that they are, overall, much more successful than those in our own culture – which relies on haphazard, romantic, encounter, as its basis. I have sympathy with this point of view.

A class mismatch is not the only problem that can occur as a result of hasty marriage.

I used, at one time, to accompany home, a lady who came to my schizophrenia fellowship support group. Then I discovered that a young man who attended the group, lived very close to her, and travelled home on the same bus – which was miles from where I lived.

To save myself the journey, I asked whether he would see her home. Next week, they came back engaged! Two months later, they married. In another month, the lady was pregnant. Eventually, they had two boys, and, needless to say, could not cope. Both suffered from severe mental illness, and they didn't even know each other. What folly, but it happens, all the time, in real life!

Look at Anita White. [Chapter 16: 'You can't go back'.] She was swept off her feet by a young man with a car – seeing him as a better prospect than her disabled husband. He turned out to be uncouth, and violent. She would have liked to return to her, suitably matched, husband, but it was too late!

Unpleasant facts have to be faced. Frequently people rationalise explanations that are palatable, rather than facing the truth. Thus Alix Martin, in 'Philomel Cottage', from the short story collection: 'The Listerdale Mystery': Agatha Christie: [Published: Collins: 1934.], although, subconsciously, knowing that her husband, whom she had married within a few weeks of meeting him, was dangerous, resorted to a plausible, and comforting explanation of the circumstances, rather than facing the unpleasant truth! Agatha Christie writes: 'This explanation [which had occurred to Alix], was so consistent with the facts, and so comforting to Alix's perturbed mind, that she embraced it eagerly.' Later, she had to disillusion herself!

Hasty marriages, and unrealistic expectations, cause problems all the time. Away from Royalty, and superstars, come down to humble you and me, our friends and families. Mismatches result in the most dire situations.

Some years ago, I had some friends. They would have been described as 'upper working class', and lived in a Council house. As a young adult, one daughter lived in a house shared by students, and young professionals.

She started courting one of her fellow-residents, a medical student, the son of rich, gold bullion merchants – multi-millionaires. He would have been described as 'upper middle class'. It worked fine while he was still a student, sharing the house. All wore identical blue jeans. All appeared to be the same!

Their subsequent marriage, once he had qualified as a doctor, and had set up in practice, lasted less than one year. Among other taunts, he described his wife as 'too fat!' What he really meant, was that she was not of his class. Needless to say, divorce ensued.

This girl's mother took her daughter's side in the affair. Good for her. One should always stand up for one's own flesh and blood. She encouraged her daughter not to accept the divorce settlement that was being offered. I sympathised, but, at the same time, as the outsider, I could see that they were on a hide into nothing.

The man did not want her daughter. He wanted a pencil thin, upper middle class, girl, from his own background. Better to accept reality, and move on, which, in time, my friend did. She went on to remarry, and have a son, Thomas.

By contrast, my youngest brother married a girl who was, almost literally, 'the girl next door'. Both from exactly the same background, the marriage worked out perfectly. This brother, the youngest of the litter, was the one of all of us who did the best financially. He set up, successfully, in business, at the age of twenty-one, and is still highly successful, forty years later, at the age of sixty-one!

Agatha Christie refers to the problem of class difference in marriage, in a number of her works.

Some readers might regard her views as snobbery, but it is not snobbery, it is realism. Agatha Christie abhorred snobbery – referring to it as having a 'hideous head', and isolating one of its victims on a permanent island of loneliness.

Agatha Christie writes: [Please see: 'A Pocket Full of Rye': Published: Collins: 1953.].

'Snobbery here raised its hideous head and marooned Mrs Emmett on a permanent island of loneliness. The necessity to talk grew upon Mrs Emmett, and on that particular day, it had burst its bounds, and Miss Marple had received the full flood of the torrent.'

On many an occasion, in the crisis house, I have occupied exactly the position of Miss Marple. The situation is not always one of a social or marital mismatch, but, for a variety of reasons, the dammed up emotion bursts its banks, and the talk becomes a flood-tide.

Sometimes, the person is babbling incoherently – so great is their need to get the words out as fast as they can. It is so important to have places where lonely people can talk – hence the need for many more crisis houses. This unbearable loneliness also indicates just how important our befriending service is.

Another example of the problems caused by social differences, is illustrated by the dilemma of Mary Gerrard in 'Sad Cypress'. [Please see: Agatha Christic: 'Sad Cypress': Published: Collins: 1940.]

Agatha Christie was a realist. Of course there is fundamental truth in the old rhyme, 'When Adam delved, and Eve spun, who was then the gentleman?' But there are class distinctions, and mismatches cause enormous problems.

In 'Death on the Nile', Miss Van Schuyler reproves Mr. Ferguson, whom, though she does not know it, is actually Lord Dawlish.

He became a communist while at Oxford, and refuses to use his title.

'There is such a thing as social position', she says. Lord Dawlish, who has proposed marriage to Cornelia, Mrs Van Schuyler's cousin, replies, 'Social position is bunk'.

To Cornelia, herself, Lord Dawlish says, 'Don't you realise, and you an American, that everyone is born free and equal?' 'They're not', said Cornelia with calm certainty.

Social position, unfortunately, isn't bunk! It is the old, old, story. It would be very nice if everyone were equal, all marriages harmonious, and life free of all mental health problems. But they are not!

In the 'ABC Murders' [Agatha Christie: Collins: 1936.], it would be very nice if, as Mr Cust has it, there were 'no wars, no plague, no sleeping sickness, no famine, and no cancer', but there are!

There is a different slant on the same theme, in 'Ordeal by Innocence': [Published: Collins: 1958]. This is where a rich, upper middle class, and childless woman, Rachel Argyle, satisfies HER need to be a mother, by running a war time nursery, and bringing up the children as though they were her own. 'But they have to go back!' [often to slum homes, and lower class biological parents], pleads her husband, but his pleas fall on deaf ears.

A similar failure to listen, and lack of insight, is also dealt with in 'The Mirror Cracked from Side to Side'. [Published: Collins: 1962.] In this instance, as with 'Ordeal by Innocence', such failure brought about tragedy.

The person IS kind, IS well-meaning, but it is fatal to interfere in other people's lives – thinking that you know what is best for them. Too frequently, in such circumstances, the person is satisfying YOUR needs! What looks like philanthropy, is, in fact, self serving, and leads to disaster.

The person becomes your victim, not your beneficiary! Do I have to point to statutory Social Services, yet again, as being guilty of this failing? I do. So many of the tragedies have occurred, because of what THEY thought, THEIR opinion, and did not take into account the realities of what was happening with the people involved.

I know, from personal experience, that people who are living in very difficult circumstances, but who are, temporarily, trapped within them, adopt coping strategies. This is the human instinct for survival, kicking in. An outsider can clomp in – in their size nineteens, and make everything a million times worse!

In the crisis house, we only advise, and intervene, when we are invited to do so. There are times when we could rip our hair out, with frustration, when we observe people doing, what we see as, stupid things. Do we know better than the people themselves? We do not!

Furthermore, although, in our twenty-five years, we have worked strenuously to help people achieve better quality lives, we are aware that, on occasions, there is no answer. Your mother was murdered. There is no answer. Your infant child died. There is no answer. Your husband prefers another woman. There is no answer. Getting up, and making the best of it, as the alternative to sitting down, and moaning for the rest of your life, is, frequently, the most realistic option to take!

PART SEVEN

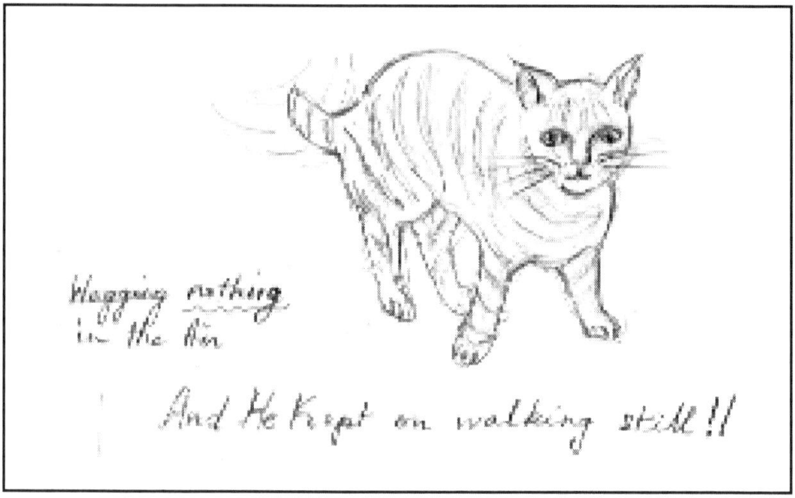

'Though He Had No Rudder There.
For All That He Didn't Care.
He Wagged His 'Nothing' In The Air,
And He Kept On Walking Still.'

Chapter 51

The Campaign For The Mentally Ill Homeless

Recently, I had a conversation with a local Police Officer. I explained, and he agreed with fervour, that the fact that our beds had closed, did not mean that they were no longer needed. If anything, the need is more desperate than ever! My letter, which follows, was published in the *Wokingham Times* Newspaper, on 19th December 2012.

Letter to the local paper - 'we need a hostel for adults in need'

"*Do any of your readers support my view that Wokingham needs a hostel for socially disadvantaged, homeless, adults?*

We have provision for youth [16-25 years] due to the 1990's campaign to set up Seaford Court. At the other end of the scale, there is also provision for the elderly [55 years and over]. But I am aware, currently, of numerous adults in Wokingham who are sleeping rough – variously – in alleys, doorways, cupboards, sheds, old cars, or on park benches.

This is the middle-aged group, for whom we have no specific provision. I am horribly conscious that they are freezing to death. When they come into our drop-in centre, they drain the hot coffee to the dregs in an attempt to get some warmth into their freezing bodies.

Our Government may well wish to support those who want to work hard and get on. We all do! But the Bible, with its timeless wisdom, tells us: 'The poor you have with you always.' They are here, in Wokingham, in the 21st Century.

These are the people who will never be able to buy the expensive houses in Wokingham, nor afford the high rents for luxury flats. Even if they do find jobs, they will probably be on minimum wages all their working lives. They don't need luxury. They are, frequently, simple people who need the simple basics – a hostel room, a bath, clean clothes, and a hot meal.

Throwing money at such people is pointless – as it is to expect them to find expensive, private-sector accommodation for rent. They always scrape enough money together for alcohol, cigarettes, and mobile phones – like children prioritizing sweets. But what they lack are the organizational skills to cope in today's complicated world, to 'put away childish things'.

With the younger age group, there might be some prospect of training them in money-management, and life-skills, but this ambition is less realistic for the middle-aged group.

I am interested in working with other local charitable organizations to set up such a hostel where homeless people could book in by the night. You would need a married couple as resident wardens, but the project need not be costly at all. In return for having free accommodation, the wardens would require only a very low wage.

Housing Benefit, which people currently claim, often for flats on their own where they cannot cope and fail to sustain, could more suitably be applied to hostel places. Nor need such a hostel be in anyone's backyard.

The Wokingham Crisis House, opposite the Station, can't be the only building in Wokingham District, which is in the heart of the community, but nowhere near any residential area. I have already floated the idea with some local groups, and I should be interested to hear from others with a view to establishing a steering committee, which could conduct a feasibility study for such a project."

In the ensuing years since my letter was published, the local campaign has gathered momentum. I recall, that when I set up the crisis house in 1991, people then thought that I should first conduct research – to see if the beds were needed. I disagreed, and went ahead without research. We started with two crisis beds, and there is not a town in the United Kingdom, that does not need such a minimum number, for community mental health. A hostel – with, say, forty beds – is a rather more ambitious project, and certainly needs research before its establishment.

We now have a forum for interested parties – set up by a researcher, who is looking at homelessness throughout Berkshire. Several local charities are involved, and there is a determination to see that the problem of local homelessness, particularly of the vulnerable, is properly addressed, and provided for.

I am particularly keen to ensure that this forum does not turn into yet another talking shop. With the advent of winter, we need homes for the homeless, not just a group of people sitting around and talking about it!

Chapter 52

Happy Memories

When I finally leave the crisis house, I shall take with me lots of happy memories of lovely, golden, summer outings to the seaside, of jolly Christmas parties, and of other, happy, events at the house.

I have lovely memories of visits to the Royal Horticultural Society's Flower Shows – at Chelsea, and at Wisley, in Surrey. So many mentally ill people, accommodated in flats, without gardens, need the opportunity to see such wonderful displays of flowers.

I shall always remember Christmas 1991 – our first at the crisis house – with Ruth, and baby Robin. Though severely mentally ill, Ruth was a devoted mother, and besotted with Robin. 'Isn't he lovely?' she would sigh ecstatically – as she handed me the damp bundle!

I used to tease her unmercifully. 'Leave Robin with me while you go to the shop' I would offer, 'If I get fed up with him, I shall throw him out of the window!' Ruth would then hug the baby even closer. Incredible to think that Robin is now twenty-five, and is a tall, strapping, man

Then I remember Christmas 1992 – with Audrey and Jessica. At just two years old, Jessica toddled around – poking her fingers into all the cakes, and then licking them with glee! Incredible to think that Jessica is now twenty-six, and got married in the summer of 2015.

In the summer of 1994, we had a trip to the seaside at Bognor Regis – taking the opportunity – as well as enjoying the sea – to visit Benita who was now a guest there – and happily settled.

In April 1995, we visited the beautiful Saville Gardens – Windsor – to look at the rare plants. Our befriender, Jane, came with her grandchildren – Victoria, aged three, and Amy, aged one-and-a half. Now, aged twenty-four, Victoria is a qualified hairdresser, and Amy, always sporty, works in a local gym.

We are fond of our wines, and made two trips to wineries. We spent a most idyllic day at a local vineyard at Henley. It was a beautiful summer's day, and , relaxing amongst the vines, we could have been in the South of France, or Italy. We also spent a lovely day at Denbigh's winery in Surrey – travelling along in their little train on a tour of the vineyard, and also being conducted around the factory itself. Such happy memories!

An amusing crisis house story about wine, is of the occasion when Murial Carsons [Chapter 24: 'Valiant 'gainst all disaster'.], was keen for us to opt for the non-alcoholic variety.

Murial was trying to persuade me as to the merits of non-alcoholic wines – Amethyst, I believe they are called. 'Pam, she said, the bottles are exactly like real wine bottles, it tastes and looks exactly like real wine!' 'Ah, I replied, but it does not have the one thing that I want in wine – the kick!'

Another amusing story about alcohol, and the crisis house, was when a senior manager from the local mental health hostel, brought some of the residents, to visit us. We gave them our usual, warm, welcome, and, since it was lunch-time, offered them all a drink from our bar.

This Manager, complained about our bar, to the Council. At a later date, she was sacked, for alcoholism! What was her problem with us? Was it jealousy? Needless to say, we changed nothing as a result of her complaint! In the DVD of the crisis house, made by Lucy and Neville, in September 2015, I describe, in detail, why our bar is such an important part of our, overall, mental health service.

Nevertheless, with regard to non-alcoholic wines, I have amended my views, in certain circumstances. If you have invited a recovered alcoholic to dinner, it is nice, at the dinner party, to provide a bottle that looks exactly like real wine – so that the person can feel part of normal, social life. They must feel demeaned, if they have to sit there with orange juice, when everybody else is sampling a choice vintage!

In September 1996, with Rob now regular driver for our minibus, we had a lovely day at Bourton-on-the-Water – the pretty, little, Gloucestershire town – with its lovely, old fashioned shops – and where the stream runs through the main street.

In the summer of 1997, we all travelled down to Selsey – where our new caravan was sited. I am convinced that it was on that day that Peter, seeing all the happy couples enjoying themselves on that sunny beach, confronted his own loneliness – trapped in the back bedroom of childhood – still in the house of his aging parents. In that moment, there was awakened in him a determination to change things, and he did!

Many further summer trips to Selsey, followed, and I can remember, in particular, meeting up with our service user, Nathan, who was enjoying a family holiday in our caravan with his daughter, son-in-law, and grandchildren. It is good to have this memory, because Nathan was with us for some years, but, sadly, passed away in 2005.

On numerous occasions when visiting Selsey, we met up with our supporters, Reg and Jean. I have been friendly with them since 1987 – Schizophrenia Fellowship days, and they were among our most enthusiastic caravanners.

In the summer of 2006, crisis house guest, Ben, though still very depressed, joined us on our annual trip to Selsey, and in the summer of 2008, Maurice, though now fully recovered, and with his life back together, nevertheless joined us for an enjoyable day out.

We have also had some happy events at the crisis house itself. In 1995, a service-user donated a, 1950's style, cocktail cabinet to the house, and this stimulated me to hold a cocktail party. We invited all our friends from the local community, and enjoyed a plethora of different, exotic, cocktails!

In May 2002, we started what became, quite regular, 'Agatha Christie' Quizzes. I am an absolute aficionado, and Chris Hoskin, who joined us in 2011, and participated in our 'Christie for Christmas', 2013 Quiz, is pretty hot stuff as well. The Agatha Christie Quizzes proved to be good fund-raisers.

Now that Toby Warfield is suffering from a severe illness, and is quite deteriorated, and in full-time care, it is good to have the memory of him chairing the quizzes, extremely smartly dressed – with dress suit, and gold cuff links.

The rumour, on the local mental health grapevine, was that the crisis house was to close on 1st October 2007 – that being the date that the break clause in the lease applied, and that the council were not renewing the lease – the local mental health establishment had succeeded in destroying us!

On 1st October 2007, I organized a huge OPEN DAY at the crisis house. I knew, but the local mental health establishment did not, that the then Leader of the Council, David Lee [who remains a friend], had visited us, seen, immediately that we are a centre of excellence, and that we had been the victim of a Social Services plot. So he had determined to keep us open.

I dressed up, as the Victorian music hall singer, Marie Lloyd, and regaled people all day long with a full repertoire of her songs! The local mental health team had thought that we were closing, and intrigued, sent a member down to find out what was going on. All day long, she lingered, hoping to get some information to take back, and all day long, I went on singing, and Maria Callas, I am not. It must have been agony! She had to endure it all day long, and still had to go away without any information.

Our twenty-fifth anniversary celebration in March 2012 - to mark twenty-five years of our work in Wokingham – well before the crisis house opened – will always remain a perfect memory. Attendance was huge, the setting – in Wokingham's Victorian Town Hall - was perfect, the food – provided by Linda's Kitchen – was marvellous, the wine was wonderful, and, then, there was the crisis house Diva, Pamela McEllen.

Throughout the evening, she sang like an angel, and was presented with orchids and roses, in the true Covent Garden tradition, by our Trustee, Maurice. I am so glad that our volunteer, Frances – who, sadly, died later that year, lived to celebrate the anniversary with us.

Christmas is always a dire time for mental health, but, every year, our stalwart Patron, Lady Elizabeth Godsal, attends our party, and distributes the presents from Santa's Sack, under the Christmas tree. Almost too sad to think about, but, nevertheless, a fact, the card, present, and party, that some service users have from us, are the only ones that they get at Christmas.

Mind you, there is another side to the 'Alone at Christmas', tragedy. At Christmas 1994, I had just one guest staying at the crisis house, and he was going to be there, alone, on Christmas Day. I felt sorry for him – making up a Christmas hamper, and explaining that the local Salvation Army always laid on a Christmas Dinner for those who would be alone.

He reassured me, that he would not be sad at all. His family were so abusive, dysfunctional, and damaging, that he was only too thankful to be on his own in the crisis house.

For Christmas 2002, we were indeed fortunate. Our guest at the time, was a trained Army chef. I provided him with money for food and wine, and he cooked and served a splendid Christmas dinner – with all the trimmings – not only for his fellow-guests, but for any of our drop-in users who would have been alone on Christmas Day.

The year 2007 had been a particularly difficult one for us – with the battle for the crisis house, so we decided to treat ourselves to a slap-up Christmas dinner – turkey with all the trimmings – and not forgetting the wine! We didn't travel far for this – to the Molly Millar Pub – next door to the crisis house. Twelve of us sat down together, for a most enjoyable meal, and since of those twelve, some have passed away, it is good to have the memory. Wonderful, happy, memories of good times at the Wokingham Crisis house.

Amongst our happy memories, our two visits to Royal Garden Parties should not be forgotten. I have described our visit to Buckingham Palace in the chapters on 'Awards'.

A second invitation came for the Diamond Jubilee Garden Party at Henley. I attended with our long-term supporter – Tony H. The Queen arrived by boat, and we had a lovely day, being lucky, once again, with the weather.

On the subject of Garden Parties, we must not forget those, to which we have been invited, by our wonderful Patron, Lady Elizabeth Godsal. These were held at her estate in Hurst, Haines Hill, and we have lovely memories of attending them with numerous other people from local charities.

Chapter 53

Twenty-Five Tips For Creating A Separatist Mental Health Crisis House

I don't wish to conclude on a negative note – that there will never be any more crisis houses. America has plenty of them. We have already adopted America's education system, and employment practices, and are well on our way to adopting their health care system.

In fact, we are rapidly adopting the American culture – which is one of self help. So there is a hopeful future for crisis houses, and I thus, conclude with my twenty-five top tips for creating them:

1. Found a separatist mental health Association, which, in its rules and constitution, bans mental health professionals from any involvement.

2. Find a property. Even a flat over a charity shop may prove suitable.

3. Make sure that the house, or flat, is easily accessible by public transport. It is no good having a beautiful house if people can't get to you.

4. Be financially independent. If one accepts any statutory money at all, it must be very minimal.

5. Find a team of people with mental health issues, their carers and friends, who are committed to the separatist, self-help, philosophy.

6. Insist that all the work is done on a totally voluntary basis.

7. Work hard on fund-raising, and get some reserves into the bank, and then go on working hard on fund-raising.

8. Make the house as beautiful as possible – with comfortable furniture, pictures, ornaments, and flowers.

9. Buy as much as you can from charity shops, and accept, with both hands, donations of furniture from the local community – in order to minimise expenditure.

10. Do as much of the work as you can, yourself, with help from volunteers. Only get paid people in, when this is essential for safety reasons – e.g. electrical work, and fire safety.

11. Make sure that you always have animals, birds, fish, and plants - flourishing living things, which are of great importance to the mentally ill.

12. Make huge efforts to see that everything in the house is very clean, well kept, and up-to-standard.

13. Always have a well-stocked mental health library, and ready internet access, so that people can get the information that they need.

14. Always, in addition, have plenty of popular fiction, popular music, and today's newspaper, so that people can feel part of ordinary life.

15. Always have clocks, kept to the right time, calendars which display the correct date, and a free land-line telephone, available, so that people can contact doctors, and benefits agencies. Also keep a stock of up-to-

date benefits leaflets.

16. Always have the best quality tea, coffee, biscuits, and house-hold products – taking advantage of supermarket offers, and always have a well-stocked bar – with a comprehensive range of both alcoholic, and soft drinks.

17. Establish a set of strict, and clear, rules, which eradicate all anti-social behaviour, and enforce them rigorously.

18. Be prepared to give a very high level of support, including befriending, advice, and financial help, if appropriate, to a person in acute crisis.

19. Make clear that you are a CRISIS service. Apart from ordinary social support, in the drop-in centre, and, the long-term befriending, ongoing, long-term care, is not within your brief.

20. Support the family of the person in crisis, as well as the individual. People live in a context, and if the family is supported as well, the long-term outcome. for the individual, is enhanced.

21. Always treat people with respect, and take their concerns seriously.

22. Involve, and interest, the local community, including its Member of Parliament, its elected representatives, its voluntary organizations, and its religious institutions.

23. Never involve yourself with the local mental health establishment. Stay completely separate, and use all your energies to make your own service excellent.

24. Never discuss your service with statutory bodies, nor attend their meetings. It is very difficult for them to attempt to control people who are not there!

25. Keep up the effort all the time. Never slacken, and never give in!

Conclusion

So my story has ended. Felix kept on walking, and keeps on walking still. My joy, is that the Crisis House is such a great success, but my sorrow, as Chris says, in his 'Foreword', is that we are, at present, but hopefully not in the future, probably unique throughout the country.

We need not have been. Were people not up against the destructive might of the mental health establishment, small crisis houses, meeting local needs, could already, using ours as a model, have been set up throughout the length and the breadth of the United Kingdom.

My hope for the future, is in my certain knowledge, that things which do not provide what society set them up to provide – eventually go. They are relegated, like the, defunct, Inner London Education Authority, of old, to the dustbin of history!

Statutory Social Services do not provide what people need – so they will go, eventually – even if not in my lifetime.

We have always been about choice, so I shall make my final point - about the only realistic, if stark, choice, that faces one in mental health.

One can choose either to sit down, and moan, for the rest of one's life, or one can choose, to get up, and make the best of it. We choose the latter! That's all folks, for now!

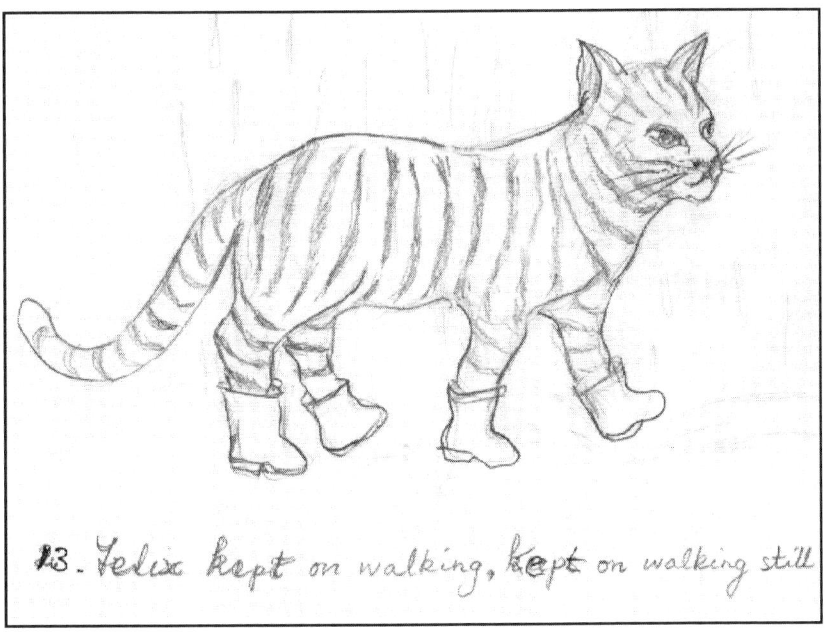

13. Felix kept on walking, kept on walking still

'On Our Own': Judi Chamberlin: MIND Publications: London: 1988.

'This is Madness: A Critical Look at Psychiatry, and the Future of the Mental Health Services': PCCS Books: Herefordshire: 1999.

Agatha Christie: 'And Then There Were None': Collins: 1939.

Agatha Christie: 'Cat Among the Pigeons': Collins: 1959.

Agatha Christie: 'Hickory, Dickory, Dock': Collins: 1955.

Agatha Christie: 'The Pale Horse': Collins: 1961.

Agatha Christie: 'Dumb Witness': Collins: 1937.

Agatha Christie: 'Five Little Pigs': Collins: 1943.

Agatha Christie: 'Sparkling Cyanide': Collins: 1945.

Agatha Christie: 'The Fourth Man' From 'The Hound of Death': Collins : 1933.

Agatha Christie: 'A Pocket Full of Rye': Collins: 1953.

Agatha Christie – 'An Autobiography': Collins: 1977.

Agatha Christie: 'Death in the Clouds': Collins: 1935.

Agatha Christie: 'The Moving Finger': Collins: 1943.

Agatha Christie: 'Three Act Tragedy': Collins: 1935.

Agatha Christie: 'They Do It With Mirrors': Collins: 1952.

Agatha Christie: 'The Flock of Geryon' From 'The Labours Of Hercules': Collins: 1947.

Agatha Christie: 'The Clocks': Collins: 1963.

Agatha Christie: 'Why Didn't They Ask Evans?': Collins: 1934.

Agatha Christie: 'The Big Four': Collins: 1927.

Agatha Christie: 'Sad Cypress': Collins: 1940.

Agatha Christie: 'The A.B.C. Murders': Collins: 1936.

Agatha Christie: 'The Body in the Library': Collins: 1942.

Agatha Christie: 'Death on the Nile': Collins: 1937.

Agatha Christie: 'Ordeal by Innocence': Collins: 1958.

Agatha Christie: 'The Mirror Cracked From Side to Side': Collins: 1962.

Agatha Christie: Short Story: 'Philomel Cottage': From 'The Listerdale Mystery': 1934.

NOTE: It was my mother who suggested that I looked out for Agatha Christie's books – when I joined the Senior Library, at the age of fourteen, just as she had suggested that I look out, for Enid Blyton, when I joined the Junior Library, at the age of seven. Thus, she introduced me to my childhood's favourite books, and also to adult life's favourite books.

Songs, Rhymes and Poetry

Abba: 'The Winner Takes it All'.

Adams, Sarah Flower: 'Nearer, my God, to Thee'.

Asaf, George and Powell, Felix: 'Pack up your Troubles'.

Ball, Michael: 'Love Changes Everything'.

Black, Cilla: 'What's it all about?'.

Blake, William: 'Jerusalem'.

Boyle, Susan: 'I Dreamed a Dream'.

Bronte, Emily: 'No Coward Soul is Mine'.

Bunyan, John: 'He who would valiant be'.

Carrol, Lewis: 'The Eldest Oyster Winked his Eye'.

Chant (Popular at Football Matches): 'Two, four, six, eight'.

Chas and Dave: 'Don't Need Nobody'.

Conner, T.W.: 'She was a Dear Little Dickie Bird'.

Crosby, Bing: 'Busy Doing Nothing'.

Disney, Walt: 'Felix Kept on Walking'.

Dylan, Bob: 'Just Like a Woman'.

Ecclesiastes: 'For everything there is a season'.

Faith, Adam: 'What Do You Want If You Don't Want Money?'.

Fields, Gracie: 'If we can't be Young and Beautiful!'

Fury, Billy: 'Don't Leave me Halfway to Paradise!'.

Gay, John: 'Youth's the Season Made for Joys. Love is Then Our Duty'.

Goldsmith, Oliver: 'The Dog is was that Died'.

Hankey, Arabella Catherine: 'Tell Me The Old, Old Story'.

Hymn (Popular): 'Just as I am, Young, Strong and Free'.

Hymm (Popular Modern): 'When I Needed a Neighbour'.

Jackson, Michael: 'Have You Seen My Childhood?'.

Jolson, Al: 'California, Here I Come'.

Jonson, Ben: 'Drink to me only'.

Juvenal: '*Mens Sana in Corpore Sano*'.

Kitt, Ertha 'I'm Just an Old-Fashioned Girl'.

Larkin, Philip: 'Annus Mirabilus'.

Magidson, Herbert: 'Enjoy Yourself. It's Later than you Think'.

Marx, Groucho: 'I Would Never Join a Club that Wanted me as a Member'.

Monsell, John Samuel Bewley: 'Fight the Good Fight'.

Music Hall: 'Oh, it's Nice to have a Home of Your Own'.

'Music, The Sound of': 'Climb Every Mountain'.

Nelson, Willie: 'And Let the Rest of the World Go By'.

Paul, St.: 'If he cannot contain, let him marry'.

Payne, John Howard: 'Home, Sweet, Home'.

Playground Game (Children's): 'In and Out of Windows'.

Presley, Elvis: 'Wooden Heart'.

Proverb Spanish: 'Take What You Want, And Pay', Says God.

Racine: '*Implacable Venus toute entière à sa proie attachée*'.

Rice-Davies, Mandy: 'Well, He Would, Wouldn't He?'.

Richard, Cliff: 'The Young Ones'.

Ridgewell, Charles and Godwin, Will 'It was only a Beautiful Picture'.

Rogers, Ginger and Astaire, Fred: 'Let's Face the Music and Dance'.

Saying (Popular): 'I'm only here for the beer!'.

Saying (Popular): 'Why did the pterodactyl become extinct?'.

Shakespeare, William: 'O, time thou must untangle this'.

Shaw, Sandie: 'I Don't Ever Want to go Home Anymore'.

Shields, Ella: 'Burlington Bertie'.

'Society, High': 'True Love'.

Song (Nursery): 'Glad to Have a Friend Like You'.

Song (Popular): 'Baby Face'.

Song (Popular): 'If Everybody's Somebody, Nobody's Anybody!'.

Song (Popular Children's): 'Knick Knack, Paddy Whack'.

Unzicker, Rae: 'To be a Mental Patient'.

Vandyke, Leroy: 'Walk on By'.

Wallis, Jay: 'All by Yourself in the Moonlight'.

Warhol, Andy: 'Everyone should be famous for five minutes'.

Watts, Isaac: 'When I Survey the Wondrous Cross'.

Wordsworth, William: 'To a Good Man of Most Dear Memory'.

Wykeham, William of: 'Manners Makyth Man'.